I0064468

Deconstructing ADHD: Mental Disorder or Social Construct?

Edited by
Eric Maisel

Deconstructing ADHD: Mental Disorder or Social Construct?
Edited by Eric Maisel

This book first published 2022
Ethics International Press Ltd, UK
British Library Cataloguing in Publication Data
A catalogue record for this book is available from the British Library

Print Book ISBN: 978-1-80441-084-4
eBook ISBN: 978-1-80441-085-1

CONTENTS

Introduction

For those of you familiar with the concerns of those who have their doubts about the ethics, tactics, logic and legitimacy of what we might call the mental health establishment, you may already know all you need to know about psychiatry as a pseudoscience and a pseudo-medical specialty, about the differences between treating actual disorders and the mere collecting of "symptoms" into "symptom pictures" which then get affixed a convenient label, about what might rightly be called medication versus mere chemicals-with-powerful-effects, and so on. But even if you know all this, you may find it convenient to hear from many voices in one place. The Ethics International Press Critical Psychology and Critical Psychiatry series is one such place.

The first two volumes in this series, *Critiquing the Psychiatric Model* and *Humane Alternatives to the Psychiatric Model*, have now appeared. This volume, Deconstructing ADHD, is the third in the series. A fourth volume, on the so-called mental disorders of childhood (with a focus on autism), will appear in 2023. We hope that further volumes will appear and tackle important subjects like psychiatry and the law, the validity of psychological testing, the logic of psychotherapy as a pseudo-medical "expert" activity, etc.

Trying to explain why the concerns explored in these volumes should be located in the territory of "ethics" would take us down paths we do not need to travel, into the definitional morasses of how to get from "what is" to "what ought to be," whose values are being promoted, and, most basically, what do we mean by "ethical"? Let me just present a few basic points as to why the concerns presented in these volumes are ethical in nature:

- If you claim that you are doing medicine, as psychiatrists do (and, by extension, every other mental health practitioner who "diagnoses and treats"), or suggest that you are doing medicine without actually making that claim, and you aren't doing medicine, that amounts to an ethical matter, wouldn't you say?

- If, as an answer to a question on a psychological test, I tell you that I prefer something, say that I like solitude, and then you repeat back to me that I prefer that something, just changing the wording and claiming, say, that I am an introvert, that is a linguistic transaction of a certain sort and not a test. What is being "tested" in that transaction? To the extent to which psychological tests are not genuine tests, or really nothing like tests at all, that is an ethical matter, wouldn't you say?

- If you claim that certain chemicals are "treating" a "disorder" but in fact they are just chemicals with powerful effects, with some of those effects perhaps sometimes desirable and many of those effects regularly undesirable, that is an ethical matter, wouldn't you say? It is not just a linguistic matter or a language game to call a chemical a "medication" when it isn't—it is also an ethical issue, yes?

- If I claim that I am "practicing psychotherapy" and that at the core of that activity is the "diagnosing and treating of mental disorders," and the whole construct is fishy, that is an ethical matter, wouldn't you say? If you are putting your psychological and emotional life in my hands, it would be nice if I knew something about the psychological and emotional life of human beings and had more in my arsenal than a symptom checklist, an ability to listen, and some rote questions, yes? To put the matter another way, if someone calls himself or herself an expert at something and isn't, that is an ethical matter, yes?

Society giving some certain people the right to electroshock you is an ethical matter. Society giving some certain people the right to incarcerate you for your unusual but not illegal behaviors is an ethical matter. Society giving some certain people the right to label you with some psychiatric label because of your political views, as part of society's tactics of oppression, because you are a child and can't defend yourself from labeling (and the chemicals that will follow), and for other social and political motives, are ethical matters. So is society denying the relationship between poverty and "poor mental health," denying the relationship between oppression and "poor mental health," denying that circumstances matter when it comes to your mental health, and in countless other ways denying that the realities of your life matter to your emotional wellbeing.

There is much that is wrong with this picture and there is much that ought to change. "Ought" is a value word located squarely in the domain of ethics. If you agree that there is a lot that ought to change with respect to our mental health paradigms and practices, then you are agreeing that we are properly in the domain of ethics. We hope that the volumes in this series prove both provocative and helpful. We welcome feedback, we hope that you will perhaps promote these books in your networks, and we look forward to hearing from you if you think that you might like to contribute to a future volume, if you might perhaps like to take on the role of editor for a future volume, or if you might like to propose a future volume.

We are happy to train a lens on any aspect of psychology and psychiatry that deserves some scrutiny. Come join us in this worthy enterprise.

Eric Maisel
Walnut Creek, California, USA.

Editor, *Deconstructing ADHD: Mental Disorder or Social Construct?*
Series Editor, *The Ethics International Press Critical Psychology and Critical Psychiatry Series.*

ADHD, ODD, Pediatric Bipolar, Oh My!

Eric Maisel

In this volume, I've invited contributors to explore, critique, and deconstruct the so-called "mental disorder" known as ADHD. I think that this is a wonderful, valuable collection of chapters and I want to thank the book's contributors. Anyone who reads these chapters will come away with a new appreciation of the gravity of the dangers associated with the wanton labeling of children with the AHDH label. They will likewise be alerted to the dangers of placing these little patients, often as young as of pre-school age, on powerful chemicals with dubious positive effects and life-altering negative effects.

In this opening chapter, I want to set the stage a little and give you a taste of this territory, the territory of the "mental disorders of childhood." This contemporary, dominant "mental disorders of childhood" paradigm is promulgated by the psychiatric profession (and, in turn, most helping professionals) and supported by mega-institutions like Big Pharma, academia, and mass media. What does this territory look like? Let's begin by picturing a child—an actual child, an actual person being his or her human self.

A child is already and really somebody. Children think, imagine, feel, dream, remember, hope, and hurt. They have that thing that we rarely talk about any more, a "personality," that unified, individual and recognizable amalgam of their original personality

---

Eric Maisel is a retired family therapist, and active creativity coach, based in California, USA.

and their formed and forming personality. To conceptualize their anger, upsets, sadness, or high energy as "symptoms" of something, as opposed to natural differences or consequential reactions to life experiences, is both to do them a dramatic disservice and to do something fundamentally illegitimate. But that is what currently occurs without a second thought. Especially in America, but increasingly worldwide, the first line of approach to dealing with a child's thoughts, feelings, behaviors, and his or her very personality is to pull out a "symptom" checklist and begin to "diagnose." This is where the train runs right off the tracks.

Little Jane is likely not sad or anxious because she has "contracted" a so-called mental disorder. Rather, she is likely sad or anxious for *reasons,* reasons that might include that her parents are harming her, that she was born easier to startle than the next child, that she just failed an exam that she expected to pass, or that performing in public terrifies her. To leap from here to there—from seeing a sad or angry child to labeling her with a so-called mental disorder like pediatric bipolar disorder or oppositional defiant disorder is both mistaken and unfair.

How exactly should we conceptualize the journey that an infant takes from birth to suicidal thoughts at fourteen or anorexia at sixteen or drug addiction at eighteen or college failure at twenty? Is it the best way—or even useful—to say, as is so often said nowadays, that it is a "biopsychosocial" process? Where is the person in that way of conceptualizing things? Is it the best way—or useful or legitimate—to say, as is so often said today, that a child with these difficulties "has a mental disorder" requiring medication? Or are there better, truer ways to conceptualize growing up as human? Is our goal to silence children's complaints and engineer their behaviors so that they fall into line with certain norms and agendas? Or is it, one hopes, to facilitate their healthiest, happiest individual life journeys?

First of all, we are faced with the current ubiquitous procedure of instantly "diagnosing" based on so-called "symptom pictures," as if a disease is the culprit causing the child's problems. This is at the heart of the current psychiatric paradigm and where the dominant system's failure begins. Let's start there.

Squirming and anger are symptoms of what?

In real medicine, you use symptoms to help you discern a cause, which then helps you pick a treatment. You take fever, fatigue, swelling, and so on as indicators of, say, a particular virus, and then you attempt to deal with the virus. If you can't discern the cause or if you can't decide between two or more causes, you run more tests and, while you are trying to identify the cause, you indeed do things that you know or suspect are likely to help relieve the symptoms.

In the meantime, as you seriously look for the cause, you work to reduce the pain or bring down the fever. You are reducing the pain and bringing down the fever while you continue to investigate what is actually causing the fever and the pain. You do not focus all of your efforts on reducing the pain or on bringing down the fever and you don't just guess what the cause is, based solely on the symptoms. Rather, you continue your investigations. You are trying to figure out what is going on. In real medicine, *your job isn't merely to treat symptoms.*

One of our neighbors recently suffered from terrible stomach pains. For a long time, on the order of two months, no conclusive diagnosis could be reached among the four contenders vying as the cause of her affliction. Finally, it was conclusively determined that it was cancer located in a certain stomach valve. Treatment began immediately. All along, she was being given relief for her symptoms—relief for the pain, help with her inability to keep food down—while the cause was being determined. Treatment for the actual affliction could only commence *once it was identified*. That is how real medicine works.

In the pseudo-medical specialty of "children's mental health," something very different goes on. There you take the report of a child's behavior—for example, that little Johnny pulled on the braids of the girl sitting in front of him—and for no reason that you can possibly justify, you call that a "symptom of a mental disorder." You collect several of these "symptoms of mental disorders"—often three, four or five are enough—and then you attach a "mental disorder" label to that "symptom picture." The label might sound like "oppositional defiant disorder," for instance, or "attention deficit hyperactivity disorder."

Once that label is provided, chemicals typically follow. Little and often no interest is shown in what is causing the behavior. Little and often no interest is shown in whether the behavior reflects something biological going on, something psychological going on, or something situational going on. Little and often no interest is shown in whether what is going on is congruent with this child's personality—rather like who she has always been—or is new, different, and incongruent. This suspiciously easy route of labeling-followed-by-chemicals is not medicine, no matter how many white coats are in evidence. It is behavioral engineering.

A child who loses his temper, argues with his parents, defies his parents' rules, and is spiteful and resentful is given, based on these four "symptoms," the pseudo-medical sounding label of "oppositional defiant disorder" and is put on chemicals to make him more obedient. This is not medicine. This is behavior control instituted to make the lives of adults easier. Why not start by asking little Johnny why he is angry and resentful? Why not step back to see if perhaps his family is in chaos? Why not look at his life and not just his "symptoms"? Why presume that a child arguing with his parents is arguing because of some impossible-to-find medical condition? Isn't it more likely—by a longshot—that he is angry with them or angry with something? Isn't is sensible to suppose that he is acting out angrily because he is angry about some very real and meaningful problem in his life?

We don't know why little Johnny is acting the way that he is acting. But we do not believe that it is cause-less, and we do not really believe that it is the result of a medical condition. Certainly, we ought to test for genuine organic problems like brain damage or neurological damage that might cause explosive rage. But in the absence of such biological challenges, we are obliged to presume that little Johnny has everyday human reasons for his anger. Once you rule out brain damage and other possible biological causes of rage, your next step ought not to be to posit a made-up, invisible medical condition. Rather, it is to treat little Johnny like a human being with everyday human reasons for his anger and resentment.

One fact alone should prove the absurdity of considering these behaviors a pseudo-medical "mental disorder." Imagine for a second that I said to you that my not being able to see any symptoms of your cancer was proof that you had cancer. Wouldn't that statement astonish you and confound you? Or imagine that I said to you that my not being able to see a break in your bone on an x-ray was proof that you had a broken bone? Wouldn't you find that a pretty odd assertion? What is fascinating is that mental health service providers are often warned that they may not get to witness any of a child's "oppositional" behaviors because a child with this "disorder" is likely not to demonstrate any defiance except exclusively with his parents and teachers!

Unlike in real medicine, where the sore is visible both at home and in the examining room, with the behaviors associated with "oppositional defiant disorder" those behaviors are likely only observable when little Johnny is *actually angry,* namely at school and at home. It is absurd but true that an indicator that you have the mental disorder of "oppositional defiant disorder" is that you do not display any signs of it when you are talking to someone you don't happen to hate. Seriously, shouldn't the fact that little Johnny is only angry around his parents suggest that little Johnny is angry with his parents?

Picture the odd thing a provider is doing here. He does not personally see any signs of little Johnny's oppositional defiant disorder. He takes not seeing them as further proof that little Johnny has an oppositional defiant disorder. He relies on reports of things that he has not observed for himself, things that are of course more logically signs of rebellion, protest, and anger than "symptoms of a mental disorder," and from those reports he "diagnoses" a pseudo-medical condition called a "mental disorder" and moves on to dispensing chemicals that act as a straitjacket in an attempt to control his behavior. He has not seen the "disorder," he has no tests for the "disorder," and he is basing his "diagnosis" in part on the fact that he has seen nothing of the "disorder"!

This is akin to the absurd claim made that proof of the presence of an attention deficit disorder is the fact that you do not display it when something interests you. Might it not be the case that you like to pay attention to things that interest you, like sports and videos games, and don't like to pay attention to things that don't interest you, like math class and your parents' dinner conversation? It is only through the looking glass that my interest in the things that interest me and that my failure to rage at someone who hasn't angered me are signs of some pseudo-medical "mental disorder."

There are many things we wish for little Johnny. We wish that he were having an easier time of it. We wish that he could stop his raging, for his own sake, since he is making everyone around him dislike him. We wish we knew what was causing his difficulties so that we could offer him help at the same level as his difficulties. If he is raging because school is too difficult for him, we might offer one sort of help, say, a tutor. If he is raging because his parents are abusive alcoholics, we might offer another sort of help, in the form of a call to child protective services. If he is raging because he can't abide his parents' strict rules, we might offer another sort of help, like, for instance, a whole-family intervention. We absolutely wish that little Johnny were having an easier time of it and we would love to help him—but not by burdening him with an illegitimate label that potentially has negative effects on his identity and by prescribing him powerful chemicals.

If a child has a medical condition, treat the medical condition. If a child is angry with his parents, do not call that a medical condition. Labeling an angry child with the pseudo-medical sounding "mental disorder" label of "oppositional defiant disorder" may serve adult needs for peace and order. But it is not medicine and it is not right. Little Johnny is making it very difficult on the adults around him, who will naturally return the favor and make it very difficult on him, perpetuating a cycle of anger. But that he is making life hard for them is not the same thing as him being mentally ill.

We must stop saying that this little Johnny is suffering from a mental disorder or that he has a medical or pseudo-medical condition. It makes no sense on the face of it to believe that an angry child is angry because he has a disease. It makes much more sense to believe that he is angry because he is angry, just as you are angry when you are angry. Maybe little Johnny is a lot angrier than you are—but that he is angrier than you are doesn't turn his anger into a disease. It also doesn't make it a disease just because his anger is problematic. As a society, we may not be equipped to deal with all of our sad, anxious, or angry children—but the answer to that shortcoming must not be to call them all diseased.

And what about pediatric bipolar disorder?

What is it that psychiatry is really trying to say when it announces that a young child has pediatric or juvenile bipolar disorder? Have you ever been around a two-year-old or a three-year-old? Don't they sometimes rush from activity to activity? Don't they sometimes melt down and have ferocious tantrums? Don't they sometimes "suffer from excesses of energy"? Can't they sometimes become inconsolably sad? Aren't they sometimes willful and defiant? Yet all of these states and behaviors, as completely normal and ordinary as they are, are now deemed "symptoms of the mental disorder of juvenile bipolar disorder." Does this make any sense?

Stuart Kaplan, author of *Your Child Does Not Have Bipolar Disorder*, explained in Newsweek:

> I have been a child psychiatrist for nearly five decades and have seen diagnostic fads come and go. But I have never witnessed anything like the tidal wave of unwarranted enthusiasm for the diagnosis of bipolar disorder in children that now engulfs the public and the profession. Before 1995, bipolar disorder, once known as manic-depressive illness, was rarely diagnosed in children. Today, nearly one third of all children and adolescents discharged from child psychiatric hospitals are diagnosed with the disorder and medicated accordingly.
>
> I believe that there is no scientific evidence to support the belief that bipolar disorder surfaces in childhood. In fact, the opposite seems to be the case. The evidence against the existence of pediatric bipolar disorder is so strong that it's

> difficult to imagine how it has gained the endorsement of anyone in the scientific community. And the effect of this trendy thinking can have devastating consequences. Such children are regularly prescribed medications that are not effective in kids and have unwelcome side effects .

To call certain childhood behaviors "manic" is to do a particular disservice to bright, sensitive, creative kids. Such kids may be restless because they're bored and under-engaged or because they have a roving curiosity that makes them play with this toy for a minute, read that book for another half-minute, and rush around from activity to activity "as if" manic or hyperactive. If a child is bright, sensitive, and creative, he or she is at a much higher risk of one day receiving a juvenile bipolar disorder diagnosis.

I've worked with creative and performing artists as a therapist and a creativity coach for more than thirty years and their concerns interest me a lot. One of those concerns is this thing commonly called "mania." People who are creative and who think a lot are more prone to so-called mania than people who do not think a lot and who aren't creative. This fact, which is indeed a fact, should alert us to the possibility that mania is not some pseudo-medical condition or some brain abnormality but rather a function of the mental pressures put on individuals who use their brains and who rely on their brains.

That intelligent, creative and thoughtful people are the ones more regularly afflicted by the thing called mania is beyond question. Research shows, for example, a clear linkage between achieving top grades and "bipolar disorder" diagnoses, between scoring high on tests and "bipolar disorder" diagnoses, and between other, similar measures of mental accomplishment and a subsequent mental disorder diagnosis. For instance, one study involving 700,000 adults and reported in the *British Journal of Psychiatry* indicated that former straight-A students were four times more likely to be "bipolar" (or "manic-depressive") than those who had achieved lower grades . Are these folks "more ill" than their C-average counterparts or are they perhaps putting their brains under considerably more pressure?

In another study, individuals who scored the highest on tests for "mathematical reasoning" were at a 12-times greater risk for "contracting bipolar disorder ." Similar studies underline the linkage between creativity and mania and we have thousands of years of anecdotal evidence to support the contention that smart and creative people often get manic (think of Virginia Woolf). Doesn't all this evidence suggest that enlisting your brain—say, to write a novel or to solve a riddle in theoretical physics—is a rather dangerous act, since it increases the pressure on a brain already pressured to deal with everyday matters like financial difficulties, psychological threats, or just finding your car keys?

"Manic-depression" and "bipolar disorder" are in quotation marks in the previous paragraphs because the current naming system used to describe "mental disorders" is weak and highly suspect. It leads to many odd, wrong-headed hypotheses, for example that "because you are bipolar you are creative" or that "perhaps mania accounts for the higher test scores." What is likely truer is that the greater a person's brain capacity and the greater a person's reliance on thinking, the greater his or her susceptibility to a racing brain. If you rev up your brain so as to think long and hard, why wouldn't your brain be inclined to then race—and maybe race out of control?

All of the characteristic "symptoms of mania" that we see in adults, including (apparently) high spirits, heightened sexual appetite, high arousal levels, high energy levels, sweating, pacing, sleeplessness and, at its severest, hallucinations, delusions of grandeur, paranoia, aggressiveness and wild, self-defeating plans, make perfect sense when viewed from the perspective that some powerful pressure, likely existential in nature, has supercharged a brain already feverishly racing along. When that particular pressurized racing begins, the "symptoms of mania" naturally follow.

And don't children already have racing brains, a feverish fantasy life, imaginary playmates, wild schemes, and all too often trauma-induced "mind pressures"? Doesn't it make sense to conceptualize "mania" in children, when it really is something different from normal childhood curiosity and distractibility, as related to the way that the mind can be pressured, in children as well as adults, to race too wildly? If it is ever fair to call a child "manic," isn't this the direction in which we should look?

Instead, in cultures dominated by the psychiatric model, the illegitimate "diagnosing" shortcut is taken and a label is affixed.

Just consider the extent to which diagnosing children with juvenile or pediatric bipolar disorder is largely an American phenomenon. Do we have more "bipolar children" in the United States? Or are we simply labeling more of our children? Peter Parry, Stephen Allison, and Tarun Bastiampillai explained in *Lancet*, in an article entitled "Reification of the paediatric bipolar hypothesis in the USA":

So why did the paediatric bipolar disorder diagnostic epidemic occur and remain mostly confined to the USA? Among more than a thousand, mostly American, articles about paediatric bipolar disorder, a few US psychiatrists and paediatricians have been vocal critics. They noted that diagnostic criteria for paediatric bipolar disorder deviate from strict DSM criteria, symptom-checklist approaches to diagnosis did not account for developmental and contextual factors, trauma and detachment disruption were overlooked, the pharmaceutical industry collaborated with key opinion leaders and researchers of paediatric bipolar disorder, and that the US health system often mandates more serious diagnoses in order to provide reimbursement, which fosters diagnostic upcoding …

A systematic literature review of articles about paediatric bipolar disorder published from 1995 to 2010 noted almost no mention of the terms 'attachment,' 'neglect,' or 'maltreatment,' and very few mentions of the terms 'trauma,' 'PTSD,' 'physical abuse,' or 'sexual abuse,' and few mentions of the terms 'verbal abuse' or 'emotional abuse' in paediatric bipolar disorder research cohorts. In an era of dominant pharmaceutical industry funding and marketing, the presumption of biomedical causes for DSM disorders filled the aetiological space .

If the "mania" part of "juvenile bipolar" is a problematic construct, so also is the "depression" part. Might not any of the following cause the thing commonly called "depression"?

- A child gets a string of bad grades and begins to feel hopeless about his chances at school.
- A child is being bullied by a sibling, learns over time that he can't come to his parents with his complaints or his pain, and feels helpless in his own home.
- A child grows up scrutinized at every turn by a stay-at-home parent who expects nothing less than perfection.
- A child is forced to live in a chaotic environment filled with marital discord, broken promises, and a lack of privacy.
- A child begins to see life as unfair and a cheat and sours on life itself.
- A child receives no permission to do any of the things that he or she actually enjoys doing and lives a life of rules and chores.

- A child has his or her efforts criticized and ridiculed in cruel and shaming ways.
- Etc.

There are countless possible non-medical, non-biological reasons for a child's despair. But despite this obvious truth, these reasons are rarely on a psychiatrist's radar. And they ought to be. It really isn't very honest to use "depression" as a pseudo-medical collection word to collect all sorts of states and behaviors, like boredom, recklessness, irritability, alcohol abuse, anger, etc. To say that a child is "depressed" when he is actually and obviously irritable and angry is to make a linguistic leap that is exactly as illegitimate as saying that you are "depressed" when you are in fact irritable and angry.

Like the other "mental disorders of childhood," the construct of juvenile bipolar disorder is extremely shaky and suspicious. A much better case could be made for severe ups and downs being caused not by faulty wiring nor by any biological malfunctioning but rather by the way plummeting naturally follows a brain's failed attempt to find good answers to life's challenges. A brain races off in search of answers—this is the "mania" part. The answers prove insufficient—despair follows. Whether this is what is actually going on or not, it has a logic to it that the construct of "bipolar" does not.

The penalty for squirming

Then, of course, there is ADHD, the subject of this volume.

The most common "mental disorder" to anoint a child with nowadays is "attention deficit hyperactivity disorder." This is the "diagnosis" you get if you squirm. This so-called diagnosis comes in different flavors—you can be "predominantly impulsive," "predominantly inattentive," and so on. What most typically follows one of these diagnoses is "treatment" in the form of powerful stimulant chemicals, very similar in molecular structure to cocaine, with serious side effects and negative livelong consequences, including the risk of addiction.

Imagine a little Bobby who squirms at school, squirms at church, squirms at home, squirms in his good clothes, squirms when given chores, squirms when he's told to sit down and chat with his aunt Rose, squirms ... a lot. But what if you lived on a huge farm, it was always perpetual summer with no mandatory schooling requirements, and you didn't need to see little Bobby from morning until night? What would little Bobby be then? Would he still have the mental disorder of "ADHD"? Or would he just be happy?

Wouldn't little Bobby zip in and out, make himself a sandwich, put a band-aide on his skinned knee, take a shower once a week or once a month, change his clothes after he fell in the pond, complain once a day about being bored, and be completely a boy? No one would be having any problems, neither little Bobby nor his parents. Where did the "ADHD" go? Where did the "mental disorder" go? Well, try sitting him down at the dinner table or in a pew at church and then it would miraculously reappear. Imagine a disease only appearing at the dinner table, at school, or in church! What sort of disease is that?

The "problem" would of course return the second you tried to impose unnatural constraints on little Bobby's energy. Try to have him sit still during a sermon in church—now you have a problem. Try to have him sit still at an authoritarian, rule-burdened dinner table—"eat your peas first, sit up straight, stop fidgeting"—and you have a problem. Try to have him not climb on something that looks promising to climb. Then you would have a problem. Have you ever seen a child NOT climb on things that were there to be climbed on? Asserting your stubborn desire to climb on everything you encounter may well get you into hot water but it should not get you a mental disorder label.

We shouldn't label children with non-existent "mental disorders." This is oppressive. Oppression of this sort goes on all the time. The psychologist David Walker, a consultant to the Fourteen Tribes & Bands of the Yakama Indian Nation since 2000, explained to me in an interview I conducted with him:

Attention Deficit Hyperactivity Disorder (ADHD) is the new way to label American Indian children as 'feeble-minded.' Tuning out and misbehaving in relation to the stultifying, manualized, test-anxiety ridden public education system is entirely understandable, and that's where ADHD kids are often first 'detected.' If one looks at the social amnesia of today's mental health system, you'll soon discover that current ideas and concepts have many historical echoes. There's little attention given to the fact that newer ideas in Western mental health are often merely updated language.

For example, during the height of the American Indian boarding school era in the 1930s and 1940s, the term 'feeble-minded' was used to describe children considered 'morally defective' as a result of being too active or impulsive, nonconformist, inattentive, or rebellious. In this way, such children were maligned and segregated from whatever limited opportunities were available to others considered to be their superiors.

When we look at today's public education system in the U.S., which has continued to fail Native children, we find the current epidemic ADHD diagnosis began in Indian Country in the late 1990s. It is only in the last ten years that the high rate of U.S. ADHD diagnosis in other children has even begun to catch up. The fact that Native children remain more than twice as likely to end up in special education classrooms than children from other ethnic backgrounds speaks to the continuity of historical segregation and their stigmatizing as uneducable by the U.S. mental health system. ADHD, therefore, continues a process that 'feeble-mindedness' began .

Family therapist Marilyn Wedge, author of *A Disease Called Childhood: Why ADHD Became an American Epidemic*, explained to me:

As a child therapist since 1987, I have seen an alarming increase in children being diagnosed with mental disorders and prescribed psychiatric drugs. For more than 25 years, I have helped children by using safe and effective family and school interventions. I have successfully treated all kinds of childhood problems--attention and focusing issues, school misbehavior, distractibility, anxiety, oppositional behavior and sadness--without ever referring them for psychiatric medication.

In 1987, when I started my practice, less than 3 percent of American children were diagnosed with what was then called ADD. By 2016, the number increased by 300 percent. Today, 12 percent of our children are diagnosed with what is now called ADHD. When I researched ADHD in other advanced countries, I found that the rates of diagnosis have remained relatively low. In France and Finland, for example, the number is 1 percent or less. If ADHD were a true biological disorder of the brain, why is the rate of diagnosis so much higher in America than it is abroad? Or is it a matter of perception—of how children and childhood are viewed in various cultures ?

Should a child learn to be orderly in school? Yes, for the sake of civil society. But that is a very different matter from whether a child should receive a mental disorder diagnosis for not being orderly in school. There the answer is no. The issue of "being orderly in school" is not a medical one. That little Bobby is squirming is not a reason to label him with a "mental disorder" label, place him on the equivalent of street drugs, and set him up for a lifetime battle with addiction.

It is easy to get lost in the weeds and argue the pros and cons of each "mental disorder of childhood" diagnosis and each chemical "treatment." Is this so-called diagnosis more legitimate than that one? Is this so-called treatment more effective or less harmful than that one? These micro-analyses have their place. But we want to make sure not to miss the forest for the weeds. The fundamental question is, "Is the current model at all legitimate?" Is it right or fair to say that an angry child, a sad child, a boisterous child, or a frightened child is, just by virtue of being angry, sad, boisterous, or frightened, mentally disordered? That is the claim that psychiatry and its collaborators are making. I hope that sounds suspicious on the face of it.

The Emperor's New Clothes: Where ADHD Gets a Real Dressing Down

Thomas Armstrong

Most people are familiar with the fairy tale classic "The Emperor's New Clothes," by Hans Christian Andersen.[1] It tells the story of an entire kingdom being duped by a couple of charlatans who convince the people that the clothes they are making for the king are the most beautiful ever made, when in fact there is nothing at all in their looms.

According to these two hoaxers, anyone who failed to see and appreciate what wonderful clothes they'd made were either stupid or unfit for their position in the kingdom. Naturally, people were afraid to admit that they saw nothing at all, including the king, because they didn't want to be considered idiots or lose their position in the kingdom.

So, the king put on the set of invisible "clothes" they had prepared for him, and walked (stark naked) in a royal procession before his adoring subjects. Everyone thought the "clothes" were the most magnificent they'd ever seen, except for one lone child, who said: "But he doesn't have anything on!" Nevertheless, the king and his subjects became more determined than ever to continue with this absurd charade.

I sometimes feel like this child when I confront the ADHD worldview. I look around and see how virtually everyone, including

---

Thomas Armstrong, Ph.D. is an educator, psychologist, and author.

[1] Hans Christian Andersen, *Andersen's Fairy Tales*, New York: New American Library, 1966, pp. 65-71.

physicians, scientists, politicians, teachers, parents, psychologists, entrepreneurs, and others, agrees that ADHD is a real psychiatric disorder. I've just never been able to see the ''clothes'' adorning the ADHD belief system. This doubt goes as far back as 1972 for me, when I wrote my first college paper on ''hyperkinetic'' children, which is what people were calling it back then. Since that time, I've seen the idea of ADHD gather force until now it has become the most common mental disorder for children, and the intervention used most often to treat it—psychoactive medications—is expected to fuel a $24.9 billion industry by 2025.[2] In my book *The Myth of the ADHD Child,* I compare ADHD to the science fiction entity known as ''the Blob'' which flows over people, houses, and communities and gets bigger and more destructive as it gathers force.[3]

The reason for this huge disparity between a point of view embraced by most authorities in the mental health field, and my own views on the subject, has to do I believe with the distinction that the Russian-British philosopher Isaiah Berlin made between the hedgehog and the fox. Quoting the ancient Greek poet Archilochus--''The fox knows many things, but the hedgehog knows one big thing''-- Berlin noted a tendency in intellectual traditions to entertain either a pluralist or a monist perspective.[4]

Let's be clear: I am looking at the *same* objective phenomena as all the ADHD advocates: hyperactivity, impulsivity, distractibility and their subordinate and associated behaviors. I have to say this because when people read my work on the subject, some of them seem to

---

[2] Grand View Research, Press Release, ''ADHD Market Size Worth $24.9 Billion By 2025,'' retrieved from https://www.grandviewresearch.com/press-release/global-attention-deficit-hyperactivity-disorder-adhd-market.

[3] Thomas Armstrong, *The Myth of the ADHD Child: 101 Ways to Improve Your Child's Behavior and Attention Span without Drugs, Labels, or Coercion*, New York: Tarcher/Perigee, 2017, p. 3

[4] Isaiah Berlin, *The Hedgehog and the Fox*, Chicago: Elephant Paperbacks, 1993.

think that I believe these symptoms don't exist. What are you, crazy? I'd have to be an alien on a strange planet to hold such a belief. I worked with these kids for several years in special education classes, so I have no illusions about the symptoms. The key difference in our perspectives is that ADHD promoters see these symptoms as due to this "one big thing," which is essentially ADHD as a fixed entity, while I apply many different perspectives to account for these same behaviors. In the rest of this chapter, I'd like to go through several of these points of view.

Developmental perspective: We don't let kids be kids anymore

Every baby displays most of the symptoms of ADHD. Over time, however, the nervous system matures, and we develop the ability to focus for longer and longer periods of time, to restrain our impulses, and gain control over our motoric movements. But kids do this at different rates, and it turns out that kids diagnosed with ADHD mature later than typically developing kids. In fact, research suggests that the brains of ADHD-labeled youngsters develop two to three years *later* than so-called normal kids.[5]

I saw this all the time in my work as a special educator: these kids acted like much younger children. Is that such bad thing? In the opinion of many people these days, yes, it is a bad thing, because we're now expecting kindergartners to do things that first and second graders used to do. In one study, in 1998, thirty-one percent

---

[5] See, for example, P. Shaw, K. Eckstrand, W. Sharp, J.L. Rapoport, et al. Attention-deficit/hyperactivity disorder is characterized by a delay in cortical maturation, PNAS, December 4, 2007, 104(49), pp. 19649-19654; and Seunggyun Ha, Hyekyoung Lee, Yoori Choi, Hyejin Kang, et al., Maturational delay and asymmetric information flow of brain connectivity in SHR model of ADHD revealed by topological analysis of metabolic networks, *Scientific Reports*, 2020, 10, Article number: 3197.

of teachers believed children in kindergarten should learn to read; by 2010 this figure had skyrocketed to eighty percent.[6]

So, here you have children being pushed to do tasks that are developmentally inappropriate for *all* kids, and on top of that, you have those kids who have developmental delay have an even a harder time catching up, which creates stress-related symptoms of ADHD in addition to their natural playfulness being regarded as part of their diagnosis.

A study published in the *New England Journal of Medicine* revealed that rates of diagnosis and treatment of ADHD are higher among children born in August than among children born in September, in states with a September 1 cutoff for kindergarten entry.[7] So the youngest children in any kindergarten class are at risk for being labeled with ADHD purely on the basis of their age. In this situation, it makes no sense to postulate an ADHD entity being responsible for the child's symptoms. Instead, we need to use a developmental paradigm (kids grow up at different rates) to make sense of these symptoms.

Media studies perspective: Mass media is rewiring our kids' brains

There's no question that the culture has speeded up in the past fifty years, due in large part to the radical changes that have occurred in media over that same time period, including advances in television,

[6] Daphna Bassok, Scott Latham, and Anna Rorem, ''Is Kindergarten the New First Grade?'' AERA Open [a publication of the American Educational Research Association], January 2016, retrieved from http://ero.sagepub.com/content/2/1/2332858415616358.

[7] Timothy J. Layton, Michael L. Barnett, Tanner R. Hicks, and Anupam B. Jena, Attention Deficit–Hyperactivity Disorder and Month of School Enrollment, *New England Journal of Medicine*, November 29, 2018, 379, pp. 2122-2130.

movies, computer technology, video games, the Internet, chat rooms and social networks, streaming entertainment, and more. The result has been a shortened attention span for all of us (one study conducted by Microsoft determined that the average attention span had declined from 12 seconds in 2000 to 8 seconds in 2015, which is shorter than the attention span of a goldfish!).[8]

Is it any wonder that we have a malady called "attention deficit disorder," emerging during this explosion in the growth of mass media? We're learning more and more about the impact of media on the brain, and there's a growing concern that among the many changes that media exposure makes to the brain, interference with proper dopamine transmission is a major issue.

We have three primary dopamine pathways in our brain that are sensitive to rewards from the outside world. When a reward is delivered (e.g. a "hit" in a video game, a "like" on Facebook, a "ding" from a smart phone, a "jolt" from a violent TV program or movie), these dopamine pathways are activated and become "wired" as the stimulation persists.[9] However, over time these pathways become habituated to the old stimuli ("been there, done that!") and ever higher levels of stimulation are required to achieve the same effect.

Advertisers and media game designers exploit these vital neuro-pathways, and try to make their latest products even more arousing. Over time, this can result in dopamine exhaustion and a situation where the individual who feels a craving for rewards seeks higher

---

[8] Kevin McSpadden, You Now Have a Shorter Attention Span Than a Goldfish, *Time Magazine*, May 13, 2015, retrieved from https://time.com/3858309/attention-spans-goldfish/.

[9] See, for example, Trevor Haynes, Dopamine, Smartphones & You: A Battle for Your Time, *Science in the News*, Harvard University, May 1, 2018, retrieved from https://sitn.hms.harvard.edu/flash/2018/dopamine-smartphones-battle-time/.

and higher levels of stimulation.[10] This is where ADHD comes in: those stimulus-seeking behaviors are indistinguishable from the holy trinity of ADHD symptoms: hyperactivity, impulsivity, and distractibility. Several recent studies have confirmed the link between media use and ADHD behaviors.[11] Fifty years ago, Canadian professor and media futurist Marshall McLuhan spoke of a generation of kids whose worldview would no longer be based on plodding, one-step-at-a-time thinking, but rather on instantaneous flashes of immediate sensory data.[12] This time seems to have come. But at what cost?

Ecological perspective: Kids need more time playing outdoors in the sun

With the advent of the environmental movement in the 1970's, people began to think of "ecology" in terms of recycling their garbage and fighting pollution in their communities. However, ecology means much more than that. In terms of this chapter, the word ecology has to do with the sum total of environmental influences in which a child or adult finds herself and the effects they have on her behavior and wellbeing.[13] While this takes in a wide range of components (including the media issues reported above), in this section I'd like to focus on three ecological components: nature, sunlight, and play.

---

[10] See Robert Kubey and Mihaly Csikszentmihalyi, Television Addiction is No Mere Metaphor, *Scientific American*, March, 2002, 286(2), pp. 74-80; The evolution of the concept of habituation in psychology is discussed in Richard F. Thompson, Habituation: *A History, Neurobiology of Learning and Memory*, September, 2009, 92(2), pp. 127–134.

[11] See, for example, I.Beyens, Patti M. Valkenburg, and Jessica Taylor Piotrowski, Screen media use and ADHD-related behaviors: Four decades of research. *PNAS*, October 1, 2018, 115 (40), pp. 9875-9881; and Sanne W. C. Nikkelen, Patti M. Valkenburg, Mariette Huizinga, and Brad J Bushman, Media Use and ADHD-Related Behaviors in Children and Adolescents: A Meta-Analysis, *Developmental Psychology*, July 2014, 5(9), pp. 2228-2241

[12] See, for example, Marshall McLuhan and Lewis Lapham, *Understanding Media: The Extensions of Man*, Cambridge, MA: MIT Press, 1994.

[13] See Urie Bronfenbrener, *The Ecology of Human Development*, Cambridge, MA: Harvard University Press, 1981.

Research suggests that when kids diagnosed with ADHD are in nature, their symptoms decrease, and the "wilder" the environment (e.g. a forest as opposed to a city park) the greater the decline in their symptoms.[14] There is also evidence that exposure to sunshine is associated with lower rates of ADHD. A map of the United States reveals that the lowest rates of ADHD are in the Southwest, the region of the country which receives the most sunshine.[15] Finally, there's evidence that the increase in the rate of ADHD in the U.S. over the past thirty years may be associated with the decrease in children's free play and "rough and tumble" activities.[16]

Richard Louv, author of the best-selling book *Last Child in the Woods: Saving Our Children From Nature-Deficit Disorder,* quotes a fourth-grade boy who said he liked to play indoors "because that's where the electric outlets are."[17] According to a Kaiser Family Foundation study, children are spending an average of seven-and-a-half hours a day engaged with mass media products.[18] The time they are spending on media is time not spent on the playground.

Neuroscientist Jaak Panksepp notes: "Play is now increasingly rule-

---

[14] Andrea Faber Taylor and Frances E. (Ming) Kuo, Could Exposure to Everyday Green Spaces Help Treat ADHD? Evidence from Children's Play Settings, *Applied Psychology Health and Wellbeing,* August, 2011, 3(3), pp. 281–303.

[15] Martijn Arns, Kristiaan B.van der Heijdenc, L. Eugene Arnold, and J. Leon Kenemans, Geographic Variation in the Prevalence of Attention-Deficit/Hyperactivity Disorder: The Sunny Perspective, *Biological Psychiatry*, October 2013, 74(8), pp. 585-590.

[16] See Thomas Armstrong, Attention Deficit Hyperactivity Disorder in Children: One Consequence of the Rise of Technologies and the Demise of Play," in Sharna Olfman (ed.) *All Work and No Play...How Educational Reforms Are Harming Our Preschoolers.* Westport, CT: Praeger, 2003, pp. 161-176; and Thomas Armstrong, Canaries in the Coal Mine: The Symptoms of Children Labeled ''ADHD'' as Biocultural Feedback, in Gwynedd Lloyd, Joan Stead, and David Cohen (eds.), *Critical New Perspectives on ADHD*, New York: Routledge, 2006, pp. 34-44.

[17] The fourth-grade boy is quoted in Richard Louv, *Last Child in the Woods: Saving Our Children From Nature Deficit Disorder*, Chapel Hill, N.C.: Algonquin Books, 2005, epigraph.

[18] Kaiser Family Foundation, Generation M2: Media in the Lives of 8- to 18-Year-Olds, January 1, 2010, retrieved from https://www.kff.org/other/poll-finding/report-generation-m2-media-in-the-lives/.

bound and organized by adults and seems increasingly lost in our evermore regulated and litigious society where too many kids have little freedom to negotiate the social terrain on their own terms."[19] Panksepp has observed that rats in his laboratories which have had their frontal lobes damaged, lose their playfulness, and that when children play they exercise their frontal lobes and establish important neural connections from the prefrontal cortex to the limbic system.[20] These are among those networks in the brain that are seen as problematic in ADHD-labeled kids according to the ADHD experts.[21] The image of children at play outdoors on a sunny day is a fond memory for many of us adults. But for too many kids today, it's gone with the wind and ADHD has come to take its place.

Cognitive perspective: Kids diagnosed with ADHD think differently and that's okay

One of the biggest problems with the ADHD world view is that there are three negatives in the label: *deficit, hyperactivity, disorder.* The failure of most (but not all) ADHD experts to acknowledge the strengths associated with this diagnosis means that all those who are charged with the responsibility of tending to the needs of ADHD-identified children are going to focus on what these kids *can't do* instead of what they *can do.*

However, there's a new voice in the childhood mental health field

[19] Jaak Panksepp, Science of the Brain as a Gateway to Understanding Play: An Interview with Jaak Panksepp, *American Journal of Play*, Winter, 2010, 2(3), p. 247.

[20] Jaak Panksepp, Can Play Diminish ADHD and Facilitate the Construction of the Social Brain? *Journal of the Canadian Academy of Child and Adolescent Psychiatry*, May, 2007, 16(2), pp. 57–66

[21] See, for example, Ana Cubillo, Rozmin Halari, Anna Smith, Eric Taylor, and Katya Rubia, A review of fronto-striatal and fronto-cortical brain abnormalities in children and adults with Attention Deficit Hyperactivity Disorder (ADHD) and new evidence for dysfunction in adults with ADHD during motivation and attention, *Cortex*, February 2012, 48(2), pp. 194-215.

which emphasizes diversity rather than disability: neurodiversity.[22] It's founded upon a wealth of recent research information that supports the identification of unique strengths associated with ADHD, autism, dyslexia, and other brain differences. ADHD experts have long pointed out the existence of a special gene mutation that is associated with novelty-seeking: the D4 dopamine receptor gene.[23]

In fact, research suggests that kids labeled ADHD have a particular mindset which thrives upon novelty (and which, conversely, eschews boredom and sameness). Brain scan studies suggest that the novelty-seeking areas of the brain light up more for children identified as ADHD than for typically developing kids when unusual or rare stimuli are flashed on a screen.[24] These kids thrive on *distractions* or information that is not considered central to a given situation. Thus, it's no surprise then, that studies have linked ADHD to creative behaviors like divergent thinking.[25] These kids are paying attention to what they're not supposed to be paying attention to. If you're a teacher demanding student's attention to a boring lecture, then you've got a problem. But we don't say that a calla lily has "petal deficit disorder," we admire its unique way of being in the world, and we need to do the same with kids identified with ADHD.

---

[22] See, for example, Thomas Armstrong, *The Power of Neurodiversity: Unleashing the Advantages of Your Differently Wired Brain*, Cambridge, MA: DaCapo Lifelong Books, 2011; and Thomas Armstrong, *Neurodiversity in the Classroom: Strength-Based Strategies to Help Students with Special Needs Succeed in School and Life*, Alexandria, VA: ASCD, 2012.

[23] See, for example, Radek Ptáček, Hana Kuželová, and George B. Stefano, Dopamine D4 receptor gene DRD4 and its association with psychiatric disorders, *Medical Science Monitor*, 2011, 17(9), pp. RA215–RA220.

[24] See, for example, Jana Tegelbeckers, Nico Bunzeck, Emrah Duzel, Björn Bonath, et al., Altered salience processing in attention deficit hyperactivity disorder, *Human Brain Mapping*, June, 2015, 36(6), pp. 2049–2060.

[25] See, for example, Bonnie Cramond, Attention Deficit Hyperactivity Disorder and Creativity: What Is the Connection? *Journal of Creative Behavior*, September, 1994, 28(3), pp. 193-210; and Martine Hoogman, Marije Stolte. Matthijs Baasd, and Evelyn Kroesbergen, Creativity and ADHD: A review of behavioral studies, the effect of psychostimulants and neural underpinnings, Neuroscience and Biobehavioral Reviews, December, 2020, 119, pp. 66-85.

Educational perspective: Kids who learn differently should be taught differently

Russell Barkley, who is one of the preeminent figures associated with the ADHD worldview, has made the comment about children identified with ADHD that, "the classroom is their Waterloo."[26] What Barkley is probably referring to here is the traditional classroom based on lecture, tests, worksheets, and textbooks. However, according to Harvard psychologist Howard Gardner, schools focus only on two of eight intelligences he has identified: linguistic and logical-mathematical.[27] If a child learns through any of the other intelligences—musical, spatial, naturalist, bodily-kinesthetic, interpersonal, etc. - then he's out of luck and may not be able to learn according to his most highly developed intelligences.

Kids identified with ADHD, for example, are often bodily-kinesthetic learners: they learn best by moving, touching, and building. If they have to sit still for any period of time, they're going to be restless, distracted, and display the core symptoms of ADHD. According to Sydney Zentall, a professor at Purdue University, these kids are understimulated in a traditional classroom. She's demonstrated that ADHD-diagnosed kids who receive a more invigorating curriculum—music, colored lights, animals, and more —perform and behave better than when they are in a "drill and kill" classroom.[28]

Another study that compared ADHD-diagnosed kids with a control group of typically developing students, found no differences

---

[26] Russell Barkley is quoted in Susan Moses, "Hypotheses on ADHD Debated at Conference," *APA Monitor* (American Psychological Association), February, 1990, p. 34.

[27] See Howard Gardner, *Frames of Mind: The Theory of Multiple Intelligences*, New York: Basic Books, 2011.

[28] See, for example, Sydney S. Zentall, Theory- and Evidence-Based Strategies for Children with Attentional Problems, *Psychology in the Schools*, 2005, 42(8), pp. 821-836.

between the two groups with regard to behavior or engagement when they were engaged in active learning (writing, reading aloud, talking with a teacher or student about the topic at hand) compared to passive learning (listening to a lecture, silently reading a book, looking at a worksheet) where the ADHD students displayed the full range of their symptoms.[29]

And this condition of "active learning" appears to me to be a bare minimum of activity compared with the wide range of options available for teaching kids, which include: projects, discussion groups, field trips, videos, the arts, experiments, role play, and much more.[30] This situation is exacerbated by a school climate that has focused far more attention on testing and accountability over the past forty years. According to one study: "... children in states with more stringent accountability laws are more likely to be diagnosed with Attention Deficit/Hyperactivity Disorder (ADHD) and consequently prescribed psychostimulant drugs for controlling the symptoms."[31] If our schools were more exciting, isn't it possible that we'd see less evidence of ADHD symptoms in our children?

The perspectives described above are only a few of the different paradigms, to use Thomas Kuhn's word, that can be cited as alternative ways of viewing ADHD symptoms.[32] One can use an *anthropological*

---

[29] Rosemary E. Vile Junod, George J. DuPaul, Asha K. Jitendra, Robert J. Volpe, and Kristi S. Cleary, Classroom observations of students with and without ADHD: Differences across types of engagement, *Journal of School Psychology*, April 2006, 44(2), pp. 87–104.

[30] For a look at a sample of the wide range of multiple intelligence-based teaching strategies available to teachers, see Thomas Armstrong, *Multiple Intelligences in the Classroom, 4th edition*, Alexandria, VA: ASCD, 2017.

[31] Quoted in Farasat A.S. Bokhari and Helen Schneider, "School accountability laws and the consumption of psychostimulants," *Journal of Health Economics*, March, 2011, 30(2), pp. 355-72.

[32] The idea of the term "paradigms" as a conceptual tool for describing developments in the history of science, is taken from Thomas Kuhn, *The Structure of Scientific Revolutions*, Chicago: IL: University of Chicago Press, 2012.

perspective to examine how an ADHD-diagnosed person might be like "a hunter in a farmer's world."[33] The traits for ADHD would have been highly adaptive in a hunting and gathering culture, where the ability to be constantly on the prowl (hyperactivity), the capacity to maintain multiple modes of attention (distractibility), and the capability to respond quickly to any stimulus (impulsivity) would have led to hunting success, thus helping to explain why these genes are still in the gene pool.[34]

A *psycho-social perspective* reveals the important influence that being raised in a family climate of adversity (substance abuse, domestic violence, mental illness, marital discord etc.) can have in fueling ADHD behaviors. Perhaps most significant of all is a *sociological perspective*, that views the ADHD worldview as a social phenomenon that has emerged since the 1970s as a convenient strategy for explaining away the tremendous changes that have rocked society over the past fifty years, as well as accounting for the emergence of a multi-billion-dollar pharmaceutical industry in fueling the growth of ADHD over the last thirty years.[35]

The core problem in my estimation is that the people who control the destinies of children and adolescents diagnosed with ADHD are not *interdisciplinary thinkers*. They have essentially been indoctrinated in the fundamental axioms of a single perspective--the ADHD worldview--and gear all of their research, treatments, and

---

[33] See Thom Hartmann, *ADHD: A Hunter in a Farmer's World, 3rd edition*, Fairfield, CT: Healing Arts Press, 2019.

[34] See, for example, P.S. Jensen, D. Mrazek, P.K. Knapp, L. Steinberg, et al., ''Evolution and revolution in child psychiatry: ADHD as a disorder of adaptation,'' *Journal of the American Academy of Child and Adolescent Psychiatry*, 1997, 36(12), pp. 1672-1679.

[35] See, for example, Peter Conrad, and Meredith R. Bergey, The impending globalization of ADHD: Notes on the expansion and growth of a medicalized disorder, *Social Science & Medicine*, December, 2014, 122, pp. 31-43.

hypotheses around that monolithic concept. With a system based on ADHD as a legitimate psychiatric disorder, it's nearly impossible for a researcher to work outside of that belief system and expect to get funded.

Every few years, the ADHD powers-that-be release a consensus statement on ADHD, and the most recent version is formidable indeed listing two hundred and eight "evidence-based conclusions" that support the legitimacy and rigor of the ADHD diagnosis.[36] However, other than references to the importance of family adversity as a contributing factor in ADHD, none of the other arguments that I've advanced in this chapter are found anywhere in the document.

While it refers to ADHD as a developmental disorder, it does not take on the argument that ADHD itself may be better explained for some kids as delayed development. Once you've built a foundation upon an idea that is conceptually shaky, people will forget to ask fundamental questions about it, and everything covering over that defect will masquerade as a truth. But of course, in this case, there are no coverings at all: the proud king stands naked for all to admire, except for those of us who can see what's right in front of our faces.

---

[36] Stephen V. Faraone, Tobias Banaschewski, David Coghill, Yi Zheng, Joseph Biederman, et al. The World Federation of ADHD International Consensus Statement: 208 Evidence-based conclusions about the disorder, *Neuroscience & Biobehavioral Reviews*, September, 2021, 128, pp. 789-818.

ADHD: It's an Industry, not an Illness

Martin Whitely

Despite the fact that its core business is selling amphetamine and amphetamine-like drugs for use by children, the for-profit ADHD Industry is an economic success story.

Since 1980, Hyperkinetic Disorder, a rarely diagnosed and treated childhood condition, has been transformed into Attention Deficit Hyperactivity Disorder, the world's most commonly diagnosed and treated childhood psychiatric disorder. In 2021, global sales of ADHD 'medications' are anticipated to total US$22.5 Billion. Sales are forecast to double by 2030.

Although no diagnostic biomarker, cause or cure has been established, the Industry has successfully marketed ADHD as a common and treatable medical condition (i.e. illness). It has achieved this by using four strategies:

1. *Medicalising* – Fostering the belief that a loosely described pattern of inattentive and/or impulsive behavior has a biological cause.

2. *Expanding* – Broadening the diagnostic criteria so that more patients (including adults) are diagnosed and treated.

3. *Alarming* – Promoting the belief that ADHD is massively underdiagnosed and that the negative consequences of untreated ADHD are severe.

Dr. Martin Whitely is a researcher and author.

4. *Pharmaceuticalising* – Exaggerating the safety and efficacy of 'medications' by emphasizing their short-term behavior-modifying effects, while understating or ignoring their risks and long-term effects.

These strategies have been integral to the industry achieving 'regulatory capture' of related policies and practices. Regulatory capture occurs when processes that are supposed to advance the public interest instead benefit commercial interests. Economists contend it is a predictable consequence of profit-maximizing behavior by well-resourced commercial stakeholders.

Professional psychiatric / psychological / teaching organizations, researchers, and patient advocacy groups all claim to act in the public interest. Opinions on the diagnosis and treatment of ADHD within these stakeholder groups are diverse. However, consistent with the concept of regulatory capture, the response of these stakeholders has typically been dominated by 'ADHD experts.' They have successfully promoted the unproven hypothesis that ADHD is a real medical condition with neurobiological underpinnings as if that was an indisputable fact.

This capture and strategic marketing, rather than scientific advancement, have been the major drivers of burgeoning ADHD diagnosis and treatment rates. As a result, the long-term implications on the wellbeing of children have received superficial consideration while the ADHD Industry has prospered.

Background

Over the last 30 years, global rates of Attention Deficit Hyperactivity Disorder (ADHD) diagnosis and treatment have soared in most developed and many developing nations.[1] The diagnosis is based on reports of dysfunctional inattentive and/or hyperactive behavior and the most commonly-used treatments are amphetamine and amphetamine-like drugs. They have numerous potentially adverse effects, including psychosis, growth retardation, cardiovascular damage and psychological and physical dependence.[2]

Selling these 'stimulant' drugs for non-medical purposes is illegal and attracts considerable criminal penalties, including extended incarceration. Yet the same drugs can be, and are, prescribed at increasing rates to both adults and children diagnosed with ADHD. Indeed, Adzenys, a fruit-flavoured chewable amphetamine pill, has been designed to encourage children to take their 'medication.'[3]

Non-stimulant drugs are less commonly used. The have the advantage of not being as addictive or as easily abused but these are generally recognized as being less effective in modifying ADHD-type behaviors and involve considerable risks, including suicidality.[4]

The obvious question is: how and why has it become commonplace for so many otherwise healthy people, particularly children, to be

---

[1] Raman S.R. et. al. Trends in attention-deficit hyperactivity disorder medication use: a retrospective observational study using population-based databases Lancet Psychiatry. VOLUME 5, ISSUE 10, P824-835, OCTOBER 01, 2018. https://www.thelancet.com/journals/lanpsy/article/PIIS2215-0366(18)30293-1/fulltext (accessed 14 August 2021)

[2] Berman, S M et al. "Potential adverse effects of amphetamine treatment on brain and behavior: a review." Molecular psychiatry vol. 14,2 (2009): 123-42. doi:10.1038/mp.2008.90 https://www.ncbi.nlm.nih.gov/pmc/articles/PMC2670101/ (accessed 29 July 2021)

[3] Persistence Market Research, Global Market Study on Attention-deficit Hyperactivity Disorder (ADHD) Therapeutics: Increasing Production of Generic ADHD Drugs to Boost Market Growth, April 2021 https://www.persistencemarketresearch.com/market-research/attention-deficit-hyperactivity-disorder-therapeutics-market.asp (accessed 15 June 2020)

[4] US Food and Drug Administration, *Public Health Advisory: Suicidal Thinking in Children and Adolescents Being Treated with Strattera (Atomoxetine)*, 17 December 2004. Available at http://www.fda.gov./Drugs/DrugSafety/PublicHealthAdvisories/ucm051733.htm (accessed 13 September 2009)

given a daily amphetamine habit in order to modify unwelcome behaviors?

Proponents of ADHD contend this is a desirable outcome resulting from increased recognition of what they claim remains an underdiagnosed and undertreated disorder.[5] An alternative explanation is that the rapid growth in treatment rates is a consequence of 'regulatory capture' where ADHD-Industry friendly voices have disproportionately influenced clinical practice.[6]

The ADHD industry

The ADHD industry is a combination of for-profit actors and not-for-profit actors who promote increased recognition and treatment of the disorder.

In 2021, global sales of ADHD medications are anticipated to total US$22.5 billion. Sales are forecast to double to US$45 billion by 2030. The majority of sales by value and volume occur in the USA, although they are rising rapidly in most developed nations. North America and Europe are anticipated to continue to remain the biggest market because of the presence of 'strong distributors and sales channels.' However, the availability of medications at lower cost is expected to drive sales in less affluent markets in the Asia/Pacific area and the Middle East and Africa.[7]

---

[5] Neelima Choahan, Australians with ADHD may be missing out on diagnosis and treatment. GP News. RACGP. 18 Sep 2018 https://www1.racgp.org.au/newsgp/clinical/australians-with-adhd-might-be-missing-out-on-prop (accessed 14 August 2021)

[6] John Abraham (2010), '*The Sociological Concomitants of the Pharmaceutical Industry and Medications*' in Chloe E. Bird, Peter Conrad, et al (eds.), Handbook of Medical Sociology, 6th edn, Nashville: pp.304-305

[7] Persistence Market Research, Global Market Study on Attention-deficit Hyperactivity Disorder (ADHD) Therapeutics: Increasing Production of Generic ADHD Drugs to Boost Market Growth, April 2021 https://www.persistencemarketresearch.com/market-research/attention-deficit-hyperactivity-disorder-therapeutics-market.asp (accessed 15 June 2020)

The sales estimates quoted above only include the revenue earned by the pharmaceutical companies that manufacture ADHD drugs (i.e. Pfizer, Novartis, Eli Lilly, GlaxoSmithKline, Mallinckrodt Pharmaceuticals, Johnson & Johnson, UCB, Hisamitsu Pharmaceutical, and Purdue and others.)[8] They do not include the retail margin earned by pharmacists and online retailers.

They also do not include the billions earned by corporations and individuals who diagnose, research and otherwise derive income from ADHD. While information on the prescribing patterns of individual clinicians is scant, the little that exists indicates that most prescribing is done by a minority of potential prescribers who specialize in ADHD and derive a significant proportion of their income from diagnosing and 'treating' the disorder.

For example, in 2015 (the latest year for which data is publicly available) in Western Australia there were 419 authorized prescribers of stimulant medication. Of these, the top 27 prescribed to more than two thirds (n=13,419) of the total number of patients (n=21,667) who received stimulants for ADHD. The top eight prescribed to more 500 patients each, with the top prescriber, a child and adult psychiatrist, prescribing to 2,074 patients, (9.6% of the total ADHD stimulant cohort).[9]

In contrast, it is very difficult to develop ADHD expertise for those clinicians who do not believe it is a valid psychiatric disorder.

---

[8] Persistence Market Research, Global Market Study on Attention-deficit Hyperactivity Disorder (ADHD) Therapeutics: Increasing Production of Generic ADHD Drugs to Boost Market Growth, April 2021 https://www.persistencemarketresearch.com/market-research/attention-deficit-hyperactivity-disorder-therapeutics-market.asp (accessed 15 June 2020)

[9] Department of Health, (2016), *Western Australian Stimulant Regulatory Scheme 2015 Annual Report*, Pharmaceutical Services Branch, Health Protection Group, Department of Health, Western Australia p 15,19, 23,39 http://ww2.health.wa.gov.au/~/media/Files/Corporate/general%20documents/medicines%20and%20poisons/PDF/StimulaThent%20Annual%20Report%202015.ashx (accessed 14 August 2021)

Opportunities to make income from specialising in not diagnosing a condition are very limited.

Similarly, it has been my experience that researchers and advocates with a critical perspective have limited opportunities to find research funding. As a result, those with a critical perspective typically rely on publicly available information and have little capacity to conduct resource-intensive original research into important underexplored issues, like the long-term safety and efficacy of ADHD medications. As with many other areas in medicine and psychiatry, some ADHD experts become Key Opinion Leaders, who are supported with pharmaceutical industry funding and promote the recognition and treatment of the disorder.[10] This is not to imply that all proponents of ADHD medication use by children are motivated by profit or other forms of self-interest. Some are undoubtedly well-intentioned and genuinely believe they are helping children.

Sometimes the lines between the for-profit and not-for-profit ADHD Industry are blurred. ADHD patient support groups, like CHADD in the U.S.A. and ADHD Australia, have the nominated intention of enhancing the welfare of individuals with ADHD. However, they have close relationships with the for-profit sector. These organisations are often controlled or heavily influenced by clinicians who derive much or all of their income from diagnosing, prescribing, researching or promoting ADHD and have received direct financial support from the pharmaceutical industry.[11]

---

[10] Watson, G.L., Arcona, A.P., Antonuccio, D.O. et al. Shooting the Messenger: The Case of ADHD. J Contemp Psychother 44, 43–52 (2014). https://doi.org/10.1007/s10879-013-9244-x (accessed 14 August 2021)

[11] For an example of this type of collaboration see Businesswire, Ironshore Pharmaceuticals Recognizes ADHD Awareness Month Through Partnership With CHADD -Company to Sponsor "Mornings Matter with ADHD" Webinar Hosted by Internationally Renowned ADHD Expert October 28, 2019 https://www.businesswire.com/news/home/20191028005208/en/Ironshore-Pharmaceuticals-Recognizes-ADHD-Awareness-Month-Through-Partnership-With-CHADD (accessed 14 August 2021)

The most prominent U.S. ADHD support group CHADD has been described as like a 'highly energised political or religious organisation.'[12] In 2003, CHADD chief executive officer E. Clark Ross admitted that the 'science' to support the validity of ADHD 'really is a matter of belief.'[13] In a similar vein in 2009, the current Chair of the Board of ADHD Australia, Professor Michael Kohn, described an article in Sydney's *Daily Telegraph* detailing extreme reactions to ADHD such as psychotic episodes and suicidal ideation as 'the latest in a series of articles *blaspheming* the use of Ritalin.'[14]

There are countless examples of not-for-profit ADHD support groups making optimistic, unsubstantiated claims about the scientific certainty of an ADHD diagnosis and/or the safety and efficacy of ADHD treatments.[15] In contrast, pharmaceutical companies are limited by law from making claims about their products that are completely false. However, when support groups exaggerate the benefits and deny the risks of medications, they increase drug company sales and profits without exposing the drug companies to any legal liability.

---

[12] Ray Moynihan and Alan Cassels, *Selling Sickness: How the World's Biggest Pharmaceutical Companies Are Turning us all into Patients*, Nation Books, New York, 2005, p. 67.

[13] Kelly Patricia O'Meara, 'Putting Power Back in Parental Hands; legislation being considered that would allow parents not schools to decide whether their children need to be medicated as a prerequisite for attending classes', *Washington Post's Insight Magazine*, 26 May 2003.

[14] Medicating our children, Reportage Online, 22 December 2009 http://www.reportageonline.com/2009/12/medicating-our-children/ accessed 29 June 2011] Professor Michael Kohn in response to an article in Sydney's Daily Telegraph detailing extreme reactions to ADHD medications reported to the TGA, such as psychotic episodes and suicidal ideation. [11. We're turning our children psychotic with ADHD medication, Kate Sikora, The Daily Telegraph October 13, 2009. http://www.dailytelegraph.com.au/lifestyle/body-soul/were-turning-our-children-psychotic/story-e6frf01r-1225786025127] (accessed 3 July 2011)

[15] Whitely MP. Attention Deficit Hyperactivity Disorder Policy, Practice and Regulatory Capture in Australia 1992–2012 [PhD]. Perth, WA: Curtin University; 2014 pp. 189-192 https://espace.curtin.edu.au/bitstream/handle/20.500.11937/1776/225953_Whitely%202014.pdf?sequence=2&isAllowed=y (accessed 17 June 2020)

Similarly, the for-profit ADHD Industry has benefitted from the uncritical publication of false claims of breakthrough discoveries by ADHD experts who purport to have discovered the biological/genetic basis of ADHD.

One of the biggest and most powerful deceptions ever in regard to ADHD occurred in September 2010 when the world media buzzed with the news that a group of British researchers had found the Holy Grail for proponents of ADHD, by proving its genetic basis.[16] [17]

One of the researchers, Professor Anita Thapar of Cardiff University, proclaimed emphatically '*now we can say with confidence that ADHD is a genetic disease.*'[18] Thapar's claim was nonsense, but by the time critics had identified the flaws in the research, the media circus had moved on and unknown millions of people around the globe had read, seen or heard the unchallenged proclamation that 'ADHD is a genetic disease.'[19]

While pharmaceutical companies have received billions in fines for dishonestly marketing other psychotropic medications in the USA,[20] it has been rare for the drug manufacturers to blatantly lie about

---

[16] Kelland, K. Study finds first evidence that ADHD is genetic, *Reuters*, 30 September 2010. http://www.reuters.com/article/2010/09/30/us-adhd-genes-idUSTRE68S5UD20100930 (accessed 22 November 2012);

[17] Landau, E. (2010) ADHD is a genetic condition, study says, *CNN Health*, 29 September 2010. Available at http://thechart.blogs.cnn.com/2010/09/29/adhd-is-a-genetic-condition-study-says/ (accessed 14 November 2012);

[18] *ABC Online News*. Study finds genetic link to ADHD, 30 September 2010. Available at http://www.abc.net.au/news/2010-09-30/study-finds-genetic-link-to-adhd/2280292 (accessed 22 November 2012)

[19] Martin Whitely, Overprescribing Madness – what's driving Australia's mental illness epidemic. Wilkinson Publishing 2021. p.p. 131-133

[20] Tiash Saha, The biggest ever pharmaceutical lawsuits, Pharmaceutical Technologies Website. 25 Jun 2019 (Updated January 31st, 2020).

https://www.pharmaceutical-technology.com/features/biggest-pharmaceutical-lawsuits/ (accessed 14 August 2021)

ADHD medications. However, as detailed below, there has been a systematic and sustained effort by pharmaceutical companies and other elements of the ADHD Industry that have strategically and often dishonestly marketed amphetamines and other similarly dangerous drugs for use by children.

While there is some limited, uncritical competition within the ADHD Industry between manufacturers producing different brands, there is unanimity of opinion in regards to the validity of the disorder and the appropriateness of a pharmaceutical intervention. In essence, the ADHD Industry is multi-layered, coordinated, well-resourced, professional and strategic, whereas critics are generally poorly-resourced, uncoordinated amateurs.

Regulatory capture

This mismatch has amplified industry friendly, 'ADHD expert' voices at the expense of critical voices. This imbalance in influence is consistent with the economic theory of 'regulatory capture.' Regulatory capture occurs if a process that is supposed to advance the public interest instead acts to benefit commercial or industry interests in ways that are contrary to or indifferent to the public interest.

Regulatory capture can relate to any actor, both government and non-government, which has the declared intention of protecting or enhancing the public good. Examples of non-government actors in the ADHD field include professional organizations, researchers, and patient advocacy groups.

Many economists consider that regulatory capture is normal because regulatory and policy processes are typically dominated by the most motivated and best resourced stakeholders.[21] The ADHD Industry has an obvious interest in capturing these processes. It is equally obvious that while potential child patients are key stakeholders, children have no capacity to influence these processes. However, the possibility that regulatory capture is a significant contributor to the rapid global growth in ADHD prescribing rates has received little systematic consideration.

In 2010, British sociologist John Abraham, based on British and U.S. experience, argued that regulatory capture is the most significant explanation of the process of pharmaceuticalisation for many health conditions, including ADHD.[22] My PhD thesis examined the relationship between ADHD prescribing rates and regulatory capture in Australia from 1992 to 2012 and demonstrated a positive relationship between regulatory capture and ADHD pharmaceuticalisation consistent with Abraham's contention. It detailed how, in Australia, ADHD had effectively become a medical speciality with the majority of prescribing done by a tiny minority of potential prescribers. These 'experts' and their allies have typically dominated not only clinical practice and regulatory processes, but also the public debate, research, and the development of diagnosis and treatment guidelines. On only rare occasions, ADHD critics have successfully competed to influence research and policy and regulatory outcomes. However, these incidents have been the exception rather than the rule.[23]

---

21 Stigler George J (1971), 'The theory of economic regulation', Bell Journal of Economics and Management Science p.3.

22 John Abraham (2010), 'The Sociological Concomitants of the Pharmaceutical Industry and Medications' in Chloe E. Bird, Peter Conrad, et al (eds.), Handbook of Medical Sociology, 6th edn, Nashville: pp.304- 305

23 Whitely MP. Attention Deficit Hyperactivity Disorder Policy, Practice and Regulatory Capture in Australia 1992–2012 [PhD]. Perth, WA: Curtin University; 2014. p. 236.https://espace.curtin.edu.au/bitstream/handle/20.500.11937/1776/225953_Whitely%202014.pdf?sequence=2&isAllowed=y (accessed 17 June 2020)

Strategies the ADHD industry use to promote child prescribing

Since 1980, the ADHD Industry has transformed a previously rare condition, Hyperkinetic Disorder, into Attention Deficit Hyperactivity Disorder, the world's most commonly 'medicated' childhood psychiatric disorder, by using four broad strategies:

1. *Medicalising* – Fostering the belief that a loosely-described pattern of inattentive and/or impulsive behavior has a biological cause.

2. *Expanding* – Broadening the diagnostic criteria so that more patients are diagnosed and require treatment.

3. *Alarming* – Promoting the alarming belief that ADHD is massively underdiagnosed and that the negative consequences of untreated ADHD are severe.

4. *Pharmaceuticalising* – Exaggerating the safety and efficacy of 'medications' by emphasising their short-term behavior-modifying effects, while understating or ignoring their risks, particularly their long-term risks.

Medicalising

Despite 30 years of hyped promises of imminent technological breakthroughs, there are no brain scans, genetic markers, blood tests, or other objective physical tests that can be used to diagnose ADHD.[24] The behavioral diagnostic criteria listed in the *Diagnostic*

---

[24] American Psychiatric Association (2013), Diagnostic and Statistical Manual of Mental Disorders. Fifth Edition, (DSM-5) pp. 59-66

and Statistical Manual of Mental Disorders (current edition DSM-5) remain the accepted basis for diagnosing the disorder. Essentially the diagnosis of ADHD is still reliant on third party (teacher and parent) reports of children often exhibiting behaviors like fidgeting, playing loudly, losing things and disliking homework to an extent that is considered dysfunctional.

The aetiology of ADHD also remains unknown. Numerous non-biological factors have been identified as being associated with an increased risk of diagnosis. For example, relative age within a classroom has been shown to strongly influence a child's chances of being diagnosed with, or medicated for ADHD – with the youngest children in a classroom being at much higher risk.[25] This global phenomenon occurs in countries with both high and low prescribing rates.[26] Critics believe that this raises concerns about perfectly normal age-related immaturity being medicalised.

Other non-biological factors that have been associated with higher rates of ADHD diagnosis and medication use include ethnicity of students and teachers [27], divorce[28], poverty[29], parenting

---

[25] Whitely M, Lester L, Phillimore J, Robinson S, Influence of birth month of Western Australian children on the probability of being treated for ADHD, Medical Journal of Australia, 2017. https://www.mja.com.au/journal/2017/206/2/influence-birth-month-probability-western-australian-children-being-treated-adhd (accessed 16 June 2020)

[26] Whitely M, Raven M, Timimi S, Jureidini J, Phillimore J, Leo J, Moncrieff J, Landman P, Attention deficit hyperactivity disorder late birthdate effect common in both high and low prescribing international jurisdictions: systematic review, Journal of Child Psychology and Psychiatry, October 2018 (accessed 15 August 2021)

[27] Schneider, H., & Eisenberg, D. (2006). Who receives a diagnosis of attention-deficit/hyperactivity disorder in the United States elementary school population? Pediatrics, 117, e601– e609.

[28] Hjern A, Weitoft GR, Lindblad F. Social adversity predicts ADHD-medication in school children--a national cohort study. Acta Paediatr. 2010;99(6):920-4. https://onlinelibrary.wiley.com/doi/10.1111/j.1651-2227.2009.01638.x (accessed 15 June 2020)

[29] Russell G, Ford T, Rosenberg R, Kelly S. The association of attention deficit hyperactivity disorder with socioeconomic disadvantage: alternative explanations and evidence. Journal of Child Psychology Psychiatry. 2014;55(5):436-45. https://acamh.onlinelibrary.wiley.com/doi/full/10.1111/jcpp.12170 (accessed 15 June 2020)

styles[30], low maternal education, lone parenthood and the receipt of social welfare[31], sexual abuse[32], sleep deprivation[33], perinatal issues[34], artificial food additives[35], mobile phone use[36], clinician speciality[37], postcode and regulatory capture.

Irrespective of this clear evidence of non-biological drivers of diagnosis and the lack of objective tests demonstrating a biological/ biochemical cause, the clinically dominant hypothesis is that ADHD is a genetically determined neurodevelopmental disorder (i.e. caused by dysfunctional brain chemistry) best treated with biochemical interventions. This dominance has not been achieved through science but through a combination of tactics detailed below.

---

[30] Johnston C, Mash EJ, Miller N, Ninowski JE. Parenting in adults with attention-deficit/ hyperactivity disorder (ADHD). Clin Psychol Rev. 2012;32(4):215-28. https://europepmc.org/article/med/22459785 (accessed 15 June 2020)

[31] Hjern A, Weitoft GR, Lindblad F. Social adversity predicts ADHD-medication in school children--a national cohort study. Acta Paediatr. 2010;99(6):920-4. https://onlinelibrary.wiley.com/doi/10.1111/j.1651-2227.2009.01638.x (accessed 15 June 2020)

[32] Weinstein D, Staffelbach D, Biaggio M. Attention-deficit hyperactivity disorder and posttraumatic stress disorder: differential diagnosis in childhood sexual abuse. Clin Psychol Rev. 2000;20(3):359-78. https://www.sciencedirect.com/science/article/abs/pii/S027273589800107X (accessed 15 June 2020)

[33] Thakkar VG. Diagnosing the Wrong Deficit. New York Times. 27 April 2013. https://www.nytimes.com/2013/04/28/opinion/sunday/diagnosing-the-wrong-deficit.html (accessed 15 June 2020)

[34] Schmitt J, Romanos M. Prenatal and perinatal risk factors for attention-deficit/ hyperactivity disorder. Arch Pediatr Adolesc Med. 2012;166(11):1074-5. Prenatal and perinatal risk factors for attention-deficit/hyperactivity disorder. https://pubmed.ncbi.nlm.nih.gov/22200325/#:~:text=CONCLUSIONS%3A%20This%20is%20the%20first,to%2040%20years%20after%20birth. (accessed 15 June 2020)

[35] McCann D, Barrett A, Cooper A, Crumpler D, Dalen L, Grimshaw K, et al. Food additives and hyperactive behaviour in 3-year-old and 8/9-year-old children in the community: a randomised, double-blinded, placebo-controlled trial. Lancet. 2007;370(9598):1560-7. https://www.thelancet.com/journals/lancet/article/PIIS0140-6736(07)61306-3/fulltext (accessed 15 June 2020)

[36] Byun YH, Ha M, Kwon HJ, Hong YC, Leem JH, Sakong J, et al. Mobile phone use, blood lead levels, and attention deficit hyperactivity symptoms in children: a longitudinal study. PLoS One. 2013;8(3): e59742. https://journals.plos.org/plosone/article?id=10.1371/journal.pone.0059742 (accessed 15 June 2020)

[37] Western Australia. Parliament. Legislative Assembly. Attention deficit hyperactivity disorder in Western Australia Perth; 2004. https://www.parliament.wa.gov.au/Parliament/commit.nsf/(Report+Lookup+by+Com+ID)/A88388l3E981CEE948257831003E9611/$file/ADD%20final%20report%20pdf%20version.pdf (accessed 15 June 2020)

Substituting consensus for science. Since its inception, ADHD's acceptance as a valid psychiatric disorder been driven by consensus processes. An American Psychiatric Association (APA) sub-committee agreed to the initial recognition of Attention Deficit Disorder (ADD) in DSM-III (1980). Similar committee processes facilitated the expansion of the definition to ADHD in DSM-IV (1994) and the further loosening of the diagnostic criteria in DSM-5 (2013). These decisions were not based on a formal analysis of robust independent science. Rather they required a consensus of like-minded experts, most of whom (like the APA) had commercial ties to pharmaceutical companies.[38]

Similar consensus processes have driven Australian ADHD policy and treatment guidelines processes. Typically, these processes have been devoid of rigorous scientific inquiry and 'ADHD experts' have by consensus developed ADHD Industry-friendly outcomes that facilitate increased diagnosis and treatment.[39]

There have also been coordinated global efforts via expert consensus to assert the validity of ADHD and reinforce the need for treatment. For example, in 2002, a self-declared 'independent consortium of eighty-four leading scientists ... who have devoted years, if not entire careers' to the study of ADHD signed the 'International Consensus Statement on ADHD.' Their statement asserted there was no more disagreement about the disorder's validity 'than there is over whether smoking causes cancer ... or whether a virus causes HIV/AIDS'.[40]

---

[38] Cosgrove L, Krimsky S. A Comparison of DSM-IV and DSM-5 Panel Members' Financial Associations with Industry: A Pernicious Problem Persists. PLoS Med. 2012. https://journals.plos.org/plosmedicine/article?id=10.1371/journal.pmed.1001190

[39] Whitely MP. Attention Deficit Hyperactivity Disorder Policy, Practice and Regulatory Capture in Australia 1992–2012 [PhD]. Perth, WA: Curtin University; 2014. p.p. 233-235 https://espace.curtin.edu.au/bitstream/handle/20.500.11937/1776/225953_Whitely%202014.pdf?sequence=2&isAllowed=y (accessed 17 June 2020)

[40] Russell A. Barkley, et al. (2002), 'International Consensus Statement on ADHD', *Clinical Child and Family Psychology Review*, Vol 5, No. 2, p.89. Available at

However, twenty years later it remains the case no ADHD expert has established a biological cause (or causes) of ADHD. So, despite the fundamentalist fervour of the authors, their assertion that ADHD 'is a real medical condition' remains at best an unproven hypothesis.

American neurologist Fred Baughman contends that any claim that ADHD is a medical condition, disease, disorder, illness or neurodevelopmental condition is fraudulent. He argues these terms imply a person 'has an objective physical abnormality' and that the absence of a biomarker means ADHD is not a real medical condition.[41]

One counter argument to Baughman's is that all psychiatric disorders, many of which are also treated with medication, are diagnosed using similar behavioral criteria. However, pointing out inadequacies in the diagnosis of other psychiatric conditions is a poor defense for the inadequacies of the ADHD diagnostic criteria. Furthermore, conditions like schizophrenia involve identifying extreme behaviors such as delusions or catatonia. In contrast, the ADHD diagnostic criteria are all normal childhood behaviors including: fidgeting, forgetting, playing loudly, losing things and disliking homework.[42]

The claim by the signatories of the International Consensus Statement that they were an 'independent consortium' is also dubious. They may not have received payment for signing the consensus statement. However, while none were disclosed in the statement, many signatories had extensive ties to pharmaceutical companies.[43] For example the first signatory, American psychologist Dr Russell Barkley, who is arguably the world's most high-profile ADHD

---

[41] Fred A. Baughman Jr., MD and Craig Hovey, *The ADHD Fraud: How Psychiatry Makes 'Patients' of Normal Children*, Trafford Publishing, Victoria BC, 2006.

[42] American Psychiatric Association (2013), Diagnostic and Statistical Manual of Mental Disorders. Fifth Edition, (DSM5) pp. 59-66

[43] Sami Timimi, et al (2004), 'A Critique of the International Consensus Statement on ADHD', *Clinical Child and Family Psychology Review*, Vol. 7, No. 1, p.59.

advocate, has extensive ties to multiple ADHD drug manufacturers.[44] And financial ties are not the only potential source of bias. There is the obvious professional credibility they have invested in validating the authenticity of a controversial disorder for those who have devoted years, if not entire careers, to its study.

Confusing cause and effect through a circular process of diagnosis and attribution. Diagnosing ADHD involves a circular process of labelling a loosely-defined pattern of dysfunctional behavior as ADHD, and then regarding ADHD as the cause dysfunctional behavior. In effect, a child (usually a boy) is diagnosed with ADHD because he misbehaves, and then the diagnosing clinician tells the boy's parents he is misbehaving because he has ADHD.[45]

The signatories of the consensus statement ignore the circularity of this process and the behavioral basis of the diagnosis process and instead claim 'those suffering the condition have a serious deficiency [that] leads to harm to the individual.'[46]

Absolving parents of responsibility by medicalising their child's poor behavior. By attributing a child's poor behavior to a 'serious deficiency' that causes a 'real medical condition.' ADHD experts offer a medicalised explanation for their behavior. This has the effect of absolving their parents of responsibility for their child's poor behavior. Typical of this absolution from parental responsibility is a 2019 WebMD article that reassures parents, 'Don't blame yourself. ADHD is a brain disorder.'[47]

---

[44] Alan Schwarz, ADHD Nation: The disorder. The drugs. The inside story. Little Brown 2016

[45] David Keirsey, 'The Great A.D.D. Hoax' at Keirsey.com. http://www.keirsey.com/add_hoax.aspx (accessed 20 March 2008).

[46] Russell A. Barkley, et al. (2002), 'International Consensus Statement on ADHD', *Clinical Child and Family Psychology Review*, Vol 5, No. 2, p.89. Available at https://www.researchgate.net/publication/259981887_Consensus_statement_on_ADHD (accessed 17 July 2021)

[47] Hope Cristol, Does Parenting Play a Role in ADHD? WebMD. 22 October 2019, https://www.webmd.com/add-adhd/childhood-adhd/parenting-role-in-adhd (accessed 29 July 2021)

Often parents are relieved when they are told that their child's real or perceived behavioral problems are not a result of their parenting. Many are persuaded that they must 'medicate' their child to ensure they don't suffer the 'debilitating' fate of undiagnosed and un-medicated ADHD sufferers.[48] Some look back at their own lives and attribute educational, social, career and relationship difficulties to their own undiagnosed ADHD and in turn become adult patients.[49]

ADHD and Identity. ADHD has become a cultural phenomenon where adult 'ADHDers' and some parents of children diagnosed with ADHD have made the label a core part of their or their child's identity. In doing so, many have accepted two contradictory messages promoted by the ADHD Industry: first, that it is a disability requiring special accommodation; and second, that it is a superpower that enables ADHDers to achieve the extraordinary.[50] [51] Equally puzzling is the acceptance of the necessity of daily medication use to manage brain chemistry among those who promote the existence of 'ADHD superpowers.'[52]

Another interesting but underexplored aspect of the explosion in ADHD diagnosis and treatment rates is the growth in the number

---

[48] Ptacek, R., Weissenberger, S., Braaten, E., Klicperova-Baker, M., Goetz, M., Raboch, J., Vnukova, M., & Stefano, G. B. (2019). Clinical Implications of the Perception of Time in Attention Deficit Hyperactivity Disorder (ADHD): A Review. Medical science monitor: international medical journal of experimental and clinical research, 25, 3918–3924. https://doi.org/10.12659/MSM.914225

[49] Daniel Lavelle, 'I assumed it was all my fault': the adults dealing with undiagnosed ADHD. The Guardian, 6 Sep 2017. https://www.theguardian.com/society/2017/sep/05/i-assumed-it-was-all-my-fault-the-adults-dealing-with-undiagnosed-adhd (accessed 29 July 2021)

[50] CHADD, Asking for Workplace Accommodations. (accessed 28 July 2021) https://chadd.org/adhd-weekly/asking-for-workplace-accommodations/

[51] CHADD, The 5 Superpowers People With ADHD Can Use to Be Better Entrepreneurs. (accessed 28 July 2021) https://chadd.org/adhd-in-the-news/the-5-superpowers-people-with-adhd-can-use-to-be-better-entrepreneurs/

[52] CHADD, Medications Used in the Treatment of ADHD. (accessed 28 July 2021) https://chadd.org/for-parents/medications-used-in-the-treatment-of-adhd/

of people who self-identify and/or describe their ADHD diagnosed children as neurodiverse (as opposed to neurotypical).[53] Despite a lack of any objective, demonstrable, diagnostic differences in brain structure or chemistry, they assert that they or their ADHD children have neurological differences that cause behavioral differences.

The term 'neurodiversity' was first coined in the 1990s by Australian sociologist Judy Singer, who wrote:

> Neurodiversity is an idea that takes into account variations in the human brain regarding learning, mood, attention, sociability, and other mental functions that doesn't pathologize the conditions, meaning they are not regarded as abnormal or unhealthy but as differences to be understood and worked with. It largely rejects the medical model of disability.[54]

Singer was encouraging the acceptance of difference. However, the subsequent completely unscientific division of the population into 'neurodiverse' and 'neurotypical' groups is arguably the antithesis of acceptance and inclusion, and encourages the medical model of disability. It sets up two groups, the normal, and the abnormal, and assumes that the cause of the abnormal behavior is abnormal brain function.

The ADHD Industry has benefitted from encouraging the simultaneous belief that those with the condition are special (neurodiverse) and gifted (with superpowers) but also disabled and in need of treatment.

---

[53] ADHD Aware Website, What is ADHD? Neurodiversity and other conditions https://adhdaware.org.uk/what-is-adhd/neurodiversity-and-other-conditions/ (accessed 15 August 2021)

[54] Singer J. *Disability Discourse*, Mairian Corker Ed., Open University Press, February 1, 1999, p 64))

Expanding

The American Psychiatric Association and Big Pharma. The current diagnostic criteria of ADHD are detailed in the American Psychiatric Association's (APA) catalogue of mental illness, the *Diagnostic and Statistical Manual of Mental Disorders 5th edition* (DSM-5).[55] An alternative framework for diagnosing mental illness, the International Clarification of Diseases (ICD), is produced by the World Health Organization (WHO).

Although there are subtle differences that result in higher diagnosis rates in jurisdictions using the DSM, the eighteen behavioral diagnostic criteria for 'Hyperkinetic Disorder' outlined in ICD-10 (the 10th edition) are virtually identical to those for ADHD in DSM-5.

Rather than being developed as competing diagnostic systems, the ICD and DSM have had different development pathways that have converged over time. In regards to ADHD, the APA has led the development of diagnostic criteria, and the WHO has followed. When ICD-11 replaces ICD-10 in January 2022, Hyperkinetic Disorder will be replaced with ADHD and the diagnostic criteria will even be marginally looser than those defined in DSM-5.[56]

With approximately 36,000 members, the APA is the dominant professional organization of psychiatrists in the USA, and the largest psychiatric organization in the world.[57] It is self-regulated

---

[55] Lisa Cosgrove, Sheldon Krimsky and Manisha Vijayaraghavan, 'Financial Ties between DSM-IV Panel Members and the Pharmaceutical Industry', *Psychotherapy and Psychosomatics*, 75, 2006, p. 154; American Psychiatric Association, *Diagnostic and Statistical Manual of Mental Disorders*, Fourth Edition, Text Revision, American Psychiatric Association, Washington DC, 2000.

[56] ADHD Institute, How is ADHD diagnosed? An educational platform developed by Takeda Pharmaceuticals https://adhd-institute.com/assessment-diagnosis/diagnosis/ (accessed 15 August 2021)

[57] American Psychiatry Association, (2012), 'About APA & Psychiatry'. Available at http://www.psychiatry.org/about-apa--psychiatry (accessed 5 June 2012)

and is led by its President and a Board of Trustees with an Executive Committee. Along with the DSM (over which it has total editorial control) the APA publishes for sale journals and other material.

Studies have revealed that the APA and most panel members of the APA committees responsible for developing diagnostic criteria in the most recent editions of the DSM (DSM III 1980, DSM-IV 1984, DSM-5 2013) have had financial ties to the pharmaceutical industry.[58] [59] On multiple occasions, over many years, senior figures within the APA have expressed the view that the relationship between American psychiatry and pharmaceutical companies is too close and potentially corrupts psychiatric practice.[60] [61]

The co-dependent relationship between the APA and pharmaceutical companies has been attributed to declining incomes for both the APA and individual American psychiatrists. Critics contend that, partly in response to increasing competition from non-medical mental health practitioners, psychiatry has increasingly become dominated by the 'pill for every ill' biomedicalised model.

They argue this close commercial relationship first emerged in the 1970s and coincided with the shift from a psychoanalytical focus in

---

[58] American Psychiatry Association, (2012), 'About APA & Psychiatry'. Available at http://www.psychiatry.org/about-apa--psychiatry (accessed 5 June 2012)

[59] Sheldon Krimsky and Manisha Vijayaraghavan, (2006), 'Financial Ties between DSM-IV Panel Members and the Pharmaceutical Industry', Psychotherapy and Psychosomatics, 75, p. 54.

[60] Steven S. Sharfstein, 'Big Pharma and American Psychiatry', *Psychiatric News*, Vol. 40, No. 16, (August 2008): p. 3.

[61] In 1985 Fred Gottlieb, APA Speaker of the House, told the APA: I do not suggest that either they [the drug companies] or we [the American Psychiatric Association] are evil folks. But I continue to believe that accepting such money is, in the long run, inimical to our independent functioning. We have evolved a somewhat casual and quite cordial relationship with the drug houses, taking their money readily…We seem to discount available data that drug advertising promotes irrational prescribing practices. We seem to think that we as psychiatrists are immune from the kinds of unconscious emotional bias in favour of those who are overtly friendly toward us…We persist in ignoring an inherent conflict of interest. Quoted in Breggin, Talking Back to Ritalin, p.216.

DSM-II (1968) to a biological focus in DSM-III (1980) and in later editions. This biological focus aligned American psychiatry with the interests of pharmaceutical manufacturers selling products that treat perceived biochemical imbalances.[62] [63]

The evolution of ADHD's diagnostic criteria. In line with this biomedicalised trend, there has been a progressive broadening in the diagnostic criteria for ADHD and the conditions that predated it.[64] The second edition of the Diagnostic and Statistical Manual of Mental Disorders (DSM II) published in 1968, included 'Hyperkinetic Disorder of Childhood' which required children to demonstrate extreme hyperactive behaviors. It was rarely diagnosed, particularly outside the USA.[65]

For DSM-III, published in 1980, the American Psychiatric Association (APA) changed the name to 'Attention Deficit Disorder' (ADD) and expanded its diagnostic criteria. The new definition was based on the assumption that attention difficulties are sometimes independent of impulse problems and hyperactivity and two subtypes were classified ADD/H, with hyperactivity, and ADD/WO, without hyperactivity or passive ADD.

With DSM-III-R (APA 1987), the revised version of DSM-III, the name of the condition was changed to the one used today, Attention

---

[62] Breggin, Talking Back to Ritalin, p.216.

[63] Robert Whitaker (2010), Anatomy of an Epidemic: Magic Bullets, Psychiatric Drugs, and the Astonishing Rise of Mental Illness in America, Crown Publishing Group, New York, pp.276–278. 68 companies.

[64] Whitely MP. Attention Deficit Hyperactivity Disorder Policy, Practice and Regulatory Capture in Australia 1992–2012 [PhD]. Perth, WA: Curtin University; 2014. https://espace.curtin.edu.au/bitstream/handle/20.500.11937/1776/225953_Whitely%202014.pdf?sequence=2&isAllowed=y (accessed 17 June 2020)

[65] Thorley G. Hyperkinetic syndrome of childhood: clinical characteristics. Br J Psychiatry. 1984 Jan; 144:16-24. doi: 10.1192/bjp.144.1.16. PMID: 6692072. https://pubmed.ncbi.nlm.nih.gov/6692072/ (accessed 2 August 2021)

Deficit Hyperactivity Disorder, and the symptoms were again merged into a single disorder without any subtypes. Specifically, DSM-III-R required a child to display six of nine inattentive behaviors and six of nine impulsive/hyperactive behaviors.[66] This diagnostic requirement did away with the possibility that an individual could have the disorder without being hyperactive. A child had to display both inattentive and hyperactive/impulsive behaviors. This change went against the long-term trend of loosening the diagnostic criteria.

Subsequent to the release of DSM-IIIR, a number of studies were published justifying the existence of passive or inattentive ADD without the hyperactivity element. In response to this backlash, the definition was changed yet again in the fourth edition of the manual published in 1994 (DSM-IV). The 1987 decision was effectively reversed as the criteria were broadened so that a 'patient' needed to display six of nine inattentive or six of nine hyperactive/impulsive behaviors.

The APA did not change the name ADHD, but the symptoms were divided into two categories: inattentive and hyperactive/impulsive. Three subtypes of the disorder were also defined: 'ADHD – Primarily Inattentive', 'ADHD – Primarily Hyperactive/Impulsive', and 'ADHD – Combined Type (both inattentive and impulsive)'. Not surprisingly, this created some confusion. Sometimes when the term Attention Deficit Disorder (ADD) is used today, it is used in its original generic sense – interchangeably with ADHD. On other occasions, it is used as a specific descriptor of passive ADHD without the H for Hyperactivity.[67]

---

[66] American Psychiatric Association (1987), Diagnostic and statistical manual of mental disorders, 3rd edn, revised, Washington, DC, American Psychiatric Association.

[67] For further detail on the evolution of ADHD in the DSM see Whitely MP. Attention Deficit Hyperactivity Disorder Policy, Practice and Regulatory Capture in Australia 1992–2012 [PhD]. Perth, WA: Curtin University; 2014. p.p. 70-72

DSM-IV Chairperson Allen Frances later acknowledged the role of expanded DSM-IV criteria in triggering a 'false epidemic for ADHD.' However, he believes this was part of a greater process of commercially-driven pharmaceuticalisation. He identified that new, more expensive drugs for ADD were brought to market 'that were no better than the old drugs,' and were aggressively marketed direct-to-consumers in the USA following a relaxing of advertising restrictions.

The epidemic started precisely when aggressive drug company marketing succeeded in 'educating' and sensitizing doctors, parents, and teachers to spot ADD in kids previously considered to be on the normal side of the spectrum's boundary. The drug company cause has been furthered by heavily-subsidized thought leaders (usually psychiatrists), by physicians (especially in primary care) who are too free in diagnosis and treatment, and by harried parents and teachers trying to figure out how best to help and manage their difficult children.[68]

The process of 'diagnostic creep.' A broadening of diagnostic criteria took another leap forward when DSM-5 was published in May 2013. The final version made it significantly easier to qualify for a diagnosis of ADHD, but it could have been even easier.

An early draft of DSM-5, released by the APA for public comment, proposed the inclusion of four extra ways of exhibiting impulsivity:

1. Tends to act without thinking.

2. Is often impatient.

---

[68] Allen Frances (March 2012), 'Attention Deficit Disorder is Over-Diagnosed and Over-Treated', Huffington Post, 5 March 2012. Available at http://www.huffingtonpost.com/allen-frances/attention-deficit-disorder_b_1206381.html (accessed 9 January 2013)

3. Is uncomfortable doing things slowly and systematically.

4. Finds it difficult to resist temptations or opportunities.

For a diagnosis of the primarily hyperactive subtype, instead of children having to display 6 of 9 (67 percent) impulsive/hyperactive diagnostic criteria, it was proposed that 6 of 13 (47 percent) would be sufficient.[69]

This early draft also proposed that, for anyone aged 17 or older, the ADHD diagnostic threshold was to be lowered further. If the proposed changes were adopted, it would be sufficient to meet as few as four (down from six) of either the nine inattentive or four of the proposed expanded 13 impulsive/hyperactive criteria.[70]

Following a considerable backlash, the final version of DSM-5 was tightened a little from what was proposed in the draft. Most notably the four extra criteria were not included. But despite the back-down, the changes between DSM-IV and DSM-5 were significant, with an emphasis on making it easier to diagnose ADHD in adults. For those aged 17 or over, the number of criteria that had to be displayed was reduced from six to five. The final DSM-5 also relaxed the DSM-IV requirement that signs of the behavior should be displayed before age seven. It is now sufficient to display some symptoms before age twelve.

Other significant loosening of the criteria from DSM-IV to DSM-5 included:

---

[69] American Psychiatric Association, 'DSM-5 Development, Proposed Revision', Attention Deficit/Hyperactivity Disorder. Was available at http://www.DSM-5.org/ProposedRevision/Pages/proposedrevision.aspx?rid=383 (accessed 25 July 2011 but is no longer available).

[70] American Psychiatric Association, 'DSM-5 Development, Proposed Revision', Attention Deficit/Hyperactivity Disorder. Was available at http://www.DSM-5.org/ProposedRevision/Pages/proposedrevision.aspx?rid=383 (accessed 25 July 2011 but is no longer available).

- The relaxation of the expectation that teachers independently provide evidence.[71]

- Replacing hyperactive actions in the wording of criteria to feelings or perceptions of 'restlessness.'

- Medicalising normal work/study-related stress by including the statement that ADHD behaviors are 'typically more marked during times when the person is studying or working' than 'during vacation'.

- The inclusion of adult-relevant examples in most of the diagnostic criteria which had previously been primarily orientated to children in a school setting.[72]

The APA only modified its original proposals after significant past users of the DSM, including the British Psychological Association and chapters of the American Psychological Association, threatened a boycott of DSM-5.[73] This supports the contention that the American Psychiatric Association's DSM development involves a process of bidding, negotiation and compromise, that is more characteristic of politics or a business deal than it is of scientific discovery.

---

[71] DSM-IV (p87) states 'The clinician should therefore gather information from multiple sources (e.g. parents, teachers) and inquire about the individual's behavior in a variety of situations within each setting'. However, DSM-5 states 'In children and young adolescents, the diagnosis should be based on information obtained from parents and teachers. When direct teacher reports cannot be obtained, weight should be given to information provided to parents by teachers that describe the child's behavior and performance at school'.

[72] For example, one of the hyperactive/impulsive diagnostic criteria in DSM-IV states; 'often leaves seat in classroom or in other situations in which remaining seated is expected'. This was replaced in DSM-5 with is 'often restless during activities when others are seated (may leave his or her place in the classroom, office or other workplace, or in other situations that require remaining seated)'.

[73] Caroline Giles, Rebecca Mathews, Diagnostic dilemmas: DSM-5 review and development. InPsych 2012. Vol 34. Australian Psychological Association. https://www.psychology.org.au/for-members/publications/inpsych/2012/feb/08-Diagnostic-dilemmas-DSM-5-review-and-developm (accessed 14 August 2021)

The global increase in sales of ADHD drugs has coincided with broadening in diagnostic criteria. Market research analysts Persistence Market Research predict 'the low threshold of diagnostic criteria' will continue 'to fuel revenue growth of the global ADHD therapeutics market.'[74]

Neurologist Fred Baughman believes this broadening of diagnostic criteria is contrary to the process of defining legitimate diseases. Normally, as a condition is studied and more is learned about it, the diagnostic signs (signs = objective abnormalities) are narrowed down to a specific set of objective criteria that can be reliably applied. With ADHD, the opposite happened.[75]

Girls and Adults as under-exploited markets. To date, the biggest market for ADHD drugs has been boys. All across the globe, boys are roughly three to four times more likely than girls to be medicated. The ADHD Industry has recognized that girls are an under-exploited market. In response, they have made a significant effort to market 'passive ADHD' (or ADD without the H for hyperactivity) as a gender equity issue. The argument is that quiet daydreaming girls are believed to be missing out, as their disability is being under-recognised.[76]

There is some evidence that the gender gap is slowly closing, but only because the prescribing rates for girls may be rising even faster than that for boys. One of the disturbing drivers of this trend may be the

---

[74] Persistence Market Research, Global Market Study on Attention-deficit Hyperactivity Disorder (ADHD) Therapeutics: Increasing Production of Generic ADHD Drugs to Boost Market Growth, April 2021 https://www.persistencemarketresearch.com/market-research/attention-deficit-hyperactivity-disorder-therapeutics-market.asp (accessed 15 June 2020)

[75] Fred A. Baughman Jr., MD and Craig Hovey, *The ADHD Fraud: How Psychiatry Makes 'Patients' of Normal Children*, Trafford Publishing, Victoria BC, 2006. p. 58.

[76] Slobodin Ortal, Davidovitch Michael, Gender Differences in Objective and Subjective Measures of ADHD Among Clinic-Referred Children, Frontiers in Human Neuroscience. VOL 13 2019 https://www.frontiersin.org/article/10.3389/fnhum.2019.00441

use, particularly by teenage girls and young women, of prescription amphetamines to get thin.[77]

Another marketing push in recent years has been in selling 'adult ADHD.' Taken in moderate doses, amphetamines make most adults feel alert, focussed and on top of their game.[78] Convincing some adults that this effect is a result of 'medicating their ADHD' and they can only be their best self with amphetamines in their system is easy and profitable. Some become passionate advocates for the validity of the 'lifelong disorder.'[79]

Alarming

Inflated prevalence rate estimates are cited to argue that ADHD is underdiagnosed and undertreated. Prevalence rates are estimates of the percentage of a population with a disease or disorder. A prevalence rate is different from a diagnosis rate, which is the percentage of the population diagnosed with a condition. For diseases like asthma, haemophilia, or leukaemia – with science-based diagnoses, real and indisputable negative consequences, and medically valid treatments – parents, policymakers and clinicians need to be concerned if prevalence rates exceed diagnosis rates because it means that real disease is going undiagnosed and untreated. For a subjective, ill-defined diagnosis like ADHD, estimates of prevalence rates are virtually meaningless.

---

[77] Low Keath, Turning to Adderall for Weight Loss, very well mind. 8 January 2020. https://www.verywellmind.com/adderall-rapid-weight-loss-speed-diet-3972108 (accessed 15 June 2020)

[78] Ilieva, I. P., & Farah, M. J. (2013). Enhancement stimulants: perceived motivational and cognitive advantages. Frontiers in neuroscience, 7, 198. https://doi.org/10.3389/fnins.2013.00198 (accessed 31 July 2021)

[79] Evan Starkman, Big Emotions From Learning You Have Adult ADHD WebMD March 2021. https://www.webmd.com/add-adhd/features/adult-adhd-diagnosis-emotions (accessed 24 August 2021)

Nonetheless there have been numerous studies to determine prevalence rates for ADHD. Not surprisingly, estimates of ADHD prevalence vary widely. An American study conducted in 1998 found that prevalence estimates vary between 1.7 per cent and 16 per cent.[80] Estimates of prevalence rates also vary across cultures, presumably influenced by cultural norms with the highest reported (29 per cent) being in India.[81] The huge range is a predictable consequence of relying on subjective and ill-defined diagnostic criteria.

Even if levels of inattention, hyperactivity and impulsivity could be objectively measured, so that children could be reliably placed on a continuum of ADHD behaviors, many parents of children who may qualify for a diagnosis would not accept the label or allow their child to be prescribed amphetamines or similar drugs. For this reason, estimates of ADHD prevalence rates inevitably exceed diagnosis and treatment rates.

Nonetheless there have also been countless examples of where criticisms that ADHD is over-diagnosed and over-medicated are defended with the claim that prevalence rates exceed diagnosis and prescribing rates, and therefore ADHD is *under*-diagnosed and *under*-medicated.

Promoting the alarming belief that the negative consequences of untreated ADHD are severe. It is very common for ADHD proponents to attribute a variety of problems to undiagnosed/untreated ADHD.

---

[80] Larry S. Goldman, Myron Genel, Rebecca J. Bezman, Priscilla J. Slanetz, for the Council on Scientific Affairs, American Medical Association, 'Diagnosis and treatment of attention-deficit/hyperactivity disorder in children and adolescents', *Journal of the American Medical Association*, 279(14), pp. 1100–07.

[81] Professor Stephen Houghton, Psychologist/University Professor, Graduate School of Education, University of Western Australia, transcript of evidence given to Inquiry into Attention Deficit Disorder and Attention Deficit Hyperactivity Disorder in Western Australia, in Perth on 26 November 2003.

For example, the International Consensus Statement states: "... there is no doubt that ADHD leads to impairments in major life activities, including social relations, education, family functioning, occupational functioning, self-sufficiency, and adherence to social rules, norms, and laws. Evidence also indicates that those with ADHD are more prone to physical injury and accidental poisonings."[82]

Even criminality and drug abuse are attributed to undiagnosed, and therefore un-medicated, ADHD.[83] The effect of this association with extreme dysfunctional behavior is to create a sense of crisis that extreme consequences will result from ADHD going untreated.

Criminal and drug-taking behavior are in themselves dysfunctional and often impulsive acts. How many problematic drug users aren't forgetful, distracted or disorganised? It is self-evident that many criminals and drug addicts tend to demonstrate ADHD behaviors and certainly live dysfunctional lives, therefore qualifying for a diagnosis of adult ADHD.

Yet arguing that ADHD, when left un-medicated, causes criminal behavior or drug abuse is to confuse cause and effect. It involves identifying dysfunction in what is already identified as a dysfunctional population. This is the equivalent of being able to bet on which horse will come last after the race has finished.

Giving children a daily amphetamine habit so they don't become drug addicts. The American Psychiatric Association (APA) acknowledges that methamphetamine and cocaine, and the stimulants prescribed

---

[82] Russell A. Barkley, et al. (2002), 'International Consensus Statement on ADHD', *Clinical Child and Family Psychology Review*, Vol 5, No. 2, p.89. Available at https://www.researchgate.net/publication/259981887_Consensus_statement_on_ADHD (accessed 17 July 2021)

for ADHD are 'neuro-pharmacologically alike'[84]. All ADHD stimulants are addictive and carry warnings for abuse. In DSM-5 the APA recognises that prescribed stimulants are diverted for illicit use and classifies the abuse of methamphetamine, cocaine and prescription stimulants in a single condition – 'stimulant use disorder'.[85]

Furthermore, in the USA methamphetamine, brand name Desoxyn, is prescribed to ADHD diagnosed children as young as six years of age.

Nonetheless, ADHD proponents repeatedly assert that treating ADHD with stimulant drugs reduces the probability a child will become a problematic drug user later in life. Fundamentally they are arguing that giving children with challenging behaviors a daily dose of amphetamines prevents them becoming drug abusers.

To justify this claim they cite numerous research items. A common thread in many of these studies is that they rely on the retrospective diagnosis of ADHD in drug-using populations. Again, the absurd circularity, of claiming that dysfunctional behavior is evidence of ADHD which in turn causes dysfunctional behavior, is ignored.

Pharmaceuticalising

There is no doubt that stimulant medications, i.e. amphetamines and amphetamine-like drugs, immediately alter behavior. There is also no doubt that extreme ADHD-type behaviors can be problematic. However, the benefits of stimulant medications are temporary,

---

[83] Department of Health, Government of Western Australia, *Inquiry into Attention Deficit Disorder and Attention Deficit Hyperactivity Disorder in Western Australia*, Legislative Assembly, Transcript of evidence taken on 27 October 2003, p. 2 (Michelle Toner).

lasting a matter of hours with 'no evidence that the medications promote or cause psychological, social, or emotional growth'.[86]

Nonetheless, the temporary behavioral effects of stimulants create the illusion of a solution to challenging and inconvenient behaviors. It is as if the deficit of attention was caused by a deficit of amphetamines. With the drugs in their system, ADHD children are regarded as 'balanced'; without them, they are considered faulty.

Emphasising the short-term benefits and ignoring the long-term outcomes. In research trials, pharmacological interventions invariably appear more effective than non-drug treatments for two reasons. First, the vast majority of the studies into the efficacy of ADHD medications are short-term research trials that last no longer than a few weeks or months and primarily focus on short-term symptom management. Second, while the behavior-altering effects of stimulants are almost universal, other forms of treatment are not. Family counselling, for example, will be of little or no benefit if the underlying cause of behavioral problems is exposure to environmental toxins.

The ADHD Drug Effectiveness Review Project was a 2005 systematic review of all 2,287 studies that were identified through a comprehensive literature search.[87] It was commissioned by fifteen US states in order to determine which ADHD medications were the safest and most cost effective. The review concluded that 'evidence on the effectiveness of pharmacotherapy for ADHD in young children is seriously lacking' and that there was 'no evidence on long-term safety of drugs used to treat ADHD in adolescents.' The review

[84] American Psychiatric Association, *Treatments of Psychiatric Disorders: a task force report of the American Psychiatric Association*, 1st ed., 1989

[85] American Psychiatric Association, Diagnostic and Statistical Manual of Mental Disorders. Fifth Edition, 2013 p. 563

also found that 'good quality evidence on the use of drugs to affect outcomes relating to global academic performance, consequences of risky behaviors, social achievements, etc., is lacking' and that overall the quality of evidence was poor.

Since the publication of this review, data has emerged raising serious issues in relation to the long-term safety and efficacy of ADHD medications. The Multimodal Treatment Study for ADHD[88] (the MTA Study) and the Preschool Attention-Deficit/Hyperactivity Disorder Treatment Study (PATS) reinforced concerns about growth retardation [89], an increased rate of substance abuse, and demonstrated that short-term behavioral benefits did not last.

The response of ADHD proponents to the MTA Study was revealing. After conducting the first fourteen months of the MTA study, the researchers concluded that 'carefully-crafted medication management was superior to the behavioral treatment and to routine clinical care that included medication.'[90] This study received widespread media coverage and was frequently cited by ADHD proponents as compelling evidence of the effectiveness of medications.

However, in 2007, after an analysis of the three-year follow-up to the MTA Study[91] one of the scientists who ran the study concluded: 'I

[88] Molina, B. S. G., Hinshaw, S. P., Swanson, J. M., Arnold, L. E., Vitiello, B., Jensen, P. S., & Cooperative Grp, M. T. A. (2009). The MTA at 8 years: Prospective follow-up of children treated for combined-type ADHD in a multisite study. Journal of the American Academy of Child and Adolescent Psychiatry, 48(5), 484–500. https://pubmed.ncbi.nlm.nih.gov/19318991/ (accessed 14 August 2021)

[89] Allegra Stratton, 'Questions raised Ritalin of no long-term benefit, study finds', The Guardian, November 12th, 2007. Available at https://www.theguardian.com/news/2007/nov/12/uknews.health (accessed 15 May 2019).

[90] The MTA Cooperative Group, 'A 14-Month Randomized Clinical Trial of Treatment Strategies for Attention-Deficit/Hyperactivity Disorder', Archives of General Psychiatry, 56, 1999, p. 1073

[91] Brooke Molina, Kate Flory, Stephen P. Hinshaw et al., 'Delinquent Behavior and Emerging Substance Use in the MTA at 36 Months: Prevalence, Course, and Treatment Effects', Journal of the American Academy of Child & Adolescent Psychiatry, Vol. 46 No. 8, August 2007: pp. 1028–1040.

think we exaggerated the beneficial impact of medication in the first study. We had thought that children medicated longer would have better outcomes. That didn't happen to be the case ... In the short run [medication] will help the child behave better, in the long run it won't. And that information should be made very clear to parents.'[92] Since then the MTA study has rarely been cited.

There is further evidence of sustained harms from ADHD stimulant use among ADHD diagnosed children from long-term data on children's health and wellbeing from Quebec, Canada and Western Australia. Both data sources indicated the academic performance of the children medicated with stimulants for ADHD relative to their peers declined significantly in the years after commencing medication.

The Quebec study also found ADHD medicated children experienced deteriorations in 'relationships with parents' and 'increases in the probability that a child has ever suffered from depression'.[93] In addition the Western Australian study found evidence of raised diastolic blood pressure persisting for a number of years after children received stimulants.[94] There are also long-term animal studies that indicate that the extended use of stimulants may

---

[92] Allegra Stratton, 'Questions raised Ritalin of no long-term benefit, study finds', The Guardian, November 12th, 2007. Available at https://www.theguardian.com/news/2007/nov/12/uknews.health (accessed 15 May 2019)

[93] Janet Currie, Mark Stabile, and Lauren Jones. Do Stimulant Medications Improve Educational and Behavioral Outcomes for Children with ADHD? https://www.ncbi.nlm.nih.gov/pmc/articles/PMC4815037/

[94] Government of Western Australia, Department of Health, Raine ADHD Study: Long-term outcomes associated with stimulant medication in the treatment of ADHD in children, Department of Health, Perth, 2010. https://www.health.wa.gov.au/publications/documents/MICADHD_Raine_ADHD_Study_report_022010.pdf

permanently impair dopamine pathways and may increase the risk of cancer.[95] [96]

With these few exceptions, there is a paucity of studies into the long-term outcomes of ADHD medication use by children. In contrast, there are literally thousands of studies reinforcing the temporary behavior-modifying effects of ADHD medications. Given that the ADHD Industry routinely promotes the message that for many it is a lifelong condition requiring ongoing treatment, the absence of curiosity as to the long-term effects of medications on children appears wilfully and profitably ignorant.

Promoting the false belief that ADHD brains respond differently to medications than non-ADHD brains. It is a common misconception that if a low-dose stimulant narrows focus or calms a child, then they must have ADHD. With a low oral dose of stimulants most people, regardless of their ADHD status, become more narrowly focussed and compliant.[97] This misconception has extended to the use of stimulants as a diagnostic tool. The erroneous logic is that if an ADHD diagnosed child's behavior is modified after taking stimulants, then this confirms the diagnosis.[98]

---

[95] Gene-Jack Wang,1,2,3,* Nora D. Volkow,4,5 Timothy Wigal,6 Scott H. Kollins,7 Jeffrey H. Newcorn,3 Frank Telang,5 Jean Logan,2 Millard Jayne,5 Christopher T. Wong,5 Hao Han,8 Joanna S. Fowler,2,3 Wei Zhu,8 and James M. Swanson6 Long-Term Stimulant Treatment Affects Brain Dopamine Transporter Level in Patients with Attention Deficit Hyperactive Disorder. Published online 2013 May 15. doi: 10.1371/journal.pone.0063023 https://www.ncbi.nlm.nih.gov/pmc/articles/PMC3655054/

[96] El-Zein RA, Abdel-Rahman SZ, Hay MJ, et al. Cytogenetic effects in children treated with methylphenidate. Cancer Lett. 2005; 230:284–291. https://www.ncbi.nlm.nih.gov/pubmed/16297714

[97] Lydia Furman, 'What is Attention-Deficit Hyperactivity Disorder (ADHD)?', Journal of Child Neurology, Vol. 20 No. 12, 2005, p. 998. https://www.researchgate.net/profile/Lydia_Furman/publication/7354308_What_Is_Attention-Deficit_Hyperactivity_Disorder_ADHD/links/5555e9b508ae6fd2d8232e29.pdf (accessed 14 August 2021)

[98] Stevens, J. R., Wilens, T. E., & Stern, T. A. (2013). Using stimulants for attention-deficit/hyperactivity disorder: clinical approaches and challenges. *The primary care companion for CNS disorders, 15*(2), PCC.12f01472. https://doi.org/10.4088/PCC.12f01472 (accessed 1 August 2021)

Amphetamine withdrawal effects mistakenly attributed to re-emerging ADHD. Stimulant behavioral effects are short-lived, lasting a matter of hours. When the medications wear off, there are often withdrawal effects that can be 'worse than the child's original or baseline behavior' even after a single dose.[99]

Witnessing the rebound effect reinforces parents' and teachers' belief that the child is chemically imbalanced without the drug and that he or she needs to keep taking medication.[100] The ADHD Industry benefit from the rebound effect their products have created, to their great profit. They now have a customer with an ongoing 'need' for their product.

Discussion

In the 59 years since the American Psychiatric Association first described the forerunner of ADHD (Hyperkinetic Disorder), no diagnostic biomarker, cause or cure has been established. While new brands and slow release versions of medications have been developed, the dominant therapeutic treatment remains amphetamine and amphetamine-like drugs.

The use of biochemical interventions is based on the speculation that ADHD is a neurodevelopmental disorder caused by faulty brain chemistry. However, viewing ADHD as a disorder, disease, or illness does not provide a satisfactory explanation of the rapid global growth in diagnosis and treatment rates.

---

[99] J. L. Rapoport, M. S. Buchsbaum, et al., 'Dextroamphetamine: cognitive and behavioural effects in normal prepubertal boys', Science, Vol. 199, No. 4323, (3 February 1978), p.561.https://www.researchgate.net/profile/Christy_Ludlow/publication/22798084_DextroamphetamineCognitive_and_behavioral_effects_in_normal_prepubertal_boys/links/5597e85708ae5d8f3933c33a/DextroamphetamineCognitive-and-behavioral-effects-in-normal-prepubertal-boys.pdf (accessed 14 August 2021)

[100] Peter R. Breggin, M.D., Talking Back to Ritalin: What Doctors Aren't Telling You about Stimulants for Children, Common Courage Press, Monroe, 1998, p. 20

The massive growth in global 'medication' sales is an obvious indicator of the success of the ADHD Industry. However, ADHD is more than just an economic success story. It is a cultural phenomenon. Its increased recognition has normalized the daily use of amphetamine by children who fidget, play loudly, run, climb, interrupt, lose things and avoid homework too 'often.'

This psychiatrization of what were previously regarded as normal if annoying childhood behaviors has resulted from a complex process of interaction between individuals, society, business and influential elements of organized biological/pharmaceutical psychiatry. Some of the factors and players driving ADHD's growth are common to other examples of psychriatrization (e.g. depression and antidepressant use).[101]

By medicalising, expanding, alarming, pharmaceuticalising, and capturing regulatory processes, the for-profit ADHD Industry has prospered. To date the implications of this growth industry on the long-term wellbeing of children has received scant consideration.
These outcomes support the contention that the rapid growth in global ADHD diagnosis and treatment rates is an example of psychiatrization, regulatory capture and effective marketing by a profit-driven industry, rather than better recognition of a valid illness.

In conclusion, economic theories that assume profit-maximizing behavior by business, offer a far more plausible explanation than 'scientific advancement' for the ADHD Industry's stunning success.

---

[101] Beeker Timo, Mills China, Bhugra Dinesh, te Meerman Sanne, Thoma Samuel, Heinze Martin, von Peter Sebastian. Psychiatrization of Society: A Conceptual Framework and Call for Transdisciplinary Research. Frontiers in Psychiatry. Vol 12 2021. https://www.frontiersin.org/articles/10.3389/fpsyt.2021.645556/full (accessed 21 august 2021)

Is ADHD a Disease?

Patrick Hahn

In November of 2018, a review published in *PLoS* reported that total health care spending on something called "ADHD" for the year 2016 in the United States topped twenty billion dollars. For that amount of money, we could pay the mid-career salaries of an extra 365,000 teachers, or 827,000 teachers' aides.[1] The justification for this state of affairs rests on the assumption that the complaints that fall under the diagnostic rubric of "ADHD" are caused by an underlying disease, which medical doctors presumably are uniquely qualified to treat.

Is ADHD a disease?

That all depends on what we mean by the word "disease." *The Oxford English Dictionary* offers this definition:

> *A condition of the body, or of some part or organ of the body, in which its functions are disturbed or deranged; a morbid physical condition; a departure from the state of health, especially when caused by structural change.*

Patrick D. Hahn is an affiliate professor of Biology at Loyola University Maryland.

Is ADHD a Disease? has previously appeared in a longer form in *Obedience Pills: ADHD and the Medicalization of Childhood* by Patrick D. Hahn. Permission to use granted.

[1] Brian J. Piper et al., "Trends in Use of Prescription Stimulants in the United States and Territories, 2006 to 2016," *PLoS One*, November 28, 2016, https://doi.org/10.1371/journal.pone.0206100.

The essential part of this definition is "a condition of the body," which implies something that can be measured, such as blood glucose levels in the case of diabetes – a point tacitly acknowledged by psychiatrists and other medical professionals when they compare ADHD meds to insulin.

But no one is claiming that ADHD is caused by a deficiency of Adderall. Have scientists demonstrated any kind of measurable biological lesion that causes ADHD? They certainly have tried. There are two categories of relevant studies here: neuroimaging studies and genetics studies. Let's take a look at each of these in turn.

Neuroimaging studies

Surprising findings

In 1978, a group of Swedish researchers used the newly-developed technology of computerized tomography to scan the brains of forty-six children referred to a clinic for suspected "minimal brain damage."[2] Fifteen of these children exhibited measurable brain anomalies of one form or another.

There was no control group, so we have no way of knowing the proportion of typically-developing children who have similar anomalies. Furthermore, for two-thirds of the MBD children, the researchers were not able to find any brain abnormality at all. Nevertheless, the authors concluded "It may be of some comfort to the parents and others to know that brain damage is the primary cause

---

[2] K. Bergstrom and B. Bille, "Computed Tomography of the Brain in Children with Minimal Brain Damage: A Preliminary Study of 46 Children," *Neuropädiatrie* 9, no. 4 (November 1978): 378-384, https://doi.org/10.1055/s-0028-1091497

of the disturbance and not, for example, social or environmental factors."[3]

They never considered the possibility that attributing these children's problems to "brain damage" (despite the complete lack of evidence of brain damage in the majority of cases) might be a preposterous distraction from focusing on the social and environmental roots of these children's problems -- which unlike brain damage, can be undone or mitigated.

Since then, a mountain of data has failed to demonstrate any anomaly of brain structure or function that reliably distinguishes patients diagnosed with ADHD from those who are not – a point that has been repeatedly emphasized in the scientific literature:

> *"Computed tomography of the brain does not appear to be a necessary screening procedure in the evaluation of the child with minimal brain damage and learning disabilities. Most children evaluated with computed tomography can be expected to have normal scans."*[4]

> *"If anatomic abnormalities are present in ADD, they are not discernible using present-day CT technology."*[5]

> *"No evidence of structural damage in the brains of children with hyperactivity has yet appeared."*[6]

---

[3] Ibid., 382.

[4] J.S. Thompson, Ronald J. Ross, and Samuel J. Horowitz, "The Role of Computed Axial Tomography in the Study of the Child with Minimal Brain Dysfunction," *Journal of Learning Disabilities* 13, no. 6 (June/July 1980): 334-337, https://doi.org/10.1177/00222/1948001300608

[5] Bennet A. Shaywitz et al., "Attention-Deficit Disorder: Quantitative Analysis of CT," *Neurology* 33, (November 1983): 1500-1503, https://doi.org/10.1212/wnl.33.11.1500

[6] Eric Taylor, "Syndromes of Attention Deficit and Hyperactivity," in *Child and Adolescent Psychiatry: Modern Approaches*, ed. Michael Rutter, Eric Taylor, and Lionel Hersov (Oxford: Blackwell Science, 1994), 285-307.

"There is no evidence at present to support psychological testing, laboratory measures of attention, electroencephalography, or neuroimaging studies in the clinical assessment of attention deficit hyperactivity disorders."[7]

"No specific abnormality in brain structure or function has been convincingly demonstrated by neuroimaging studies."[8]

"MRI is not currently diagnostically useful in the routine assessment or management of ADHD."[9]

That last quote was from a 2001 review article by psychiatrist F.X. Castellanos and his colleagues at the National Institute of Mental Health on neuroimaging studies of ADHD. The studies reviewed had reported a dizzying variety of anomalies of brain structure and function said to correlate with a diagnosis of ADHD, but most of the sample sizes were small – which is especially problematic given the high degree of variability in brain structure even in typically-developing subjects. Moreover, all of these differences were quantitative rather than qualitative – that is to say, no abnormality of brain structure and function had ever been shown to distinguish children with a diagnosis of ADHD from those who had no such label.

Even if such an abnormality were ever to be discovered, it would be an open question as to whether that anomaly was the *cause* of

---

[7] James J. McGough and James T. McCracken, "Assessment of Attention Deficit Hyperactivity Disorder: A Review of Recent Literature," *Current Opinion in Pediatrics* 12, no. 4 (August 2000): 319-324, https://doi.org/10.1097/00008480-200008000-00006

[8] Alan Baumeister and Mike F. Hawkins, "Incoherence of Neuroimaging Studies of Attention Deficit/Hyperactivity Disorder," *Clinical Neuropharmacology* 24, no. 1 (2001): 2-10, https://doi.org/10.1097/00002826-200101000-00002

[9] Jay N. Giedd et al., "Brain Imaging of Attention Deficit/Hyperactivity Disorder," *Annals of the New York Academy of Sciences* 931, (June 2001): 33-49, https://doi.org/10.1111/j.1749-6632.2001.tb05772.x

ADHD. We know that experience changes the brain – indeed, that is the whole point of having a brain. Any commonalities between the brains of children labeled ADHD might reflect common experiences associated with that label.

Moreover, as Dr. Castellanos and his co-authors themselves pointed out, most of the studies have not adequately controlled for drug effects[10] – even though, again, there is overwhelming evidence that psychotropic drugs cause measurable structural and/or functional changes in the brain. How could it be otherwise? If a drug did not have an effect on the brain, it would not be considered "psychotropic."

In order to fill this gap in knowledge, Dr. Castellanos and his co-workers published a paper in the October 2002 issue of *JAMA* describing the results of a ten-year study conducted at the NIMH of 152 children diagnosed with ADHD, including forty-nine never-medicated kids, and 139 controls.[11] The researchers found that the brains of children diagnosed with ADHD were smaller than those of typically-developing kids. But perhaps the most surprising finding was that the unmedicated children had significantly smaller white matter volumes compared to both the controls and the medicated ADHD subjects.

None of these differences was diagnostic, and there was considerable overlap between the data sets. Nevertheless, these findings were greeted enthusiastically by the popular media. The headline in the *New York Times* proclaimed "Brain Size Tied to Attention Deficit Hyperactivity Disorder."[12]

---

[10] Ibid., 45.

[11] Francis Xavier Castellanos et al., "Developmental Trajectories of Brain Volume Abnormalities in Children and Adolescents with Attention-Deficit/Hyperactivity Disorder," *JAMA* 288, no. 14 (October 9, 2002): 1740-1748, https://doi.org/10.1001/jama.288.14.1740

[12] Erica Goode, "Brain Size Tied to Attention Deficit Hyperactivity Disorder," *New York Times*, October 9, 2002.

Education Week informed readers "ADHD Drugs Unrelated to Smaller Brain Sizes,"[13] while the Detroit Free Press gushed "Ritalin is safe – and it works: Research dispels fears that drug hurts kids, and finds that it actually helps brains grow."[14]

There was just one problem: the unmedicated ADHD kids in the NIMH study were, on average *more than two years younger* than the medicated ones,[15] and presumably shorter and lighter. Both brain size and white matter volume are known to correlate with age, so it's not surprising that both of these were smaller in the undrugged kids.

Dr. Castellanos and his colleagues claim to have controlled for that confounder by means of a secondary analysis of twenty-four unmedicated patients with ADHD, fifty medicated patients, and fifty-four unmedicated controls, and they reported that "all measures remained essentially unchanged."[16] But since the authors don't give us any details about this secondary analysis, we just have to take their word for it.

The following year, the Castellanos paper was the subject of a withering review[17] by psychiatrist Jonathan Leo and David Cohen, a Professor of Social Work at Florida Atlantic University, who asked:

> *Why is the control group two years older, taller, and heavier than the group of unmedicated patients? It seems odd that, given ten*

---

[13] Lisa Fine Goldstein, "Study: ADHD Drugs Unrelated to Smaller Brain Sizes," *Education Week* 22, no. 7 (October 16, 2002).

[14] *Detroit News*, "Ritalin Is Safe – and It Works," December 12, 2002.

[15] Castellanos et al., "Trajectories," 1743.

[16] Ibid., 1745.

[17] Jonathan Leo and David Cohen, "Broken Brains or Flawed Studies? A Critical Review of ADHD Neuroimaging Research," *Journal of Mind and Behavior* 24, no. 1 (Winter 2003): 29-55.

years and the resources of the NIMH, these experienced researchers could not have found a more appropriate control group.[18]

Drs. Leo and Cohen also re-reviewed the brain imaging studies cited in the 2001 review paper by the Castellanos group. Of thirty-three studies, twelve did not report the medication history of the subjects. Of the remaining ones, in eleven of them all of the subjects had a prior history of ADHD medication treatment, while in seven more a majority of them had. Only two of the studies had been conducted on undrugged patients.[19]

A 2013 review paper[20] by Dr. Castellanos and a colleague concluded:

Based primarily on lesion studies in animals and humans, the imaging community initially embraced a prefrontal-striatal model of ADHD which expanded to include cerebellar involvement ... This model has been largely supported by an ever-increasing number of structural and functional imaging studies.[21]

The paper made no mention of the potential confounding role of drug effects.

Big data

Meanwhile, a group of scientists, including Dr. Castellanos, formed the ADHD-200 Consortium to coordinate efforts to find the still-

---

[18] Ibid., 47.

[19] Ibid., 34-41.

[20] Francis Xavier Castellanos and Erica Proal, "Large-Scale Brain Systems in ADHD: Beyond the Prefrontal-Striatal Model," *Trends in Cognitive Science* 16, no. 1 (January 2012): 17-26, https://doi.org/10.1016/j.tics.2011.11.007

[21] Ibid., 17.

elusive biomarkers for ADHD. On 1 March 2011, they released a large-scale database consisting of 776 fMRI scans collected at eight independent imaging sites, along with phenotypic information including ADHD diagnostic status, ADHD symptom measures, age, sex, IQ, handedness, and medication history. They held a competition, inviting researchers to use the data from brain scans along with the phenotypic data to construct an algorithm that could be used to distinguish kids diagnosed with ADHD with typically-developing kids. This algorithm would then be tested against an additional 197 datasets which were released without providing ADHD diagnostic status.[22]

The winners were a team from the Johns Hopkins Medical Institutions, who devised an algorithm which was accurate sixty percent of the time.[23] For calibration, they could have achieved fifty-five percent accuracy by just guessing "typically-developing" one hundred percent of the time.[24] Moreover, the algorithm correctly diagnosed only twenty-one percent of the ADHD kids.[25]

Another team from the University of Alberta ignored the brain scan data entirely and formulated an algorithm using only the phenotypic data. While this was inconsistent with contest rules, the algorithm they submitted had an accuracy rate of sixty-two percent – surpassing that of the one created by the Hopkins team.[26] This

---

[22] ADHD-200 Consortium, "The ADHD-200 Consortium: A Model to Advance the Translational Potential of Neuroimaging in Clinical Neuroscience," *Frontiers in Systems Neuroscience* 6, Article 62 (September 2012): 1-5, https://doi.org/10.3389/fnsys/2002.00062

[23] Ibid., 2.

[24] Matthew R.G. Brown et al., "ADHD-200 Global Competition: Diagnosing ADHD Using Personal Characteristic Data Can Outperform Resting State fMRI Measurements," *Frontiers in Systems Neuroscience* 6, (September 28, 2012): 1-22, https://doi.org/10.3389/fnsys.2012.00069

[25] ADHD-200 Consortium, "Neuroimaging," 3.

[26] Brown et al., "Diagnosing," 13.

suggests that any commonalities in brain activity of the ADHD kids may be just correlates of the phenotypic variables – age, sex, and so forth – which are known to correlate with ADHD, rather than manifestations of some disease process.

But rather than conclude that this is not a profitable line of inquiry, the ADHD-200 Consortium researchers wound up by calling for more funding for even larger studies.[27]

Bigger data

On 15 February 2017, *Lancet Psychiatry* published the results of a "mega-analysis" conducted by the ENIGMA ADHD Working Group of brain scans of 3,242 individuals, including 1,713 persons diagnosed with ADHD and 1,529 controls.[28] This was the largest such analysis ever conducted, and the researchers found that overall brain volume, as well as the volume of several specific brain regions, was smaller in subjects diagnosed with ADHD than those who were not.

The paper's eighty-two authors concluded:

> *Data from our highly powered analysis confirms that patients with ADHD do have altered brains and that ADHD is a disorder of the brain. This message is clear for clinicians to convey to parents and to patients, which can help to reduce the stigma that ADHD is just a label for difficult children and caused by incompetent parenting.*[29]

---

[27] ADHD-200 Consortium, "Neuroimaging," 4.

[28] Martine Hoogman et al., "Subcortical Brain Volume Differences in Participants with Attention Deficit Hyperactivity Disorder in Children and Adults: A Cross-Sectional Mega-Analysis," *Lancet Psychiatry*, published online February 15, 2017, https://doi.org/10.1016/S2215-0366(17)30049-4

[29] Hoogman et al., "Brain Volumes," 316.

This message was dutifully picked up by the mainstream media. *Newsweek* told its readers "Study Finds Brains of ADHD Sufferers Are Smaller."[30] CNN reported "People diagnosed with attention deficit hyperactivity disorder have smaller brain volume than those without the disorder."[31] Other outlets quickly followed suit:

> *"ADHD is a brain disorder, not a label for poor parenting."*[32]

> *"Children with ADHD have some smaller brain regions, study shows."*[33]

> *"These findings revealed that those with ADHD had smaller brain volume compared to people without ADHD."*[34]

The *Lancet Psychiatry* study was the target of a withering broadside by author Robert Whitaker in his Mad in America blog, co-authored by educational psychologist Michael Corrigan.[35] Whitaker and Dr. Corrigan noted the differences between the ADHD subjects and controls were not categorical differences, but rather were average

[30] Conor Gaffey, "Study Finds Brains of ADHD Sufferers Are Smaller," *Newsweek*, February 16, 2017, https://www.newsweek.com/brains-adhd-sufferers-are-smaller-suggesting-it-physical-disorder-study-557372

[31] Susan Scutti, "Brains of Those with ADHD Show Smaller Structures Related to Emotion," CNN, February 16, 2017, https://www.cnn.com/2017/02/15/health/adhd-brain-scans-study/index.html

[32] Henry Bodkin, "ADHD is a Brain Disorder, not a Label for Poor Parenting," *Daily Telegraph*, February 16, 2017, https://www.telegraph.co.uk/science/2017/02/15/adhd-brain-disorder-not-label-poor-parenting-say-scientists/

[33] Vic Adhopia, "Children with ADHD Have Some Smaller Brain Regions, Study Shows," Canadian Broadcasting Corporation, February 16, 2017, cbc.ca/news/health/adhd-brain-structures-1.3983919

[34] Jennifer Lea Reynolds, "Are Brains Different for Kids Who Have ADHD?" *US News and World Report*, June 16, 2017, https://usnews677-yahoopartner.tumblr.com/post/161890476983/are-brains-different-for-kids-who-have-adhd

[35] Robert Whitaker and Michael W. Corrigan, "*Lancet Psychiatry* Needs to Retract ADHD Brain Scan Study," Mad in America, April 15, 2017, https://www.madinamerica.com/2017/04/lancet-psychiatry-needs-to-retract-the-adhd-enigma-study/

differences – and tiny ones, at that. *There was a more than ninety-two percent overlap in brain size between the ADHD subjects and the controls.*

In plain English, nearly half the ADHD subjects had larger-than-average brain sizes. Nearly half of the control subjects had smaller-than-average brain sizes. And this relationship was true not just for overall brain size, but for every one of the brain structures the researchers looked at. The study produced no findings that could be used to distinguish the brain of a person diagnosed with ADHD from that of someone who was not.

In fairness, the CNN article did acknowledge this point – although that admission was buried in paragraph number thirty-seven. None of the other laudatory news stories mentioned the matter at all. Indeed, the article in *Newsweek* featured an impressive color photograph of sections of plastinated brains on display at the Plastinarium in Guben, Germany. The article never actually said that doctors can diagnose ADHD by looking at a patient's brain, but it's hard to imagine why they included that particular picture if they did not wish to leave their readers with that impression. This kind of mendacity is quite common in news stories about ADHD and other "mental illnesses."

The authors of the *Lancet Psychiatry* paper found no clinically significant differences whatsoever between the brains of subjects diagnosed with ADHD and those who were not, although they did find some statistically significant differences. What could be the cause of those differences? Could it be a drug effect? The researchers themselves flatly ruled out that possibility, stating "The brain differences we have reported are not caused by medication effects."[36]

---

[36] Hoogman et al., "Brain Volumes," 316.

The researchers did not find proof of a drug effect – but they don't seem to have looked very hard. All they did was compare those who had taken ADHD meds for at least four weeks with those who had never taken them. In other words, people who took the drugs for just four weeks were lumped in with those who had taken them for years and years – a tactic guaranteed to blur any drug effect. Would a more fine-grained level of analysis, looking for a dose-dependent relationship, have found something? The study authors don't seem interested in finding out.

Whitaker and Dr. Corrigan started a petition demanding that the paper be retracted. The petition garnered over 800 signatures, but to this day *Lancet Psychiatry* has refused to do so.

A distributed network-based pathology

On 18 February 2019, the journal *Neuroscience and Biobehavioral Reviews* published a meta-analysis titled "Brain Alterations in Children/Adolescents with ADHD Revisited: A Neuroimaging Meta-Analysis of 96 Structural and Functional Studies." The authors of the meta-analysis concluded:

> *To the best of our knowledge, this study is the largest meta-analysis of structural and functional neuroimaging experiments in children/adolescents with ADHD. We found* ***no significant convergence*** *across structural and functional regional alterations in ADHD, which might be attributable to clinical heterogeneity, experimental and analytical flexibility, and positive publication bias, but could also point towards a more distributed, network-based pathology lacking a consistent expression at any particular location.* (Emphasis added.)

The possibility that "ADHD" is not even a coherent diagnostic category was not considered. At this point, the existence of an underlying brain pathology seems more an article of faith than a testable hypothesis.[37]

Genetics studies

Nobody's fault

Is ADHD genetic?

Perhaps a better question would be "What difference would it make if it were?" If it were ever demonstrated unequivocally that ADHD was a genetically-based condition, it still would not follow *logically* that it was more tractable to drug treatment rather than to social or psychological interventions.

But it seems safe to say most people would tend to assume so. In a 2012 talk, psychologist Russell Barkley told listeners "ADHD is due to neurogenetic deficits, and that means that medication is absolutely justifiable."[38]

This type of thinking goes back a long way. In a 1996 commentary, psychologist Steven Faraone, one of the world's leading experts on ADHD genetics and a member of the Biederman group, advised that telling parents that ADHD is a genetically-based disorder is a good way to get them to give their kids the drugs:

> *Many parents are reluctant for their children to take psychotropic medication and others find it difficult to maintain the prescribed*

---

[37] Fateme Samea et al., "Brain Alterations in Children/Adolescents with ADHD Revisited: A Neuroimaging Meta-Analysis of 96 Structural and Functional Studies," *Neuroscience and Biobehavioral Reviews* 100 (May 2019): 1-8, https://doi.prg/10.1016/j.neubiorev.2019.02.011

[38] Russell Barkley, "This is How You Treat ADHD Based off Science," September 23, 2014, https://www.youtube.com/watch?v=_tpB-B8BXk0&t=189s

regimen. Many parents hold naïve beliefs about the etiology of their children's problems; they are quick to attribute them to life circumstances, events in the past, or parental inadequacies ... For many psychiatric disorders, genetic data provide the quickest and most convincing means of showing patients how biology plays a role in their condition.[39]

This idea was expanded to book length by Harold S. Koplewicz, a Professor of Psychiatry at New York University and author of *It's Nobody's Fault: New Hope and Help for Difficult Children.*[40] Dr. Koplewicz begins by heaping scorn on those benighted souls who still believe that a child's problems have anything to do with the actions of his parents:

The fact is, when a child has a brain disorder, it is not the parents' fault. A brain disorder is the result of what I call 'DNA Roulette.' In the same way that a child comes into the world with a tendency to go gray in his twenties, or, like Kenny, beautiful hazel eyes and deep dimples, a child is born with a brain that functions in a particular way because of its chemical composition ... ***It is brain chemistry that is responsible for brain disorders, not bad parenting.***[41] (Emphasis in the original.)

Dr. Koplewicz goes on to explain:

If bad parenting is what is causing a child's disease, it stands to reason that good parenting can make it better. Unfortunately, that's

---

[39] Steven V. Faraone, "Discussion of 'Genetic Influence on Parent-Reported Attention-Related Problems in a Norwegian General Population Twin Sample,'" *Journal of the American Academy of Child and Adolescent Psychiatry* 35, no. 5 (May 1996): 596-598.

[40] Harold S. Koplewicz, It's *Nobody's Fault: New Hope and Help for Difficult Children* (New York: Times Books, 1996).

[41] Ibid., 5-6.

> *not how it works. Parents don't cause the disorders, and they can't cure them either.*[42]

No doubt that kind of statement is a siren song in a society which has sadly undermined parental authority to the point where many parents feel like their children's frazzled servants. It is also a formulation that effectively slams the door on any serious inquiry into the social and psychological roots of children's problems.

So, what is the cause of these children's distress? Dr. Koplewicz sets his readers straight on that point, too:

> *ADHD has nothing to do with diet or bad parenting.*[43]

> *ADHD is a disorder of the brain.*[44]

> *Neuroimaging techniques – especially magnetic resonance imaging (MRI), positron emission tomography (PET) scans, and single photon emission computer tomography (SPECT) – have demonstrated that children with ADHD have brains that are different from the brains of kids that don't have it.*[45]

Fortunately, Dr. Koplewicz and his colleagues stand by, ready to help:

> *There are more than 200 studies showing that a stimulant called Ritalin (generic name: methylphenidate) works wonders for children with ADHD.*[46]

---

[42] Ibid., 14.
[43] Ibid., 79.
[44] Ibid., 79.
[45] Ibid., 79.
[46] Ibid., 80.

At this point the reader may be wondering if we are setting up the child for a lifetime of failure by saddling him with the idea that he was born with a broken brain that requires long-term treatment with powerful stimulant drugs. This fear is not shared by Dr. Koplewicz, who regales his readers with the tale of Ned, who was "having a terrible time in school." His academic performance was poor, his teacher was complaining about his behavior, none of the other kids wanted to play with him, and even his own parents didn't like having him around.[47]

But all that changed, thanks to Dr. Koplewicz. After young Ned began taking his prescribed forty milligrams of Ritalin a day, his grades were now "terrific," he had lots of friends, and his parents found him a joy to be with. To express his gratitude, Ned invited Koplewicz to his elementary school graduation where the boy was awarded the prize for the best science project. Afterwards, he introduced the good doctor to his grandparents thusly: "This is Dr. Koplewicz. He's my … my friend."[48]

Are these results typical? Dr. Koplewicz never explicitly says so, but he certainly does nothing to disabuse his readers of this notion.

The book is chock-full of heartwarming little tales like this one. Apparently, none of Dr. Koplewicz's patients ever suffers from mania, tics, akathisia, or any of the myriad other toxic effects psychiatric drugs have been shown to exert on developing brains.

In fairness to Dr. Koplewicz, the book isn't just about drugs. He does leaven his work with some child-rearing advice, which seems

---

[47] Ibid., xv.

[48] Ibid., xvi.

to center mainly on giving children gold stars for good behavior.[49] (Does anyone really want a child who can be manipulated by giving or withholding gold stars? It's a measure of how beleaguered some parents today feel that the answer is probably Yes.)

Dr. Koplewicz was one of twenty-two notional authors of SmithKline Beecham's notorious Study 329 of Paxil published in the *Journal of the American Academy of Child and Adolescent Psychiatry*, which reported that the drug was safe and effective for treating major depression in adolescents, even though their own data showed no difference between Paxil and placebo for any of the eight original outcome variables, and that one out of eight youths given the drug suffered from suicidality or self-harming behavior. So, the sincerity of his professed concern for "difficult children" like Ned may be open to question. But never mind that for now.

The question is: is ADHD really a genetically-based condition? A 1992 paper by Drs. Faraone and Biederman and several of their colleagues claimed to demonstrate that ADHD is caused by a single co-dominant gene with a low rate of penetrance.[40] No one today, including Faraone and Biederman, believe this. A 2019 review article on the genetics of ADHD by Faraone and another colleague did not even mention the 1992 paper.[51]

Today, psychiatric-oriented genetics experts conceptualize of ADHD as a polygenic disorder, affected by numerous genes, each contributing a tiny bit to one's risk of developing this condition.

---

[49] Ibid., 84.

[50] Stephen V. Faraone et al., "Segregation Analysis of Attention Deficit Hyperactivity Disorder," *Psychiatric Genetics* 2, no. 4 (1992): 257-275, https://doi.org/10.1097/00041444-199210000-00004

[51] Stephen V. Faraone and Henrik Larsson, "Genetics of Attention Deficit Hyperactivity Disorder," *Molecular Psychiatry* 24, (2019): 562-575, https://doi.org/10.1038/s41380-018-0070-0

The psychiatric literature is replete with statements to the effect that "ADHD is seventy percent [or eighty percent, or ninety percent] inherited."[52] But what does it even mean to say that?

"Heritability" means the proportion of population variance in a trait due to genetic variability, as opposed to environmental variability. The concept of heritability was invented by the geneticist Sewall Wright to give agricultural scientists a way to predict the results of controlled breeding experiments on plants and animals on factory farms. But it is an open question as to whether the concept even means anything when applied to human beings.

The figure of ADHD having a heritability of seventy percent (or eighty percent, or ninety percent) comes from family studies, twin studies, and adoption studies. But the same kinds of studies have "proven" that pellagra, tuberculosis, and "hysteria" are also hereditary disorders, so a bit of skepticism seems in order here. Elsewhere I have argued that all of these studies are fatally flawed,

---

[52] E.g., Dawei Li et al., "Meta-Analysis Shows Significant Association between Dopamine System Genes and Attention Deficit Hyperactivity Disorder (ADHD)," *Human Molecular Genetics* 15, no. 14 (2006): 2276-2284, https://doi.org/10.1093/hmg/ddl152; J. Gordon Millchap, "Etiologic Classification of Attention-Deficit Hyperactivity Disorder," *Pediatrics* 121, no. 2 (February 2008): 358-365, https://doi.org/10.1542/peds/2007-1332; Ian R. Gizer, Courtney Ficks, and Irwin D. Waldman, "Candidate Gene Studies of ADHD: A Meta-Analytic Review," *Human Genetics* 126, (2009): 51-90, https://doi.org/10.1007/s00439-009-0694-x; Oussama Kebir et al., "Candidate Genes and Neuropsychological Phenotypes in Children with ADHD: Review of Association Studies," *Journal of Psychiatry and Neuroscience* 34, no. 2 (2009): 88-101; Benjamin M. Neale, "Meta-Analysis of Genome-Wide Association Studies of Attention-Deficit/Hyperactivity Disorder," *Journal of the American Academy of Child and Adolescent Psychiatry* 49, no. 9 (September 2010): 884-897, https://doi.org/10.1016/j.jaacp.2010.06/008; Mauricio Arcos-Burgos and Maximillian Muenke, "Toward a Better Understanding of ADHD: LPHN3 Gene Variants and the Susceptibility to Develop ADHD," *ADHD Attention Deficit Hyperactivity Disorder* 2, no. 3 (November 2010): 139-147, https://doi.org/10.1007/s12402-0030-2; Stephen V. Faraone, "Epidemiology of Attention Deficit Hyperactivity Disorder," in *Textbook in Psychiatric Epidemiology 3rd Edition* ed. Ming T. Tsuang, Mauricio Tohen, and Peter Jones (New York: John Wiley and Sons, 2011), 449-467; B. Franke et al., "The Genetics of Attention-Deficit/Hyperactivity Disorder in Adults, a Review," *Molecular Psychiatry* 17, no. 10 (October 2012): 960-987, https://doi.org.10.1038//mp/2011/138

in ways that cannot be fixed, and none of them adequately control for environmental variability.[53]

Granted, this is a minority view, but the new science of molecular genetics seems poised to put an end to this controversy once and for all. In 1998, clinical psychologist Russell Barkley boldly stated, "The day is not far off when genetic testing for ADHD may become available and more specialized medications may be designed to counter the specific genetic defects of the children who suffer from it."[54] How have promises like this worked out for us in real life?

There are two categories of molecular genetics studies we are interested in: copy-number variant studies and genome-wide association studies.[55] Let's take a look at each of these in turn.

Copy-number variant studies

In October of 2010, the Lancet published the results of a study of rare

---

[53] The fundamental assumption of family studies – that familial equals genetic – is false. The fundamental assumption of twin studies – the Equal Environment Assumption – is false. The fundamental assumption of adoption studies – that adoption randomizes environmental variation – is false. See chapters 2-5 of my book, *Madness and Genetic Determinism*. On these matters I am deeply indebted to Jay Joseph, a clinical psychologist who has been writing and publishing critiques of psychiatric genetics for the past more than twenty years. For Dr. Joseph's devastating review of family, twin, and adoption studies of ADHD, see "Not in Their Genes: A Critical View of the Genetics of Attention-Deficit Hyperactivity Disorder," *Developmental Review* 20, (2000): 539-567, https://doi.org.10.1006/drev/2000/0511; see also his follow-up paper, "ADHD and Genetics: A Consensus Reconsidered," in *Rethinking ADHD: From Brain to Culture*, ed. Sami Timimi and Jonathan Leo (New York: Palgrave MacMillan, 2009), 58-91; for a discussion of the inherent problems of psychiatric genetics studies in general, see his other voluminous writings on the subject.

[54] Barkley, Russell A., "Attention-Deficit Hyperactivity Disorder," *Scientific American* 279, no. 3 (September 1998): 66-71.

[55] I have elected to omit linkage studies and candidate-gene studies, which have failed to produce any clinically significant findings and which now are considered obsolescent modes of inquiry anyway. For a review of these studies, see Stephen V. Faraone and Henrik Larsson, "Genetics of Attention Deficit Hyperactivity Disorder," *Molecular Psychiatry* 24, (2019): 562-575, https://doi.org/10.1038/s41380-018-0070-0

large copy number variants said to be associated with ADHD.[56] The term copy number variants (CNV's) refers to repeated sequences of DNA in which the number of copies varies between individuals. The researchers scanned the genomes of 366 children diagnosed with ADHD and 1,047 controls, and found the number of large CNV's (i.e., more than 500 kb in length) was significantly greater in the ADHD kids than in the controls.

Some of these CNV's had previously been found to be associated with schizophrenia and autism as well – which seems to contradict the notion that these conditions are properly regarded as discrete disorders. Nevertheless, the paper was greeted enthusiastically by the media. Headlines proclaimed:

> *"ADHD is a genetic condition, study says"*[57]
>
> *"Hyperactive children may suffer from a genetic disorder, says study"*[58]
>
> *"Study finds genetic link to ADHD"*[59]

The stories also repeated the comforting "It's nobody's fault" mantra. The *Guardian* proclaimed "Parents of hyperactive children should not be blamed for failing to bring up their offspring properly,"[60] while

---

[56] Nigel M. Williams et al., "Rare Chromosomal Deletions and Duplications in Attention-Deficit Hyperactivity Disorder: A Genome-Wide Study," Lancet 376, no. 9750 (October 23, 2010): 1401-1408, https://doi.org/10.1016/S0140-6736(10)61109-9

[57] CNN, "ADHD is a Genetic Condition, Study Says," September 29, 2010, thechart.blogs.cnn.com/2010/09/29/adhd-is-a-genetic-condition-study-says/

[58] Sarah Boseley, "Hyperactive Children May Suffer from Genetic Disorder, Says Study," *Guardian*, September 29, 2010, https://www.theguardian.com/society/2010/sep/30/hyperactive-children-genetic-disorder-studya

[59] Kate Kelland, "Study Finds Genetic Link to ADHD," Australian Broadcasting Company, September 30, 2010, abc.net.au/news/2010-09-30/study-finds-genetic-link-to-adhd/228092

[60] Boseley, "Hyperactive Children.

Reuters informed readers "The research should help dispel myths that ADHD is caused by bad parenting."[61] Such formulations may make troubled children and their parents feel better momentarily – but they also exculpate the rest of us from doing something about crowded, underfunded schools and offering meaningful help to exhausted and overextended parents.

What exactly did the researchers find? They found that fourteen percent of the ADHD kids had one or more large CNV's, as opposed to seven percent of the controls.[62] In other words, the vast majority of ADHD kids had no CNV's, while some of the controls did. They certainly did not find any kind of genetic anomaly that could be used to diagnose ADHD.

What's more, the index and control groups were not comparable. Thirty-three of the ADHD kids also suffered from intellectual disability, defined as an IQ below seventy, and the rate of CNV's was much higher in these children (thirty-six percent) than in the rest of the ADHD kids. When these thirty-three children were dropped from the analysis, along with fourteen more for whom IQ data was unavailable, the relationship between CNV's and a diagnosis of ADHD persisted, although it was greatly attenuated.

The researchers didn't have any IQ data for the controls, but presumably it was the same as that of the general population, which by definition is one hundred. Even after the children with intellectual disability were dropped from the analysis, the average IQ of the remaining ADHD kids was only eighty-nine.[63] Low IQ is a well-

---

[61] Kelland, "Study."

[62] Williams et al., "Chromosomal Deletions," 1404.

[63] Ibid., 1404.

known risk factor for a diagnosis of ADHD,[64] but the researchers did not adequately control for this, instead engaging in a rhetorical sleight of hand – substituting a categorical variable (presence or absence of intellectual disability) for an incremental one (IQ).

Since then several more such studies have been carried out,[65] without producing any findings of clinical significance. None of the CNV's they have found associated with ADHD are found in any more than a tiny minority of index cases, and many of these can be found in normal controls as well. None of the studies adequately controls for IQ – they usually exclude index cases with IQs below some arbitrary cutoff, but none of them employs a set of controls matched to the ADHD subjects for IQ.

It seems likely that if these researchers have discovered anything here, it was a correlation between CNV's and low IQ, with the ADHD label coming along for the ride.

Anyone who knows anything about life as it is lived knows that kids vary in the speed at which they learn, and that a child forced to sit through classes run at a pace too rapid for him is likely to stop

---

[64] Julia J. Rucklidge and Rosemary Tannock, "Psychiatric, Psychosocial, and Cognitive Functioning of Female Adolescents with ADHD," *Journal of the American Academy of Child and Adolescent Psychiatry* 40, no. 5 (May 2001): 530-540, https://doi.org/10.1097/00004583-200105000-00012

[65] Klaus-Peter Lesch et al., "Genome-Wide Copy Number Variation Analysis in Attention Deficit/Hyperactivity Disorder: Association with Neuropeptide Y Gene Dosage in an Extended Pedigree," *Molecular Psychiatry* 16, no. 5 (May 2011): 491-503, https://doi.org/10.1038/mp.2010.29; J. Elia et al., "Genome-Wide Copy Number Variation Study Associates Metabotropic Glutamate Receptor Gene Networks with Attention Deficit Hyperactivity Disorder," *Nature Genetics* 44, no. 1 (December 4, 2011): 78-84, http://doi.org/10.1038/ng.1013; Nigel M. Williams et al., "Genome-Wide Analysis of Copy Number Variants in Attention Deficit Hyperactivity Disorder: The Role of Rare Variants and Duplications at 15q13.3," American Journal of Psychiatry 169, no. 2 (February 2012): 195-204, https://doi.org/10.11176/appi.ajp.2011.11060822; I. Jarick et al., "Genome-Wide Analysis of Rare Copy Number Variations Reveals PARK2 as a Candidate Gene for Attention-Deficit/Hyperactivity Disorder," *Molecular Psychiatry* 19, no. 1 (January 2014): 115-121, https://doi.org/10.1038/mp/2010.29

paying attention and/or start acting out – thereby earning himself a diagnosis of "ADHD." Wouldn't hiring more teachers (to enable more individualized learning opportunities for kids) be preferable to continuing to pour money into this kind of research?

Genome-wide association studies

In genome-wide association studies, entire genomes of large numbers of individuals are scanned for the presence of single-nucleotide polymorphisms, or SNP's. A typical study might look at hundreds, thousands, or even tens of thousands of index and control subjects, and as many as a million or more SNP's, to find ones that are correlated with the condition of interest. In order to eliminate false positives, levels of significance typically are set at $p = 10^{-8}$, corresponding to the customary level of $p = 0.05$, divided by one million. These techniques have enabled researchers to go over the human genome with a fine-toothed comb. And what have the researchers found?

The first GWA studies of ADHD found no DNA variants of genome-wide significance. Even a 2010 meta-analysis of studies failed to find any significant results.[66] But in November of 2018, the journal *Nature Genetics* reported the discovery of the first genome-wide significant risk loci for ADHD.[67] The paper listed seventy-one individual authors along with the ADHD Working Group of the Psychiatric Genetics Consortium, the Early Lifecourse and Genetic Epidemiology Consortium, and the 23andMe Research Team. The researchers sequenced the DNA of 20,183 index subjects and 35,191 controls and found twelve genetic loci correlated with a significantly increased risk of a diagnosis of ADHD.

---

[66] Benjamin M. Neale et al., "Meta-Analysis."

[67] Ditte Demontis et al., "Discovery of the First Genome-Wide Significant Risk Loci for ADHD," *Nature Genetics* 51, no. 1 (January 2019): 63-75, https://doi.org.10/1038/s41588-018-0269-7

Once again, these findings were greeted with enthusiasm. The *Daily Mail* repeated a familiar trope: "Don't blame the parents. ADHD is in our genes."[68] The Guardian declared "The findings could help shed light on the biological mechanisms behind ADHD, potentially aiding the development of new drugs,"[69] while the Economist informed readers:

> *These findings will not, therefore, lead directly to genetic tests. What they do do, though, is dispel the idea that ADHD is merely bad behavior, or even a mythical condition. And that, of itself, may help to change attitudes toward children who have it, and towards their parents.*[70]

Again, what exactly did the researchers find? The odds ratios for these "significant risk loci" were on the order of 1.198 or even less, meaning a 19.8 percent increase in risk (or even less). Now, the published estimates for the incidence of ADHD vary wildly, but a meta-analysis by Stephen Faraone and Joseph Biederman and several of their colleagues came up with a figure of 5.3 percent,[71] so let's go with that. Multiply 5.3 percent by 19.8 percent and you get a figure of 0.0105, or a little over a one in a hundred increase in absolute risk. Can a gene associated with a one in a hundred increase in risk serve as a target for drug development?

The piece in the *Guardian* quoted one of the senior authors of the study, Anders Børglum of Aarhus University in Denmark, as follows:

---

[68] *Daily Mail*, "Don't Blame the Parents. ADHD is in Our Genes," November 27, 2018, 5.

[69] Nicola Davis, "Scientists Find Genetic Variants That Increase the Risk of ADHD," *Guardian*, November 26, 2018, https://amp.theguardian.com/society/2018/nov/26/scientists-find-genetic-variants-that-increase-risk-of-adhd

[70] *Economist*, "Attention Please: Psychiatric Genetics," 429, no. 9120 (December 1, 2018).

[71] Guilherme Polanczyk et al., "The Worldwide Prevalence of ADHD: A Systematic Review and Metaregression Analysis," *American Journal of Psychiatry* 164, no. 6 (June 2007): 942-948, https://doi.org/10.1176/ajp.2007.164.6.942

"Among all the causes that can lead to ADHD, genetic factors account for between 70% and 80%,"[72] presumably a reference to the figures obtained from family, twin, and adoption studies. Dr. Børglum added that all the loci put together accounted for just one percent of the population-wide increase in risk, and, deploying a theme that has become commonplace in psychiatric genetics, averred that the missing genes *must* be there, somewhere, still waiting to be found:

> *"Those 12 regions are just representing the tip of the iceberg," he said, noting there were likely thousands more to be discovered.*[73]

The possibility that the figures obtained from family, twin, and adoption studies were wildly inflated was not considered. Nor did the article mention that if "thousands" of genes are somehow involved in the development of ADHD, their individual effect sizes must be orders of magnitude tinier than the already puny figure of one in a hundred, or less. This is stretching the notion of cause and effect into meaninglessness.

These genes are not disease genes, as genes for cystic fibrosis or sickle cell anemia or Huntington's disease are. These are simply part of the normal range of human genetic variation.

What do we mean by "A gene for...?"

As every high school biology student knows, the laws of genetics were discovered by Gregor Mendel, through his tireless experiments with pea plants. Mendel never defined what he meant by a gene for a given trait – he just used an "I-know-it-when-I-see-it" definition.

---

[72] Davis, "Genetic Variants."

[73] Ibid.

(Actually, the word "gene" had not even been coined back then – Mendel used the term *anlagen*, but that clearly corresponds to our modern notion of a gene.)

In a 2005 paper,[74] Kenneth Kendler, one of the world's leading experts in psychiatric genetics, proposed the following criteria for identifying a gene for a specific trait:

1. Strength of association: If a pea plant has two copies of the gene for wrinkled seeds, it will produce wrinkled seeds, under any of a wide range of conditions – provided it is able to produce seeds at all. The odds ratio, if you like, is infinity, or at least astronomically large. Dr. Kendler proposed a minimum odds ratio of 100:1 for identifying a gene for a specific trait.

2. Specificity of association: The genes that Mendel worked on had very specific effects: one gene affected seed color but not shape or stem length, while another affected seed shape but not color or stem length.

3. Noncontingency of association: The relationship between the gene and the trait is not dependent on other factors, such as exposure to a particular environment or the presence of other genes.

4. Causal proximity: There must be a direct causal link between the gene and the trait in question.

5. Appropriate level of explanation: The formulation "X is a gene for Y" must address the phenomena in question at the most

[74] Kenneth S. Kendler, "'A Gene For…': The Nature of Gene Action in Psychiatric Disorders," *American Journal of Psychiatry* 162, no. 7 (July 2005): 1243-1252, https://doi.org/10.1176/appi.ajp.162.7.1243

> appropriate level. Dr. Kendler provides a hypothetical example: suppose there were a gene that conferred its owner with perfect pitch. Such a gene might well predispose its owner to enjoying the music of Mozart. Would it be appropriate to call this "a gene for liking Mozart?" Hardly. This hypothesized gene could just as easily increase the likelihood of one enjoying the music of Hayden, Beethoven, and Brahms as well. Calling it a gene for perfect pitch is both more parsimonious and has greater explanatory power.

Genes for monogenic disorders such as Huntington's disease, cystic fibrosis, and sickle-cell anemia, pass all five of these tests with flying colors. However, not one of the genes said to be associated with ADHD can pass even one of them. The same is true for the genes associated with any of the other "functional disorders" listed in the *DSM*.

Follow the money

There is no abnormality of brain structure that can be used to diagnose ADHD. There is no abnormality of brain function that can be used to diagnose ADHD. There is no gene for ADHD. And there is no credible evidence that the brains of children labeled "ADHD" are different from those of other children.

So, to get back to the original question, "Is ADHD a disease?", it just depends on how you define the word "disease." It certainly is not a disease in terms of having any measurable signs.

And how could there be? There are literally hundreds of reasons why a child might have problems with inattention or hyperactivity – lack of discipline, lack of outdoor free play time, a curriculum that is too challenging, or not challenging enough, hunger, fatigue, a chaotic home life, or any of a large number of untreated medical conditions. How could there be a common gene, or a common neural substrate, underlying all these disparate problems?

We have seen that the popular press (which is heavily dependent on drug company advertising) has been all too ready to hail the latest findings of neuroimaging and genetics research as proof of the supposed biological basis of "ADHD" – a paradigm that has proven enormously lucrative for the drug companies and their paid agents. However, despite the billions of dollars that have been spent on this research, not one patient in a clinic anywhere in the world has benefitted. No new treatment, or cure, or even a new diagnostic test has come about as a result.

One may wonder about the clinical utility of phenomena whose mere existence can be demonstrated only after spending enormous sums of money and generating untold petabytes of data – and sometimes not even then. At what point do we start asking whether we really want to continue pouring more billions down this particular black hole? If not now, when?

Debunking the Science Behind ADHD as a "Brain Disorder"

Albert Galves and David Walker

In 2001, The Society for the Advancement of Psychotherapy (Division 29 of the American Psychological Association) partnered with Celltech Pharmaceuticals, a producer and marketer of Ritalin, an amphetamine that is used in the treatment of Attention Deficit/Hyperactivity Disorder, to produce a pamphlet which contained the following statements:

1. ADD/ADHD is generally considered a neuro-chemical disorder.

2. Most people with ADD/ADHD are born with the disorder, though it may not be recognized until adulthood.

3. ADHD is not caused by poor parenting, a difficult family environment, poor teaching or inadequate nutrition.

Dr. Galves sent a letter to Alice Rubenstein, President of Division 29, complaining that there was not sufficient scientific evidence to support those statements. Dr. Rubenstein asked Drs. Robert

---

Al Galves, Ph.D., is a psychologist based in Las Cruces, New Mexico.

David Edward Walker, Ph.D., is a liberation psychologist, writer, and musician.

This chapter is an updated, adapted version of the article Galves, A. and Walker, D. (2012). Debunking the science behind attention deficit/hyperactivity as a "brain disorder". *Ethical Human Psychology and Psychiatry*, 14(1), 27-40

Resnick and Kalman Heller to provide Dr. Galves with the evidence supporting the statements. Drs. Galves and Walker reviewed the evidence provided by Drs. Resnick and Heller and wrote the following article in reply.

ADD/ADHD is generally considered a neuro-chemical disorder

Although ADD/ADHD may be generally considered by popular opinion to be a "neuro-chemical disorder," there is no scientific evidence to back this claim. The scientific record contains only equivocal and inconsistent evidence that the brain physiology of individuals diagnosed with ADD/ADHD is different from that of individuals not diagnosed with the disorder (Goldstein and Goldstein, 1998; Barkley, 1990; Ross and Ross, 1982). Even if there were more solid and conclusive evidence, it would not support the implication that ADD/ADHD is **caused** by these biological dynamics.

All that can be derived from a careful review of the literature is that there is evidence of a ***correlation*** between the biological dynamics and the ADHD category. Because this evidence is entirely correlational and the brain is a living, functioning organ constantly responding to its environment with complex neurochemical and other neurofunctional changes, it is just as likely (and perhaps more likely) that the biological dynamics are a **result** of an interplay of emotions, thoughts, intentions and behavior experienced by the diagnosed individuals. The following research findings support such a perspective:

- Jeffrey Schwartz et.al of UCLA (1996) found that a group of people suffering from obsessive-compulsive disorder had "abnormalities" in their brains. Half of the group received drug therapy; the other half received cognitive behavioral "talk therapy." All of the patients improved and, when Schwartz checked their brains, he found that their brains had changed in the same ways. Presumably, the cognitive-behavioral therapy had the same impact on the physiology of the brain as did the biological therapy.

- With more frequent diagnosis of ADHD among children in the United Kingdom, Visser and Jehan (2009) reviewed existing evidence for the "veracity" of the disorder as a "biomedical entity," particularly studies originating from the biopsychiatric perspective using neuroimaging and behavioral genetics as their methods. They appropriately point out the limitations of neuroimaging scanning research in being inconclusive due to only capturing changes in transient blood flow in the brain.

- Jackson (2006) has critiqued the theory of neurovascular coupling (the idea that blood flow illustrates neural activity) upon which neuroimaging methodology is premised, both for its reliance on summing scans in order to obtain an "average image" of alleged differences between ADHD and non-ADHD brains as well as researchers' failures to mention the equivocal nature of such methods in providing evidence for a theory of neurovascular *decoupling* (in which blood flow into one brain area might suggest an inhibition of neural firing that is just as meaningful).

- Mark Rozensweig et.al. (1972) found that the brains of monkeys raised in rich environments had a greater number of neurons and more complex interneuronal connections than the brains of monkeys raised in more impoverished environments.

- Franz Alexander (1984) found that the people who had been deprived of support, affirmation and ample time while growing up were much more likely to suffer from overactive thyroids than people who were brought up in more nourishing environments.

- James Pennebaker (2000) found that students who were assigned the task of writing about traumas they had suffered and about their fears, relationships and desires had stronger immune systems and were healthier than students who were assigned to write about less emotionally charged topics.

- A study by Cornell researchers found that a two-week course in remedial reading significantly changed the brain physiology of dyslexic students (Rappaport, 2003).

- A study by Seattle psychiatrist Arif Khan (Khan et al., 2002) indicated a large overlap in effect between placebo and antidepressants in the original FDA trials of these drugs. Leuchter and fellow UCLA researchers (Leuchter et al., 2002) found that these placebo effects result in detectable changes in brain function. Similar studies which would confound the finding that ADHD is caused by brain abnormalities have not been undertaken with ADD/ADHD subjects.

- Jonathan Leo and David Cohen (2002) found that many of the subjects of ADD/ADHD studies had been taking stimulant medication for significant amounts of time, thereby confounding the finding that brain abnormalities caused the symptoms of ADD/ADHD.

- Baumeister and Hawkins (2001) undertook an exhaustive review of efforts to substantiate a neuroanatomical site or sites related with ADD/ADHD through structural and functional neuroimaging techniques such as PET, single positron scanning, MRI, and electrophysiological measurement. These researchers

> stated that while "[t]here seems to be a consensus among experts today that ADHD is associated with structural and/or functional abnormalities in the brain," they could only conclude that "the present review indicates that the neuroimaging literature provides no convincing evidence for the existence of abnormality in the brains of persons with ADHD" (p. 7-8).

The above evidence contradicts the statement that ADD/ADHD is a neuro-chemical disorder. The scientific principle of parsimony compels us to arrive at a completely different conclusion, i.e. that the biological dynamics which are cited as correlating with ADD/ADHD at the brain level **can be more accurately depicted as a result of psychological and environmental variables** than a neurodevelopmentally damaged, diseased, or dysfunctional brain.

The mind-body dynamic that has been most thoroughly researched in this regard is the human stress response. The human stress response is a profound, complex biochemical and physiological dynamic that is preceded by a perception of threat and a cognition that the threat is real and needs to be dealt with. The psychological variables of the human stress response precede and likely cause the physiological variables, rather than the converse (Everly, 1989; Selye, 1974).

Calling ADHD a "neurochemical disorder" with a "biological cause" implies that it has nothing to do with how a child thinks, feels, reacts, intends, perceives, adjusts and responds. It implies that the behaviors are not under the control of the child or those within the child's world and have nothing to do with how the child finds and makes meaning in that world. That is a fundamental error contradicted by those who work very closely with children and families every day.

"Most people with ADD/ADHD are born with the disorder, though it may not be recognized until adulthood."

The implication here is that ADD/ADHD is a genetic disorder. There is a body of research that purports to demonstrate that this disorder is essentially a result of genetic factors. Most of that research has used studies that compare interclass correlations between the rates of the disorder in monozygotic twins and dizygotic twins. Virtually all of this research has found significantly higher correlations between monozygotic twins than between dizygotic twins (Goodman & Stevenson, 1989; Pauls, 1991; Biederman et al., 1992; Gillis et al., 1992; Edelbrock et al., 1995; Sherman et al., 1997). However, this research suffers from the following serious deficiencies:

- All of this research is based on the assumption that monozygotic twins and dizygotic twins are raised in equivalent environments. That assumption is erroneous. As Jay Joseph (2003) has explained, identical twins spend more time together than fraternals, and more often dress alike, study together, have the same close friends and attend social events together. James Shields, in his 1954 study of normal twin school-children found that 47% of the identical twins had a 'very close attachment' which was true for only 15% of fraternal twins.

According to Kringlen's (1967) survey, 91% of identical twins experienced "identity confusion in childhood" which was true for only 10% of fraternal twins. Kringlen also found that identical twins were more likely to have been considered as alike as two drops of water (76% vs. 0%), "brought up as a unit" (72% vs. 19%) and "inseparable as children" (73% vs. 19%). Sixty-five percent of identical twins were found to have an "extremely strong" level of closeness which was true for only 19% of the fraternal pairs (p. 60). Since the equal environment assumption is not valid, the correlations between monozygotic twins are just as likely a result of environmental factors as of genetic factors.

- Findings of genetic influence over behavior are confounded by the fact that genes direct the synthesis of protein and protein synthesis can be affected by environmental factors such as stress, trauma and lack of parental responsiveness (Hubbard & Wald, 1993). The process of gene expression is much more complex than is suggested by stories in the popular press (Commoner, 2002). Thus, the process through which genes influence the behavioral characteristics of a person is itself greatly influenced by environmental factors.

- In order to scientifically demonstrate genetic etiology for any trait, the precise genetic mechanism involved must be identified. As Ross and Ross (1982) point out: "The only procedures that can precisely define a genetic mechanism are segregation studies which could only be done with humans under very unusual circumstances and linkage studies which would require the identification of the genetic marker associated with hyperactivity ... and these are possibilities for which there is as yet no evidence." (p. 73, 74)

The evidence of a correlation between genetic factors and ADHD has not been sufficiently replicated to make it convincing:

- Brookes-Keeley and his colleagues (2005) found that the correlation between the dopamine receptor DRD4 and ADHD failed to replicate in a large clinical sample of Taiwanese youth or urban Mexican youth diagnosed with ADHD.

- Martinez-Levy (2009) and colleagues contend that studies of "Latin Americans have failed to show an association" between ADHD "with the 10R allele of DAT1 and the literature surrounding the 7R allele of the DRD4 is inconsistent." (p. 259). They caution that their findings "highlight the importance of cross-ethnic research." (p. 257).

- M. Martel (2011) and colleagues use their comparative study of over 300 ADHD youth and nearly 200 non-ADHD-diagnosed youth to challenge a "main effect" for genes in favor of a more classic interaction between gene (G) and environment (E): "The current study provides novel findings of GxE interaction in ADHD. The results are consistent with a theory of regulation breakdown via the interaction between genes influencing brain neuromodulatory systems in prefrontal cortex (where DRD4 is widely expressed) and socially-mediated family processes on which the development of self-regulation is presumed to depend" (p.7).

These researchers include as "socially-mediated family processes" inconsistent parenting, marital conflict, and child self-blame. Instead of describing a gene-environment relationship for ADHD using DRD4, their findings seem to support more well-established and accepted research on temperament and activity in infancy (Thomas, Chess & Birch, 1968) which incorporates concepts of fit, lack of fit, and the reciprocal socialization processes of the child, parents, and family.

- Wheeler (2010) felt Visser and Jehan did not go far enough in their critique of evidence for biomedical factors in ADHD, pointing out that parents may seek an ADHD diagnosis in order to "prove that their child's challenging behavior is not their fault" (p. 260). She mentions that while a sociological stance regarding ADHD might endorse evolutionary selectivity for genetically-based hypervigilance and "response-readiness" among some children, it seems likely that: "Changes in society and a weakening of traditional family structures contribute toward difficulties experienced by children. In today's world more children have short attention spans and instant gratification offered in modern culture means that children are not being taught to control their impulses" (p. 262).

These flaws cast doubt on the validity of the research that purports to show a genetic etiology for ADD/ADHD. Even without considering these powerful contaminating factors and obstacles, the research on genetic factors in ADHD accounts for no more than 50 % of the variance. This is hardly a reasonable basis for a declaration that ADD/ADHD is present at birth.

A second approach to demonstrating genetic etiology is by using research on the correlation between infant temperament (Thomas and Chess, 1977) and later diagnosis of ADD/ADHD. Some theorists have suggested that such temperament factors as activity level, threshold of responsiveness, intensity of reaction, distractibility and attention span and persistence of these elements might be associated with characteristics of behavior disorders such as ADD/ADHD later on.

Thomas and Chess (1977) indicated, for example, that "features of temperament played *significant roles* [emphasis added] in development of childhood behavior disorders." However, those same researchers concluded that, "in no case did a given pattern of temperament, as such, *result in* [emphasis added] behavioral disturbance. Deviant development was always the result of the *interaction* [emphasis added] between a child's individual makeup and significant features of the environment." (p. 40).

Indeed, the most carefully administered study of this factor found that "the contributions of family characteristics and pre-natal/ perinatal characteristics are outweighed by the contribution of constitutional factors (hyperactivity in the family, chronic illness as a child and temperament characteristics) *and by the home environment domain (measures of achievement press, provision of early learning activities and parent-child interactions)* [emphasis added]" (Lambert & Harsough, 1984)

A third approach to inferring genetic etiology of ADHD is research that compares the incidence of ADHD and other psychiatric disorders in the relatives of children diagnosed with ADHD with the incidence of such disorders in relatives of children not diagnosed with ADHD (Safer, 1973; Biederman et al., 1986; Pauls, 1991). This research is confounded by the failure to control for the many environmental factors that could also explain the intergenerational transmission of mental disorders in families. Research on attachment dynamics and trauma demonstrate the profound influence that parent-child relationships in the first months of life have on the mental health of individuals. (Holmes, 1995; Bretherton, 1995; Crittenden, 1995; Lewis, Amini & Lannon, 2000; Herman, 2000; van der Kolk, McFarlane & Weisath, 1996). None of the research on the incidence of ADHD in families controls for these crucial factors.

Research and common sense confirm that genetic inheritance must have some influence over temperament and, therefore, over the behaviors that characterize ADHD. However, research also demonstrates that genetic influence is not a major factor. As three psychiatrists, Lewis, Amini and Lannon (2000) put it:
"Genetic information lays down the brain's basic macro-and microanatomy; experience then narrows still-expansive possibilities into an outcome. Out of many, several; out of several, one ... While genes are pivotal in establishing some aspects of emotionality, experience plays a central role in turning genes on and off. DNA is not the heart's destiny; the genetic lottery may determine the cards in your deck, but experience deals the hand you can play ... From their first encounter, parents guide the neurodevelopment of the baby they engage with. In his primal years, they mold a child's inherited emotional brain into the neural core of the self." (pp. 149-153)

A balanced review of this research indicates that there is no scientific evidence that ADD/ADHD is present at birth and that genetic factors are, at best, a minor influence over the behaviors that characterize ADD/ADHD.

"ADHD is not caused by poor parenting, a difficult family environment, poor teaching or inadequate nutrition."

In fact, a preponderance of the scientific evidence demonstrates that ADHD is *significantly associated* with unmet needs for nurturance in childhood, difficult family environments and inhumane and oppressive school and community environments. Researchers have found an association between the behavioral characteristics of ADHD and the following characteristics of parenting and family environments:

- Family instability, differences in praise for achievement in the family, provision for early learning, disciplinary practices, interest in the child's schooling, negative and pessimistic perception by parents of the child's academic and intellectual competencies accompanied by decreased expectation levels and decreased desire to participate with the child in learning activities. (Lambert and Harsough, 1984)

- Parents feeling threatened and inadequate; parents unconsciously rejecting the child; and parents blaming children for the extra problems they present. (Lambert, 1982)

- Mothers' use of criticism and general malaise in parenting (Goodman and Stevenson, 1989).

- Mothers who rate the causes of oppositional and inattentive-impulsive child behaviors as more stable and global (Johnston, Chen and Ohan, 2006).

- Problematic family functioning including greater stress within the family, higher rates of parental psychopathology and conflicted parent-child relations (Deault, 2010).

- Family environments that are less organized and higher in family conflict. (Schroeder and Kelley, 2009)

- Father's hypercritical and destructive attitude, inconsistent, impatient and pressuring parenting approach and mothers who are judged to be emotionally disturbed (Thomas and Chess, 1977).

- Maternal anxiety and attitude toward pregnancy (Sameroff & Chandler, 1975).

- Mothers who are more directive, commanding and negative; parents with depression, alcoholism, conduct disorder, anti-social behavior and learning disabilities; mothers who are less responsive to positive or neutral communications of their children (Barkley, 1990)

- A negative, critical and commanding style of child management (Campbell, 1990)

- Parental distress, hostility and marital discord (Cameron, 1977)

- Greater familial anger during conflicts, more disengagement from each other and repeated disputes over school issues and issues pertaining to siblings; parents who adhered to rigid beliefs about their teens' bids for autonomy and who attributed misbehavior to malicious intentions (Robin, Kraus, Koepke and Robin, 1987)

- Parents who use aggressive behavior, indiscriminate aversiveness and submissiveness or acquiescence toward their children during management encounters (Patterson, 1982).

- Disharmony in early mother-child relationships (Battle and Lacy, 1972).

- Experiences of high level of stress in parenting and feelings of lower self-esteem (Goldstein and Goldstein, 1990)

- Mothers who were critical of their difficult babies during infancy and showed lack of affection for them, continued to be disapproving, and tended to use severe penalties for disobedience during the primary school years and assessed their children's intelligence as low (Ross and Ross, 1982).

There are two other areas of research that have clearly demonstrated the impact of early familial experience on the behaviors characteristic of ADHD: *attachment and trauma.*

Attachment researchers have found significant relationships between the quality of mother (and father) – child relationships in the first months of life, the quality of attachment (secure, disorganized or avoidant) at one year of age, and the school performance, sociability, levels of anxiety and general health of children in primary and secondary school (Goldberg, Muir and Kerr, 1995). As J. Holmes (1995) puts it, "Attachment research has shown that a school-age child's sense of security is greatly influenced by the consistency, responsiveness and attunement he or she experienced with his or her parents in infancy." Certainly, the behavior that is used to diagnose ADHD can be seen as the normal and understandable reaction of an insecure child to a stressful situation.

Researchers who have studied trauma have found that traumatic experiences early in life have a great impact on the ability of victims to modulate their emotions and to react effectively and appropriately to stressful and frustrating experiences (van der Kolk, McFarlane

& Weisaeth, 1996; Herman, 2000). Trauma victims tend to become easily activated by threat and adversity, to react impulsively; or they protect themselves by shutting down and retreating into themselves. Both of these are behaviors that are used to diagnose ADHD. Traumatic experiences do not have to be life-threatening to have such an impact. They can consist of deficits in love, support, nourishment, affirmation that are experienced as being life-threatening.

Deutsch et al. (1982) found that adopted children are much more likely to be diagnosed with ADHD than non-adopted children. This is understandable in view of the fact that all adopted children have suffered the trauma of being separated from their birth mothers.

This research, which demonstrates the relationship between attachment and trauma in early life and the kinds of behavior used to diagnose ADHD, contradicts the statement in question.

The statement denies the impact of "poor teaching" on ADHD. While "poor teaching" may, indeed, not be "to blame" for the rise of ADD/ADHD, the rigid, stultifying environment of the typical public school as a primary factor is undeniable. Current educational curriculums are stuffed down the passively-receptive throats of students through repetitive, boring worksheets, one-size-fits-all, standardized methodologies, and minimal or no opportunity for active learning.

Seldom is a child asked what he or she wants to learn or how she or he wants to learn it. Children are subjected to a skewed value system in which primary emphasis is placed on linguistic and mathematical intelligence at the expense of other intelligences that are just as important: musical, spatial, mechanical, kinesthetic, interpersonal and intrapersonal. If children become bored, frustrated, and complain about it, they are told to be quiet or go to the principal's office.

The lead author has tried numerous times to encourage teachers of students diagnosed with ADHD to become more flexible and find ways of accommodating the different learning styles or desires of these students. None of the teachers has been willing or able to do that. Unfortunately, these children may be shuffled into the special education diagnostic category of ADD/ADHD and placed in "less over-stimulating" classrooms. In such circumstances, it is the children who are now pathologized as the "problem" and "abnormality," rather than a major societal system that fails to serve them.

Many scholars have testified to the ways in which the typical school hurts children by failing to encourage them to develop into the unique, separate, creative beings they crave to be (Leonard, 1968; Holt, 2000; Gatto, 2001). Others have noted that ADHD is diagnosed by watching the behavior of children in a typical classroom and that, if the same children are observed in a less oppressive environment, they don't engage in such behaviors. So, Alfie Kohn (2000) wonders if we are diagnosing the child or the learning environment. And Willerman (1973) asks, "Should we classify a high level of activity and a low tolerance for being forced to pay attention to something one doesn't want to pay attention to as a disorder?"

Even the ADHD researchers who support the statements in question have found evidence of the school environment's impact on diagnosis of ADHD:

- Inattention is most dramatically seen in situations requiring the child to sustain attention on dull, boring, repetitive tasks in which there are minimal immediate consequences of completion (Barkley, 1990)

- Task failure or a sudden reduction in anticipated reward or reinforcing feedback may severely disrupt behavior (Barkley, 1990);

- Pre-school hyperactive children were notably more restless, difficult and off-task than their nonhyperactive peers when required to engage in academic-type pursuits such as sitting at a table and listening but were indistinguishable from their peers in free play (Ross & Ross, 1982);

- Onset of hyperactivity often coincides with the point of school entry (Ross and Ross, 1982);

- Hyperactive children perform best on self-paced tasks and their behavior often deteriorates on 'other-paced' tasks (Ross & Ross, 1982);

- Hyperactive children have a difficult time in school, particularly in adolescence, when school work becomes more demanding and achievement becomes an important goal--this situation improves in adulthood when they can select for themselves a job in which they can succeed. (Ross and Ross, 1982).

Are we diagnosing a child or are we diagnosing a learning environment that is intolerable and damaging to a particular cohort of children with certain characteristics who are then called "mentally ill" (ADD/ADHD) only because some choose to call them that?

We can think of many reasons why a child would resist being forced to pay attention to something that doesn't meet his or her need or that diverts him or her from something that is considered more important at that moment:

- She may have some deep concerns that are so troubling that she doesn't have space for anything else:

    - Will I ever have any friends who I can really depend on and feel safe with?

- Is there something I can do to help my parents be happier so they can do a better job of nurturing me?

- Why is it that I have so much trouble doing this work and the other kids seem to be able to do it with ease?

He may have a burning desire to express a talent or drive that is not being honored. When he was ten years old, Picasso's teachers were concerned because all he wanted to do was paint.

For practitioners of professional psychology to treat such concerns as a "mental illness" and respond with a "prescribing predisposition" is a disservice to a child whose individual crisis needs to be understood and used as an opportunity for learning—not how to read, write and do math but how to manage his emotions, thoughts and intentions and how to get along with other children without losing himself.

That ADD/ADHD is generally considered to be a neuro-chemical, genetic disorder with little relationship to parenting and environment is a case of popular opinion being at odds with scientific evidence.

The matter we are discussing here is of the utmost importance to psychology and to the people who are treated by psychologists. If we see the hyperactivity, impulsivity and "disinhibition" that characterize ADHD as driven by genetics and random biological dynamics, we call it a disorder and treat it with drugs and techniques of operant conditioning. If we see that same behavior as a functional response of the child to a situation that is difficult, off-putting, oppressive, abusive, irrelevant, discounting, disaffirming, and/or inhumane, we can call it a normal and understandable reaction and treat it by helping the child, family, and caretakers to fashion a better, more adaptive and life-enhancing response.

References

Alexander, F. (1984). Psychological aspects of medicine. *Advances, 1*: 53-60

Armstrong, T. (1997). *The myth of the ADHD child.* New York: Plume Books.

Barkley, R.A. (1990). *Attention deficit-hyperactivity disorder: A handbook for diagnosis and treatment*. New York: Guilford

Battle, E.S. & Lacy, B. (1972). A context for hyperactivity in children, over time. *Child Development*, 43, 757-773

Baumeister, A. & Hawkins, M. (2001). Incoherence of neuroimaging studies of attention deficit/hyperactivity disorder, *Clinical neuropharmacology*, 24:1, 2-10.

Biederman, J., Munir, K, Knee, D, Habelow, W., Armentano, M, Autor, S, Hoge, S.K., & Waternaux, C. (1986). A family study of patients with attention deficit disorder and normal controls. *Journal of Psychiatric Research*, 20, 263-274

Biederman et al. (1992). Further evidence for family-genetic risk factors in attention deficit hyperactivity disorder. *Archives of General Psychiatry*, 49, 728-738

Bretherton, I (1995). The origins of attachment theory: John Bowlby and Mary Ainsworth. In *Attachment Theory: Social, Developmental and Clinical Perspectives.* S. Goldberg, R. Muir & J. Kerr (Eds.). Hillsdale, NJ: The Analytic Press

Brookes-Keeley, J., Xui, X., Chen, C.K., Huang, Y.S., Wu, Y.Y. & Asherson, P. (2005) No evidence for the association of DRD4 with ADHD in a Taiwanese population within-family study. *BMC Medical Genetics* 2005, 6, 31

Cameron, J. R. (1977). Parental treatment, children's temperament, and the risk of childhood behavioral problems: I. Relationships between parental characteristics and changes in children's temperament over time. *American Journal of Orthopsychiatry*, 47, 568-576

Campbell, S. B. (1990). *Behavior Problems in Preschoolers: Clinical and Developmental Issues*. New York: Guilford Press

Caplan, P. (1996). *They say you're crazy: How the world's most powerful psychiatrists decide who's normal*. Cambridge, MA: Perseus.

Carey, W. (1998, November 16-18). Is ADHD a valid disorder? Invited address to the National Institute of Health, Consensus Conference on ADHD. Available from William Carey, MD, 511 Walnut Lane Swarthmore, PA 19081-1140.

Commoner, B. (2002). Unraveling the DNA myth: The spurious foundation of genetic engineering. *Harper's, 304*, 39-47

Crittenden, P.M. (1995). Attachment and psychopathology. In *Attachment Theory: Social, Development and Clinical Perspectives*. S. Goldberg, R. Muir & J. Kerr (Eds.) Hillsdale, NJ: The Analytic Press

Deault, L.C. (2010). A systematic review of parenting in relation to the development of comorbidities and functional impairments in children with ADHD. *Child Psychology and Human Development*, 41(2), pp. 168-192

Deutsch, C.K., Swanson, J.M., Bruell, J.H., Cantwell, D.V. (1982). Over-representation of adoptees in children with attention deficit disorder. *Behavioral Genetics*, 12, 231-238

Edelbrock et al. (1995). A twin study of competence and problem behavior in childhood and early adolescence. *Journal of Child Psychology and Psychiatry*, 36, 775-786

Everly, G. (1989). *A clinical guide to the treatment of the human stress response*. New York: Plenum Books.

Gatto, J.T. (2001). *The Underground History of American Education*. Oxford, NY: Oxford Village Press

Gillis et. al. (1992). Attention-deficit disorder in reading disabled twins: Evidence for a genetic etiology. *Journal of Abnormal Child Psychology*, 20, 303-315

Goldberg, S., Muir, R. & Kerr, J. (Eds.) (1995). *Attachment Theory: Social, Developmental and Clinical Perspectives*. Hillsdale, NJ: The Analytic Press

Goldstein, S. & Goldstein, M. (1998). *Managing attention deficit-hyperactivity disorder in children: A guide to practitioners*. New York: John Wiley & Sons

Goodman, R. & Stevenson, J. (1989). A twin study of hyperactivity – II. The aetological role of genes, family relationships and perinatal adversity. *Journal of Child Psychology and Psychiatry*, 30(5), 691-709

Herman, J. (2000). *Trauma and Recovery*. New York: Basic Books

Holmes, J. (1995). "Something there is that doesn't love a wall:" John Bowlby, attachment theory and psychoanalysis. In *Attachment Theory: Social, Developmental and Clinical Perspectives*. S. Goldberg, R. Muir & J. Kerr (Eds.). Hillsdale, NJ The Analytic Press

Holt, J. (2000). *How Children Fail*. New York: Perseus Books

Hubbard, R & Wald, E. (1993). *Exploding The Gene Myth*. Boston: Beacon Press

Jackson, G. (2006). A curious consensus: 'Brain scans prove disease?'. *Ethical human psychology and psychiatry*, 8(1), 55-60.

Jensen, J. Cardello, F. & Baun, M (1996). Avian companionship in alleviation of depression, loneliness and low morale in older adults in skilled rehabilitation units. *Psychological Reports*, 78, 339-348

Johnson, S.L. & Roberts, J.F. (1995). Life events and bipolar disorder: Implications from biological theories. *Psychological Bulletin*, 117(3), 434-449

Johnston, C, Chen, M. & Ohan, J. (2006). Mothers' attribution of behavior in non-problem boys, boys with Attention-Deficit Hyperactivity Disorder and boys with Attention-Deficit Hyperactivity Disorder and Oppositional Defiant Behavior. *Journal of Clinical Child and Adolescent Psychology*, 35(1), pp. 60-71

Joseph, J. (2003). *The Gene Illusion: Genetic Research in Psychiatry and Psychology Under the Microscope*. Ross-on-Wye, UK: PCCS Books

Khan A., Leventhal, R. M., Khan, S. R., & Brown, W. A. (2002). Severity of depression and response to antidepressants and placebo: An analysis of the Food and Drug Administration database. *Journal of Clinical Psychopharmacology, 22*, 40-45.

Kohn, A. (2000). *Schools Our Children Deserve: Moving Beyond Traditional Classrooms and "Tougher Standards."* New York: Houghton Mifflin

Kramer, P.D. *Listening to Prozac*. New York: Penguin

Kreger, D.W. (1995). Self-esteem, stress and depression among graduate students. *Psychological Reports, 76*, 345-346

Lambert, N.M. (1982). Temperament profiles of hyperactive children. *American Journal of Orthopsychiatry, 52* 458-467

Lambert, N.M. & Harsough, C.S. (1984) Contribution of predispositional factors to the diagnosis of hyperactivity. *American Journal of Orthopsychiatry, 54* 97-109

Lehmicke, N & Hicks, R. (1995). Relationship of response-set differences in Beck Depression Inventory among undergraduate students. *Psychological Reports, 76*, 15-21

Leo, J.T. & Cohen, D. (2002). Broken brains or flawed studies? A critical review of ADHD neuroimaging research. *The Journal of Mind and Behavior, 24*, 29-56

Leonard, G. (1987). *Education and Ecstasy*. Berkeley: North Atlantic Books

Leuchter AF, Cook IA, Witte EA, et al.: Changes in brain function of depressed subjects during treatment with placebo. *American Journal of Psychiatry* 2002; 159:122-129.

Lewis, T. Amini, F & Lannon, R. (2000). *A General Theory of Love*. New York: Random House

Martínez-Levy, G., Díaz-Galvis, J., Briones-Velasco, J., Gómez-Sánchez, A., De la Peña-Olvera, F., Sosa-Mora, L., Palacios-Cruz, L. Ricardo-Garcell, J., Reyes-Zamorano, E. & Cruz-Fuentes, C. (2009). Genetic interaction analysis for DRD4 and DAT1 genes in a group of Mexican ADHD patients, *Neuroscience letters*, 451, 257-260.

Martel, M. M., Nikolas, M., Jernigan, K., Friderici, K., Waldman, I., & Nigg, J. T. (2011). The dopamine receptor D4 gene (DRD4) moderates family environmental effects on ADHD. *Journal of Abnormal Child Psychology*, 39(1), 1-10.

McCutcheon, L. (1995) Further validation of the Self-defeating Personality Scale. *Psychological Reports, 76*, 1135-1138

Patterson, G.R. (1982) *Coercive Family Process*. Eugene, OR: Castalia

Pauls, D.L. (1991). Genetic factors in the expression of attention-deficit hyperactivity disorder. *Journal of Child and Adolescent Pharmacology, 1*, 353-360

Pennebaker, J.W. (2000). The effects of traumatic disclosure on physical and mental health; The values of writing and talking about upsetting events. In *Posttraumatic Stress Intervention: Challenges, Issues and Perspectives*. J. Volanti & D. Paton (Eds.)

Rappaport, J. (2003). Cornell improves the brain. *Stratiawire.com*, February, 2003

Robin, A.L., Kraus, D, Koepke, T. & Robin, R.A. (1987). *Growing up hyperactive in single versus two-parent families*. Paper presented at the 95th annual convention of the American Psychological Association, New York

Rosenzweig, M.R., Bennett, E.L. & Diamond, M.C. (1972). Brain changes in response to experience. *Learning and Memory*, 8: 294-300

Ross, D.M. & Ross, S.A. (1982). *Hyperactivity: Current issues, research and theory* (2nd Ed. New York: Wiley & Sons

Safer, D.J. (1973). A familiar factor in minimal brain dysfunction. *Behavioral Genetics*, 3, 175-186

Sameroff, A.J. & Chandler, M.J. (1975). Reproductive risk and the continuum of caretaker causality. In *Review of Child Development Research, Vol. 4*. F. B. Horowitz (Ed). Chicago: University of Chicago Press

Schroeder, V. M. & Kelley, M. L. (2009). Associations between family environment, parenting practices and executive functioning of children with and without ADHD. *Journal of Child and Family Studies, 18(2)*, pp. 227-235

Schwartz, J.M., Stoessel, P.W., Baxter, L.R., Karron, M. et.al. (1996) Systematic changes in cerebral glucose metabolic rate after successful behavior modification treatment of obsessive-compulsive disorder. *Archives of General Psychiatry, 53(2)*: 109-113

Seligman, M. (1975). *Helplessness: On Depression, Development and Death*. San Francisco: Freeman

Selye, H. (1974). *Stress Without Distress*. Philadelphia: J.B. Lippincott

Sherman, D.K., Iacono, W.G. & McGue, M.K. (1997). Attention-deficit hyperactivity disorder dimensions: A twin study of inattention and impulsivity-hyperactivity. *Journal of the American Academy of Child and Adolescent Psychiatry, 36(6)*, 745-753

Thomas A. & Chess, S. (1977). *Temperament and Development*. New York: Brunner-Mazel

Thomas, A., Chess, S. & Birch, H. (1968). *Temperament and disorders in children*. New York, New York University Press.

van der Kolk, B., McFarlane, A. & Weisath, L (Eds) (1996). *Traumatic Stress*. New York: Guilford

Visser, J. & Jehan, Z. (2009). ADHD: A scientific fact or a factual opinion? A critique of the veracity of Attention Deficit Hyperactivity Disorder, *Emotional and behavioral difficulties, 14*, 127-140.

Wheeler, L. (2010). Critique of the article by Visser and Jehan: 'ADHD: A scientific fact or a factual opinion? A critique of the veracity of Attention Deficit Hyperactivity Disorder,' *Emotional and behavioral difficulties, 15,* 257-267.

Willerman, L. (1973). Activity level and hyperactivity in twins. *Child Development, 44,* 388-293

ADHD: What We've Been Told Ain't Necessarily So

Burton Norman Seitler

We are told that attention deficit hyperactivity disorder (ADHD) is diagnostically characterized by excessive and pervasive behavioral symptoms of inattention and/or hyperactivity. Further, we are informed that it originates in childhood and often persists into adulthood. Moreover, we are advised that it results in significant lifelong impairments in social, emotional, and cognitive functioning and development (American Psychiatric Association, 2013). Likewise, the American Psychiatric Association developers of the DSM arbitrarily placed ADHD in the category of neurodevelopmental disorders, even though, *by their own admission*, they knew that "it could just as easily have been placed within disruptive, impulse-control, and conduct disorders" (2013, p. 11).

Multiple name changes

Historically, what we now call ADHD has been referred to by a number of different names. It was once called "minimal brain damage," then "minimal brain dysfunction." After this no longer satisfied, "minimal cerebral dysfunction" was invented, which was followed by "minor cerebral dysfunction." Soon thereafter, "minimal cerebral insult" was substituted. Curiously, all of the above names seem to emphasize a neurological origin, despite little or no evidence at that time to support that speculation.

Burton Norman Seitler, Ph.D. is a psychoanalyst/clinical psychologist in private practice.

Although no "hard" neurological signs were ever found (e.g., lesions, tumors, malformations, diseases, and so forth), the idea persisted that there must be a neurological component in there somewhere. Even when the above neurological-sounding names were finally changed to a more behavioral-appearing designation, the implicit notion still held sway of the existence of faulty brain mechanisms (possibly acting in league with "biochemical imbalances").

Reflecting this somewhat modified perspective, more and more name changes occurred. "Hyperkinesis," was replaced by "hyperactivity," which was then followed by "attention deficit disorder," which too, was modified to provide an option for the inclusion or omission of hyperactivity. Years later, "executive functioning deficit" almost supplanted ADHD, but, for some reason, it did not seem to catch on.

In view of all these terminological alterations, how can an objective observer who reads such inconstant psychiatric nomenclature (often couched in "scientific language" that is made to look like the final word on the subject), ever feel confident in what otherwise appears to be a *toss it against the wall and see what sticks* process?

Multiple definitional changes

Along with multiple name changes, definitions fluctuated as well. Justman (2015) comments on the widespread, ever-changing conjectures abut ADHD:

> *The tangled history and mutating specifications of the disorder alternately known as ADD or ADHD make it clear that the disorder (call it ADHD) is not a specific entity given in nature but a construct, and by the same token, its prevalence is highly subject to interpretation (p. 28).*

Connors agrees that the definition of ADHD has failed to remain uniform. Rather than see this as moving the goal posts until you finally get the results you had in mind, he says:

> *Formal diagnostic criteria for the disorder underwent rapid changes as new syntheses and accumulation of data from field trials took place. The fact that the concept of ADHD has evolved with changing evidence should be taken as a strength, not as a sign of unreliability or vague conceptualization (p. 21).*

Interestingly enough, Connors' statement almost cavalierly glosses over the fact that while the ever-changing definitions were "evolving," there was no commensurate change in bio-psychiatric treatment, which continued to promulgate the use of powerful stimulant medications like Ritalin, Adderall, Strattera, or the like. Considering Connors' reputation for being detail-oriented, his statement seems to represent a rather conspicuous omission of the above fact. Not only that, one has to wonder how studies can be undertaken if what one is studying has not been carefully, consistently, and consensually defined, even by the likes of that august document, the DSM?

As George Gershwin wrote in *Porgy and Bess* (1933):

> It ain't necessarily so
> It ain't necessarily so
> The t'ings dat yo' li'ble
> To read in de Bible,
> It ain't necessarily so.

What I am referring to as the "Bible," is the honorific often accorded to the Diagnostic and Statistical Manual (DSM) and the multiple incarnations of the various versions of the DSM referred to above (Horwitz, 2021). Simply put, if the authors of the DSMs got it right the first time, why the need for so many emendations and shapeshifting?

This is not the first time that the authors of the various DSMs made major revisions. For example, it seems as though one day Asperger's was regarded as a disorder, and then, on another day, it was deleted from the DSM and "folded" within the "autism spectrum." Again, one day, shyness was not included in the DSM, but on the next, it was officially pronounced as a pathological condition. The same is true with respect to a number of other so-called disorders or timelines for when a particular behavior meets the "criteria" for being regarded as a disorder (and thus becomes eligible to be included in the DSM), such as grief reaction, and so on. This makes the renderings of the DSMs somewhat suspect. Even the NIMH has, for all intensive and practical purposes, withdrawn its support of and funding for the DSM 5 because of "its lack of validity" (Lane, 2013). And yet, many still follow its writings, tenuous as their previously-noted assertions might ultimately be.

With special respect to so-called ADHD, the question arises, does it even exist, or is it an aggregation or compilation of a variety of symptoms (Carey, 1998)? Even though biopsychiatry has made firm proclamations about ADHD being a real thing, in the minds of a host of other researchers and practitioners alike, a substantial number of questions remain unanswered. For example, Carey (1998) questioned the rush to judgment by biopsychiatry as to the existence of ADHD. He maintained:

> *There does seem to be general agreement on the existence of a small group of readily recognizable "hyperkinetic" children ... But even for this group, it is generally not clear whether the symptoms come from abnormal brains or adverse environments (p. 33).*

He examines the literature on the subject and raises several points regarding differences in temperament between so-called "normal" children and children said to have ADHD. Summarizing Levy, Hay, McStephen, et al's work (1997), he notes:

> *No solid research data support the current cutpoints, where normal high activity and inattentiveness leave off and abnormal amounts begin … But even at their extremes, these traits do not necessarily lead to dysfunction unless other factors are present (p. 34).*

Carey elaborates on this by observing that the diagnostic questionnaires which are commonly utilized to determine the diagnosis are often vague, impressionistic, and highly subjective, resulting in poor inter-rater reliability, misdiagnosis, over-diagnosis, and over-inclusiveness of other diagnostic categories (as seen in the co-morbidity issue, a confounding variable which may distort the whole picture, p. 34). He indicates that the traits associated with the overt behavioral symptoms of ADHD, rather than their being signs of brain damage, ought to take into account their evolutionary adaptive value. He goes on to say:

> *… an evolutionary perspective informs us that the ADHD traits may have been highly adaptive in primitive times but less so now (Jensen, Mrazek, Knapp, et al., 1997).*

Support for this is seen in Stolzer's work (2005). She provided a bioecological analysis of ADHD. However, Carey's final point may have the most consequence.

Diagnosis of ADHD stigmatizes

Carey declares that ADHD stigmatizes children by implying that they have defective brains. In addition, Carey maintains that ADHD:

> *offers no articulation of the individual's problems and strengths and no suggestions for specific management other than medication … The label may be harmful and stigmatizing by stating or implying brain malfunction when it is unproven (p.35).*

Soren Kierkegaard insightfully observed that once you label me, you negate me (1976). We do the same, iatrogenically, with our diagnostic labels and pseudoscientific terms. As Anu Garg pointedly remarked: "If you torture words long enough, they will confess to anything."

ADHD, real entity or hypothetical construct?

At this point in our arguably imperfect understandings of ADHD, would it not be better to take a more moderate stance? An alternative position would be to regard it as a hypothetical construct, instead of an actual entity (Amaral, 2007; Mather, 2012; Campayo, Diez, & Gascon, 2012, Harwood, Jones, Bonney, & McMahon, 2017). In that manner, it could be treated as a piece of incomplete knowledge requiring further research, rather than something about which certain authorities, mainly, but not exclusively, from the biopsychiatry camp, reached a foregone, absolutistic conclusion.

Honkasilta & Koutsoklenis (2022) say: "the frequent changes in the diagnostic criteria for ADHD do not reflect any real scientific progress." Instead, ADHD represents an example of a myriad number of difficulties. By treating ADHD as a concrete entity, it reifies its existence as a disorder, which, in turn, leads to a natural assumption that it must therefore be physical in nature and hence, related to or having a neurological and/or biochemical origin.

This puts the emphasis on conducting certain types of research to the neglect of others. Thus, physiological research (mostly involving neurological investigations), has been favored—and funded—to a significantly greater degree than psychosocial studies. This minimizes the importance and impact of the environment and neglects or even completely turns a blind eye to psychosocial research and findings.

In fact, that is what has happened. There have been a plethora of investigations which mostly focused on finding a physical substrate or underlying biological cause of ADHD (Biederman, et al., 1992; Biederman, et al., 1986; Biederman, et al, 1992; Cornforth, C., Sonuga-Barke, E., & Coghill, D, 2010; Barkley, R.; Chronaki, G., et al., 2010; Kutcher, S. et al. 2004; Spencer, T. et al. 2006; Spencer, T., Wilens, T. et al. 1995), but which have devoted considerably less money, energy, and attention to environmental conditions, psychological factors (both internal and external), and social influences that contribute to what manifests behaviorally as ADHD (Baughman, 1993; Baughman & Hovey, 2006, Belitski, 2017; Breggin, P. 1998, 2002; Conway, F.,2014; Conway, Oster, M. & Szymanski, 2011; Seitler, 2006.; Seitler, 2008; Seitler, 2011; Seitler, 2017; Sonuga-Barke, et al., 2006; Stolzer, 2005).

Even worse than ADHD being reified as an actual entity, a considerable amount of research in certain quarters has taken it for granted that there is general agreement about its neurological origination. However, the fact is that there is no such unanimity or consensus. Rather, there is a great deal of dispute regarding what ADHD is, or is not, as well as a variety of ways to approach the topic, conceptualize it, and ultimately treat it.

As I indicated, biopsychiatry has decided, I think a bit prematurely, that ADHD is physiological in nature. That position has led to the use of powerful drugs, usually stimulants, to help modify the behavior of individuals who have been given that diagnosis. In short, if the belief on the part of biopsychiatry is that the ADHD phenomenon has a biological basis, there is no need to look further for anything beyond that. The long and the short of it is that biopsychiatry has by-passed the intersection of environmental, interpersonal, social, and intrapsychic routes, in favor of neurological, genetic, or biochemical itineraries.

But is their roadmap accurate, or are they unwittingly (or otherwise) blinding themselves to other research which contradicts their neurobiochemical premise? I believe so, based on the following information that supports my contention, and the subsequent case study that I will present shortly, which graphically illustrates not only how I conceptualize the issue, but also my treatment approach (without the use of drugs) to a particular youngster independently diagnosed "with ADHD."

It should be noted that there is no biological marker that is diagnostic for ADHD (Baughman, 2006; Thapar and Cooper, 2016). Barkley (1998) states that doubts have been raised by "neuropsychological studies [which] demonstrate a clear heterogeneity in samples of ADHD defined solely by symptom criteria" (Conners, 1997). Barkley (1998b) wondered about "the possibility that inattention and hyperactivity-impulsivity reflect separate disease entities" (p. 23). Connors claims that as a result of this lack of agreement, there have been excesses regarding the use of medications. He adds:

> *The embarrassment of riches from neuroimaging studies reflect a poor understanding of any specificity for the neural basis of ADHD. The high levels of comorbidity of ADHD with oppositional, conduct, and mood disorders also call in question the specificity of the definition of the disease and whether current criteria are sufficient to allow further understanding of the neurology of the syndrome (p. 23).*

Over-diagnosis

The Centers for Disease Control indicated that ADHD was diagnosed in 15% of high school-aged youths, adding that the incidence of children receiving stimulant medications for ADHD rose dramatically from 600,000 in 1990 to over 3.5 million in 2013. When Connors was interviewed by the New York Times, in December of 2013, he referred to this as "a national disaster of dangerous proportion." He added, "The numbers make it look like an epidemic. Well, it's not. It's preposterous."

Subsequently, he proclaimed "This is a concoction to justify the giving out of medication at unprecedented and unjustifiable levels."

In Great Britain, less than 5000 children were diagnosed with ADHD prior to the 1990s. In 2003, that number had risen to 200,000 children who were given that label (Newnes, p. 161). In addition, the sale of stimulant medications for ADHD quintupled just from 2002 to 2012. University students, believing that their test scores would be greatly enhanced by stimulants, added to their skyrocketing use. Even more so, Watson, Arcona, & Antonuccio (2015) asserted: "There is no evidence that stimulant medications used for ADHD increase intellectual functioning or scholarly contributions." Their work contradicts what we have been told about the benefits of stimulants on academic work and social adjustment:

> *Compelling new evidence indicates that ADHD drug treatment is associated with deterioration in academic and social-emotional functioning (p. 10).*

Medication aftereffects

As I have written elsewhere (Seitler, 2017), "medications have been shown to have serious after-effects" (p. 396). This has been borne out by a number of researchers (Baughman, 1993, 2006; Jackson, 2005, 2009; Breggin & Breggin, 1995; Barkley, et al., 1993). I purposely refer to the results of taking stimulants as *aftereffects*, rather than side-effects, because "side-effects" implies that the effects are either rare or minimal. Research tells us something far more unsettling about the after-effects of stimulants (Jackson, 2005, 2009; Lambert,

1998, 2005; Lambert & Hartsough, 1998; Raine, et al, 2009, 2010). [see Tables I and II below for a list of after-effects]

Longitudinal investigations

The Raine research studies are a series of longitudinal investigations (which are still ongoing) that initially followed Australian children who were receiving stimulant medication for 8 years. A brief summary of their findings is at once informative and, at the same time, rather alarming:

- long-term cardio-vascular damage (i.e., significant increases in diastolic blood pressure, as compared to matched children who did not receive stimulants).

- school failure—despite the long-held (and what turns out to be false) belief that children concentrate better and have higher achievement when on stimulants.

- children receiving stimulants have a 10.5 times greater chance of being identified by a teacher as performing below grade level.

- inattention and hyperactivity slightly worsened over the long term (contrary to what the general public believes and what some professionals have opined).

In a very large study recently conducted by Pelham, et al. (2022), children diagnosed as ADHD who received stimulant medication showed no increment in academic learning, contrary to what had largely been assumed for years and to the study's own initial predictions. The authors examined their results and concluded: "Children learned the same amount of subject-area and vocabulary content whether they were taking OROS-MPH (Osmotic Release Oral System Methylphenidate) or placebo."

Thus, this study provides controlled, experimental, preliminary evidence that fails to support the expectation that medication will improve academic achievement in children with ADHD (p. 376).

Faced with the results of the earlier Raine longitudinal research, advocates for the use of drugs contended that the medicated children in the Raine study must have had more severe forms of ADHD. But, in truth, when the children were first being included in the Raine study, the medicated group and non-medicated group were compared with each other on developmental, behavioral, and health measures, producing **no** significant differences between the two groups at the outset. This seems to put the kibosh on the "severity of the disorder" argument and relegate it to the junkheap of denials.

But the Raine studies are not alone in pointing out the significant dangers of being prescribed stimulant medications. Lambert (2005) and earlier, Lambert & Hartsough (1998) in their own longitudinal studies (in the United States) observed that children on stimulants over a course of time have a significantly greater chance of becoming addicted to other stimulants--ranging from cigarettes to cocaine. Carpentier (2012) points to a causal link between ADHD and addiction:

> *"The high prevalence of ADHD in adults with substance use disorders (SUDs) points to the causal role of the disorder in the development of addiction" (p.285).*

Regrettably, there is still an insinuation that the ADHD "caused" the ensuing addictive behavior, rather than it being caused by the use of the drugs that were prescribed for the ADHD. Does it matter whether the drugs are licit—because they are prescribed—or if they are illicit street drugs? I think not, especially since the prescribed medications (i.e., stimulants) are regarded by the U.S. Drug Enforcement Agency as Schedule II drugs (2022) and as the equivalent of cocaine and amphetamine.

Interestingly enough, the World Health Organization (WHO) went so far as rejecting the listing of methylphenidate (Ritalin) on its official Essential Medicine List, according to researchers Storebø & Gluud (2018) writing in the British Medical Journal of Evidence-Based Medicine. They take issue with its use: "Even though methylphenidate has been used for over 60 years, the evidence concerning the benefits of this medication in children, adolescents and adults with ADHD is uncertain." The decision of the committee was not to include methylphenidate in the WHO Model List of Essential Medicines "due to uncertainties in the estimates of benefit, and concerns regarding the quality and limitations of the available evidence for both benefit and harm" (Storebø & Gluud, 2020). This confirms earlier research by the Cochrane Database System review (Storebø, Pedersen, Ramstad, et al., 2018) and other studies (Storebø, Faltinsen, Zwi, et al., 2018).

Nevertheless, the reification of the ADHD terminology, which treats the "it" of ADHD as a real thing, rather than a theoretical construct, holds "it" responsible for subsequent behavior, including addictions. But "it" is simply a name that has been given to a set of behaviors. The manner in which those behaviors are treated (i.e., with drugs) effect 'it," rather than the other way around. However, the upstart of it all is the strange logic that is invoked to "help" people in the throes of addiction, which is to administer drugs, as if the "legal" drugs will be curative, ostensibly because they are legal.

In the previous case, there is no consideration of even the most remote possibility that the "legal" drugs (methylphenidate) might have led to the use of illegal or street drugs, like cocaine, which curiously enough, resemble methylphenidate. In other words, the child who receives methylphenidate makes the connection that the drug underlies and effects his behavior, rather than understanding that his/her feelings may give rise to the behavior. As a result, s/he makes the connection that drugs are the solution. And so, the possibility that his/her feelings might be responsible for the resulting behavior is lost.

As for the "chemical imbalance" notion that has been bandied about for quite some time, it too is bogus, despite the fact that the public has been led to believe that low serotonin, for example, or a chemical imbalance, causes depression, as a case in point (Lacasses & Leo, 2005). Moncrieff, et al. (2022) say telling patients that their feelings and their behavior are due to chemical imbalances in their brains unfortunately communicates the following unconstructive reactions: the message that we are powerless to change ourselves or our situations. When things go wrong, it persuades us we need a pill to put them right. This approach may appeal to some people, and I am in no way disparaging those who chose to follow it. But it is important that everyone knows how little evidence there is to support it.

Pies (2019) also decries the chemical imbalance notion and refers to it as "The theory that never was." He ascribes its prevalence to direct-to-consumer advertising by the pharmaceutical companies. He states: "SSRIs were accorded a rock-star status as effective anti-depressants that they did not deserve. Most troubling from the standpoint of misleading the general public, pharmaceutical companies heavily promoted the chemical imbalance trope in their direct-to-consumer advertising."

Moncrieff's research (2020) on chemical imbalances with respect to depression found: "no support for the hypothesis that depression is caused by lowered serotonin activity or concentrations." Twenty years earlier, Valenstein (2002) bared the runs in the superficially attractive nylon stockings that supported the biochemical imbalance theory underlying emotional problems. Presciently and provocatively, he raised the hackles on our collective backs to alert us to the fact that our need for a quick-fix made us fair game for being duped by, and dependent upon Big Pharma and their magical pills to help cure our alleged serotonin shortages (propaganda which they had produced, promoted, and propagated).

Genetics as a cause of emotional problems

Similarly, genetic causes were claimed to be at the bottom of ADHD. However, the well documented studies of Joseph (2006, 2009, 2014, 2017) and Fosse, Joseph & Richardson (2015) strongly refute the genetic causality of emotional disorders. Research on genetic variation (Pelham, et al. 2022), encompassing tens of thousands of patients, including the putative gene for serotonin transport, found no difference in the genes of patients with depression and healthy subjects. This counters any previous genetic association between serotonin and depression. What is more, the researchers examined the effects of excessively stressful events in everyday living and found that individuals who experienced such stressors had a greater probability of becoming depressed, or anxious, or dysregulated in some fashion or other.

By claiming that ADHD is neurological or biochemical, or genetic in origin, the examination of other possible factors is dodged. One such factor has to do with what happens internally to individuals said to manifest this disorder. In other words, what do such individuals feel? And, do their feelings contribute in any way to what ultimately manifests itself in the symptomatology of ADHD? Later on in this chapter, the agitation associated with the relationship between inner feelings of sadness and external behavioral manifestations of ADHD will be discussed.

Corrigan (2014) adds his own strong warning about ADHD and the use of medications: "Despite the fact that manufacturers of ADHD drugs readily admit to not knowing what their products actually do to children's brains or development, an abundance of research documents the drugs' contribution to harmful, irreversible neurological and developmental conditions in children" (p. 57).

More recently, Honkasilta & Koutsoklenis (2022) questioned the very basis of what is called ADHD. After reviewing the evidence, they concluded: "In other words, there is no scientific evidence to support the claim that ADHD is a condition within the individual—something individuals have, owing to which they are [italics theirs] vulnerable to various risks the condition exposes them to. Asserting that ADHD is a neurodevelopmental disorder is a scientific conceit, on the one hand, and reflects the DSM's political, cultural, and financial role in the psychiatrization of children's everyday lives, on the other.

A number of other researchers also took issue with specific factors said to underlie ADHD (Travell and Visser, 2006; Gallo & Posner, 2016; Pittelli, 2002; Joseph, 2000; Perez-Alvarez, 2012). They showed that genetic evidence on ADHD is inadequate and peppered with ambiguous interpretations, that no biological marker is diagnostic for ADHD (Thapar & Cooper, 2016), that there are no biological tests to diagnosis it, and that its supposed underlying mechanisms are still unknown (Cortese, 2012: Matthews, et al, 2013). They are not the only ones who acknowledge its dubious neurodevelopmental origination. As I pointed out earlier, even the authors of the DSM 5 admit that the classification of ADHD as a neurodevelopmental disorder, could just as easily have been placed within the disruptive, impulse-control and conduct disorders category (p. 11).

If it were not for these negative aftereffects, the idea of a combo of medications and other approaches (presumed to be effective and safe) would seem to be the most logical solution. However, logic is no substitute for facts. And, the facts are that stimulants are neither benign nor as effective in the long term as we have been told. But, as I said in my introduction, the things that we have been led to believe, "ain't necessarily so."

Thus, if the use of drugs poses serious dangers, as the above literature indicates, what other alternatives exist for parents, schools, and society in general, other than psychoactive medications? Fortunately, we are not solely limited to a bio-psychiatric approach or restricted to the utilization of powerful prescription drugs in order to help children with various kinds of behavioral issues, including ADHD.

Non-medication options

The above literature and tables detail the deleterious effects of psychoactive drugs for ADHD. So, if drugs, such as stimulants, are harmful, what alternative approaches are there? As it turns out, there are quite a few options available that do not involve prescribed psychoactive medications or result in the damage--noted above--associated with such drugs. Because of space limitations, I will merely list a few of them, recognizing that this is an incomplete compilation and that even more alternatives exist.

Because I believe that children and adolescents who exhibit symptoms ascribed to be signs of ADHD do so because of underlying problems that manifest as ADHD symptoms, I highly recommend individual psychotherapy, play therapy and family psychotherapy. By the way, the World Health Organization indicates that before medication is invoked, some sort of behavioral intervention (including psychotherapy) ought to take place. Still other alternatives to medication can be employed.

The case has been made by Sonuga-Barke, et al (2006) for specialized parent training, in particular, the utilization of the New Forest Parenting Package. Exercise has also shown efficacy without the pitfalls of medication (unless one believes that aches and pains, or an occasional charley-horse count). In addition, yoga, meditation, diet (Rojo-Marticella, et al. 2022), the use of nutraceuticals, all have been shown to be beneficial with little or no disadvantages. Now, I would like to move from the theoretical to an actual case.

Harry, an identical twin diagnosed with ADHD

The following is an example of individual psychoanalytic psychotherapy treatment of a ten-year old boy, who I will call Harry. Harry was referred by his parents because, as his mother said, "from the time he was born, his head was always in the clouds. He did not listen, and, unlike his identical twin brother [we'll call him Larry] he was always in motion, and always got into trouble." As an example, they said that he even was expelled from pre-school because "he was too boisterous."

Clinical interview of Harry's Parents

Before seeing Harry, I met with his parents—Mr. and Mrs. Y—in order to get together with them, try to know a little bit about them, listen to what their concerns were about, and take in what they were experiencing with Harry. Let me start with the developmental history they reported (mainly derived from Harry's mother).

Developmental history

Harry was the first born of identical twins (by 2 minutes). The pregnancy was long awaited and planned. At first, Mrs. Y was unable to get pregnant, despite numerous attempts over a two-year period. Shortly after fertility drugs were administered, pregnancy was finally achieved, and Mrs. Y was able to carry the pregnancy to term. Remarkably, when the doctor informed her that she was going to have twins, she was surprised. The course of her pregnancy was relatively unremarkable. There were no untoward problems.

At birth, each twin weighed about 6 pounds. Because of the weight of the twins in utero, she did, however, require a Caesarian section. Other than that, the birth was fairly trouble-free. Mrs. Y said that all developmental milestones, like making eye contact, rolling over, sitting up, babbling and cooing, sleeping through the night, walking, talking and toilet training, etc., were within age-appropriate limits.

However, Mrs. Y said that when she thought about it further, she recalled having great difficulty breast feeding. She said, "I felt like it was torture after a while, as if I was being sucked alive by a vampire. For some reason, I don't why he did it, but it was Harry that latched onto me. He wouldn't let go." When I asked her about this, she said, "I know he was just an infant, but even then, it showed that he was determined to do whatever he wanted to."

On one hand, she recognized that he was merely an infant, but almost in the same breath, she over-rode her tender feelings of compassion toward him and attributed adult qualities to him (i.e., being "determined"). I wondered to myself whether that is what she herself might have gone through as a child. I did not have long to wait to find out, as you will soon see.

Impressions

As an adjunct to working with Harry, and with my encouragement, his parents agreed to come in on a periodic basis (usually once per month, but more often, as needed). On several occasions, Mr. Y was unable to attend, due to his out-of-town work assignments.

However, when he did come in with his wife, it seemed as if other matters occupied his thoughts. At one point, I said to him "it looks like something is troubling you? Is it related to what we are talking about (his son, Harry)?

He replied that he was thinking about work and his upcoming assignment. Mrs. Y added, "He usually has work on his mind. He has a very responsible position in the company and is always on the go." He matter-of-factly explained that he and his wife had an understanding regarding work and home. "We have a division of labor. I take care of work and the finances, and she takes care of the kids." He added, "That seems to work out just fine."

On the occasions when he was unable to attend our meetings, I got to know Mrs. Y better. She initially gave the appearance of a very strait-laced, proper, almost starchy woman, who sat with perfect posture and spoke with perfectly punctuated gentility. In response to questions about her own childhood, she was quite open.

She revealed that her mother was extremely strict, sometimes painfully so. She described her mother as an intolerant, dominant and domineering nurse, who brooked no disagreement or interference with her aims. Mrs. Y added, "You had to do things right or there would be hell to pay." Mrs. Y described her older brother as an alcoholic. But, rather than see his alcoholism in the context of what might have been going on in the family that contributed to his drinking, she simply dismissed her brother as "weak-minded."

My impression was that Mrs. Y knelt to authority by identifying with the aggressor. This may have been so because she saw what happened to her brother and (despite any conscious disdain she overtly expressed towards him) she recognized—on some level—that she had better be obedient because otherwise, she was likely to suffer his fate. Similarly, I suspected that because she learned to be obedient, she expected Harry and Larry to be prim and proper, just like her.

When viewed on many levels, she got her wish. She portrayed Larry in glowing terms. As she described Larry, an image came to my mind of a well-trained, dutiful, meek child. This contrasted dramatically with her depiction of Harry as a wild, noncompliant, curious, ever-inquisitive child, and as one who often diverged from the family's tried and true expectations.

At face value, it appeared that Mrs. Y's wish was met by Larry, but was opposed by Harry's reputed defiance. Conversely, as I discovered, superficial appearances are frequently deceiving. Over the course of our meetings, I got to know Mrs. Y and her husband better. I discovered that underneath her poised, highly dignified persona, was a very sensitive, exquisitely delicate, fragile essence, a woman who was easily slighted and even more easily wounded.

It did not matter if the slight was unintentional or if she perceived a hurt when none had occurred. Typically, she would react internally as if she had been physically slapped and humiliated. It is probably no coincidence that her mother actually did those things to her. As a child, she embarrassed and degraded Mrs. Y, often in public. Mrs. Y struck me as fragile, delicate, easily slighted and easily wounded. Accordingly, she required tremendous patience and steady empathy.

As I became more familiar with Mrs. Y, I wondered to myself whether she got her wish met by Harry too. Considering the fact that she was not permitted to rebel against her exceedingly stern mother, was it inconceivable that Harry might have been a symbolic stand-in for a possible unconscious desire on her part to mutiny? If this possibility was so, it would accomplish several aims. She could safely "act out" through Harry's "misbehavior," and, in so doing, take vicarious pleasure from his noncompliance. At the same time, she could identify with her mother by punishing him for his "misdeeds."

I found Harry to be spunky, a little bit mischievous, energetic and desperately wanting to be heard, yet feeling that nobody really listened to him or understood him. He said that he joked around with other kids, but they regarded his jokes as silly and rebuffed and rejected him as a clown. It seemed to me that his jokes were entreaties to others to accept him, based on a wish for them to see beyond the jokes themselves and recognize that these were simply his way of trying to connect, awkward as they may have been.

Ironically enough, Harry's mother, much like her own mother, did not get his sense of humor. She was very exacting with, and quite critical of Harry's deportment. Even Larry told her that she was too strict with Harry. Despite the moments when she briefly became aware of how tough she was on Harry, her expectations were rarely in keeping with how most children his age act. It was as though she was terribly ashamed of him.

In some ways, Harry served as her own personal safety valve by which she could externalize her own childhood shame onto Harry, while at the same time vicariously experiencing what she could not do, dared not do, but probably wished to do—that Harry's exuberance necessitated that he must do. In other words, on an unconscious level, I believe that she took pleasure in Harry's "acting out" her (unconscious) wishes, while simultaneously re-enacting the punishment that her own mother inflicted on her.

For Harry's part of the equation, I believe that he accurately read his mother's unconscious wish to rebel. Unfortunately, for Harry, it contained a double message, filled with an unconscious wish for rebellion, but also a conscious one—to conform--messages which Harry could never get right. If he did behave properly, she became moody, depressed, and detached. At such times, he felt abandoned and completely alone. Harry hoped his father would intervene, or at least pay more attention to him, but he felt that he was never around.

Harry simply could not win. So, he chose the path of least resistance, even though it came with an obvious downside. Contrary to what would ordinarily seem to be logical, Harry's misbehavior at least offered him a modicum of connectedness. That is, it got his mother's attention, toxic as her reactivity might have been. Nevertheless, he felt unheard and alone. It was his so-called ADHD misbehavior that kept him going. His "hyperactivity" allowed him to stay in motion momentarily, just long enough so that he did not have to experience the deep sadness of being all by himself—amidst a crowd of unhearing listeners.

In essence, I had two patients, Harry and his mother, and one could not get better without the other. Their fate was intertwined, neither parasitic (although that was the Mrs. Y's early fantasy), nor fully merged, but definitely enmeshed. However, when I was able to act on her behalf as her personal interlocutor, and when she felt heard, she was eventually able to get mad at her mother (at least posthumously). At first, there was an understandable boomerang effect whenever she expressed angry fantasies toward her mother in our sessions, fantasies that she had harbored as a child. These consisted of terrible pangs of guilt. Interestingly enough, what allowed her to express some of those feelings—much of them interlaced with murderous rage—was humor.

Harry had it right after all, he just did not know how to use humor in a way that it could pull his mother out of her anger-toward-herself-depression. Instead, he called attention to himself, to take the spotlight off of her. In that regard, he acted like the Christ child who sacrificed himself so that she might live. This is quite common for children to act like this, as a way of distracting a parent (or sometimes both parents) from the parent's personal pain.

After considerable work over an extended period of time, she was eventually able to appreciate Harry's valiant efforts (all quite unconscious) on her behalf. He became less of a "bad" object onto whom she displaced her displeasure, but rather seemed to "transform" in her loyal son, who wanted nothing more than to preserve his mother. Success in the latter endeavor, of course, meant that he could finally get his needs met. It also meant that she too, could finally be seen—and heard. Her mind had changed. It now was acceptable for children to be seen and heard.

In the process of our interaction and the relationship that we had developed, Harry was able to express his feelings. He was able to move from action to putting his emotions into words. There were many stops and often fitful starts to this process. At first, his affect was fraught with uncontained and uncontainable agitation. Each time we had a setback (and there were quite a few) I felt that it was important for me to be empathic to his plight, whatever it was, and to remain consistently low-keyed and non-judgmental. It was especially crucial for me to maintain a sense of equanimity even if he got angry with me. This ultimately enabled him to (1) release his intense feelings without fear of rejection or retaliation, (2) to identify with my ability to keep my cool in the face of his barrage and (3) to begin to replace impulsive action with expressive conversation.

As his agitation eased, a modicum of sadness emerged. Initially, this dismayed him and sometimes discouraged him from wanting "to tell me about it." Nevertheless, perhaps after recognizing that I was not put off or overwhelmed by his upsetness, and that I did not withdraw from him, he was able to "take a chance" and attempt to describe what he felt inside. After one particularly difficult session, in which his feelings poured out of him in an emotional torrent, he looked up at me and said "thank you." I replied, "I know this was not easy for you to talk about." Choking back his remaining tears, he said, "You listened and didn't get mad at me." I asked, "After all that, how do you feel now?" He answered, "I can't explain it. It doesn't make any sense. I feel better." I then responded, "That's what talking and being listened to does."

As time went on, Harry's agitation decreased as his ability to speak about what he noticed was going on inside him increased. As this was happening, he felt less desperate in his efforts to make friends and less impulsive or impelled to take action if his attempts to connect were thwarted.

Attention deficit in the truest sense

Harry's improvement was not the result of a magical incantation nor was it due to the use of psychoactive medications, any more than his behavior was the result of biochemical imbalances or genetic causes (Joseph, 2014).

His progress occurred because of a concerted effort on his part to want to be heard, accepted and understood. It also occurred because Mrs. Y had very similar needs that had not been addressed when she was growing up. Treating both of them concurrently, allowed each of them to grow at their own rate alongside of each other.

More than that, it filled a need that each of them had for attention from an interested, protective, constant object. For example, it is likely that Harry may not have received a sufficient quantity or quality of attention from his father. The same may have been true for Mrs. Y with respect to her husband. In both cases, this was due to his frequent business trips away from the home. In short, it was a different relationship that they were able to have with me---and then with each other—that turned the tide.

References

Amaral, O.B. (2007). Psychiatric disorders as social constructs: ADHD as a case in point. *Amer. J. Psychiat.* doi: 10.1176/ajp.2007.164.5.712-DOI-PubMed

Barkley, R. (1998a). The prevalence of ADHD: Is it just a U.S. disorder? The *ADHD Report*, 1-6.

Barkley, R. (1998b). *ADHD and the Nature of Self-Control.* NY: Guilford Press.

Barkley, R. (2006). *Attention-Deficit Hyperactivity Disorder: A Handbook for Diagnosis and Treatment (Third Edition).* NY: Guilford Press.

Barkley, R., Fischer, M., Edelbrock, C., & Smallish, L. (1990). The adolescent outcomes of hyperactive children diagnosed by research criteria I: An 8-year old prospective follow-up study. *J. Amer. Acad. Child Adolesc. Psychiat.*, 29, 546-557

Baughman, F. (1993). Treatment of attention-deficit disorder. *JAMA*, 269, 2368.

Baughman, F. & Hovey, C. (2006). The ADHD Fraud: *How Psychiatry Makes "Patients" of Normal Children.* Victoria, BC: Trafford Publishers.

Belitski, M. (2017). Literature review and integration of biomedical and psychodynamic conceptualizations of ADHD: Toward a theoretical synthesis of a complex multifactoriala syndrome. Doctoral dissertation, *California Institute of Integral Studies.*

Biederman, J.; Munir, K., Knee, D., Habelow, W., Armentano, M., Autor, S., Hoge., S.K. & Waternaux, C. (1986). A family study of patients with attention deficit disorder and normal controls. *J. Psychiat. Res.*, 20, 263-274.

Biederman, J. et al. (1992). Further evidence for family-genetic risk factors in attention deficit hyperactivity disorder. *Arch. Gen Psychiat.*, 49, 728-738.

Bloch, M.H. & Mulqueen, J. (2014). Nutritional supplements for the treatment of ADHD. *Child Adolesc. Psychiat. Clin. N. Am.* 23, 883-897.

Breggin, P. (1998). Risks and mechanism of action of stimulants. *NIH Consensus Development Conference*, 105-120.

Breggin, P. (2002). *The Ritalin Fact Book: What Your Doctor Won't Tell You About ADHD and Stimulant Drugs.* Cambridge, MA: Perseus Books.

Breggin, P. & Breggin, G. (1995). The hazards of treating "Attention deficit/ hyperactivity disorder" with methylphenidate (Ritalin). J. Coll. Student Psychother 10(2), 55-72.

Campayo, J.C., Diez, M.A., & Gascón, S. (2012). *Trastorno por deficit de atención en la infancia y la adolescencia: del constructo social al calvinismo farmacologico.* Attention deficit/hyperactivity disorder in childhood and adolescence: From the social construct to pharmacological Calvinism. *Aten Primaria*, 44(3), 125-127.

Carey, W. B. (1998). Is ADHD a valid disorder? *NIH Consensus Development Conference on Diagnosis and Treatment of Attention Deficit Hyperactivity Disorder*, p. 33-36.

Carpentier, P. (2012). *Drug Abuse and Addiction in Medical Illness.* [Eds.] Joris C. Verster, Kathleen Brady, Marc Galanter & Patricia Conrod. NY: Springer, 285-96.

Connors, K. (1998). Overview of Attention Deficit Hyperactivity Disorder. *NIH Consensus Development Conference on Diagnosis and Treatment of Attention Deficit Hyperactivity Disorder*, p. 21-24.

Conway, F., Oster, M.A. & Szymanski, K. (2011). ADHD and complex trauma: A descriptive study of hospitalized children in an urban psychiatric hospital. *Journal of Infant, Child, and Adolescent Psychotherapy*. 10(1), 60-72.

Conway, F. (2014). ADHD, Real Neurological Disorder or Psychosocial Symptomatic Behaviors? In, *Attention Deficit Hyperactivity Disorder: Integration of Cognitive, Neuropsychological, and Psychodynamic Perspectives in Psychotherapy*. {Francine Conway, Ed.]. London: Routledge Books.

Cornforth, C. Sonuga-Barke, E. & Goghill, D. (2010). Stimulant drug effects on attention deficit/hyperactivity disorder: A review of the effects of age and sex of patients. Current Pharmaceutical Design.

Corrigan, M.W. (2014). *Debunking ADHD: !0 Reasons to stop drugging kids for acting like kids*. Lanham, MD: Rowman & Littlefield Publishers.

Cortese, S. (2012). The neurobiology and genetics of attention-deficit/ hyperactivity disorder (ADHD): What every clinician should know. *Eur. J. Paediatr*. Neurol., 16, 422-433.

Drug Enforcement Agency (2022). *Controlled Substances Act (CSA) CSA Schedules*. Medically reviewed by Leigh Ann Anderson, Pharm.D. www.drugs.com/schedule-2-drugs.html

Fosse, R, Joseph, J. & Richardson, K. (2015). An assessment of the Equal Environment Assumption of the Twin Method for Schizophrenia genetic effects. *Frontiers in Psychiatry*, 6, 62.

Gallo, E.E., & Posner, J. (2016). Moving towards causality in attention-deficit hyperactivity disorder: Overview of neural and genetic mechanisms. *Lancet Psychiatry*, 3, 555-567.

Garg, A. (2009). The philomath speaks: An interview with Anu Garg. National Assoc. of Scholars. https://libquotes.com.anu-garg

Gershwin, G. & Gershwin, I. (1935). It Ain't Necessarily So. From the American Opera, Porgy and Bess. Music by George Gershwin, Lyrics by Ira Gershwin.

Harwood, V., Jones, S., Bonney, A. & McMahon, (2017). Heroic struggles, criminals and scientific breakthroughs: ADHD and the medicalization of child behaviour in Australian newsprint media 1999-2009. Int. J. Qualitative Studies and Well-being, 12(S1), doi:10.1080/17482631.2017.1298262

Honkasilta, J. & Koutsoklenis, A. (2022). The Un(real) existence of ADHD-Criteria, functions, and forms of the diagnostic entity. *Frontiers of Sociology,* doi: 10.3389/fsoc.2022.814763.PMID: 35707639; PMCID: PMC9189308.

Horwitz, A.V. (2021). *DSM: A History of Psychiatry's Bible.* Balt., MD: Johns Hopkins University Press.

Jackson, G. (2005). *Rethinking Psychiatric Drugs: A Guide for Informed Consent.* Bloomington, IN: AuthorHouse Press.

Jackson, G. (2009). *Drug Induced Dementia: The Perfect Crime.* Bloomington, IN: AuthorHouse Press.

Jensen, P.S., Mrazek, D., Knapp, P.K., et al. (1997). Evolution and revolution in child psychiatry: ADHD as a disorder of adaptation. *J. Amer. Acad.* Child Adolesc. Psychiat., 36, 1672-1679

Joseph, J. (2004). *The gene Illusion: Genetic research in psychiatry and psychology under the microscope.* Algora Press.

Joseph, J. (2006). *The Missing Gene.* Algora Press.

Joseph, J. (2014). *The Trouble with Twin Studies: A Reassessment of Twin Research in the Social and Behavioral Sciences.* Routledge

Joseph, J. (2017). *Schizophrenia and Genetics.* BookBaby.

Joseph, J. (2009). ADHD and genetics: A consensus reconsidered. In, *Rethinking ADHD: From Brain to Culture.* [Eds] J. Leo & S. Timimi. London: Palgrave, 58-91.

Justman, S. (2015). Attention Deficit/Hyperactivity Disorder: Diagnosis and stereotypy. *Ethical Human Psychology and Psychiatry,* 17(2), 135-144.

Kierkegaard, S. (1976). In, *Journal of Marriage and Family Counseling*, 2, 33.

Kutcher, S., Aman, M., Brooks, S.J., Buitelaar, J., van Daaleen., Fegert, J., Findling, R.L., Fisman, S., Greenhill, L.L., Huss, M., Kusumakar, V., Pine, D., Taylor, E. & Tyano, S. (2004). International consensus statement on attention-deficit/hyperactivity disorder (ADHD) and disruptive behavior disorders (DBDs: Clinical implications and treatment suggestions. *European Neuropsychopharmacology*, 14, 11-28.

Lacasse, J.R. & Leo, J. (2005). Serotonin and depression: A disconnect between the advertisements and the scientific literature. PLoS Med.: e392. doi: 10.1371/journal.pmed.0020392.Epub2005Nov8

Lambert, N.M. (1998). Stimulant treatment as a risk factor for nicotine use and substance abuse. Overview of Attention Deficit Hyperactivity Disorder. *NIH Consensus Development Conference: Diagnosis and Treatment of Attention Deficit Hyperactivity Disorder.* Bethesda, MD: 19-200.

Lambert, N.M. (2005). The contribution of childhood ADHD, conduct problems, and stimulant treatment to adolescent and adult tobacco and psychoactive substance abuse. *Ethical Human Psychology and Psychiatry*, 7(3), 187-221.

Lambert, N.M. & Hartsough, C. (1998). Prospective study of tobacco smoking and substance dependence among samples of ADHD and non-ADHD subjects. *J. Learning Disabil. 6, 533-544.*

Lane, C. (2013). The NIMH withdraws its support for DSM-5: The latest development is a humiliating blow to the APA. Psychologytodayhttps://www.psychologytoday.com/intl/blog/side-effects/201305/the-nimh-withdraws-support-dsm5

Lane, C. (2007). Shyness: How Normal Behavior Became a Sickness. New Haven: Yale University Press.

Levy, F., Hay, D.A., McStephen, M., Wood, C., & Waldman, I. (1997). Attention-deficit hyperactivity disorder: A category or a continuum? Genetic analysis of a large-scale twin study. *J. Amer. Acad. Child. Adolesc. Psychiat.* 36(6), 737-744.

Mather, B.A. (2012). The social construction and reframing of Attention-Deficit/Hyperactivity Disorder. Ethical Human Psychology and Psychiatry.

Matthews, M., Nigg, J.T. & Fair, A. (2013). Attention deficit hyperactivity disorder. *Curr. Topics Behav. Neursci.*, 16, 235-266.

Moncrieff, J., Cooper, R.E., Stockmann, T., Amendola, S., Hengartner, M.P. & Horowiyz, M.A. (2022). *Molecular Psychiatry.* https://www.nature.com/articles/s41380-022-01661-0

Newnes, C. (2009). Clinical psychology and attention deficit hyperactivity disorder. In, S. Timimi and J. Leo [Eds.] *Rethinking ADHD: From Brain to Culture.* Basingstoke, UK: Palgrave Publishers, 160-168.

Pelham, W.E., Altszuler, A.R., Merrill, B.M., Raikert, J.S., Macphee, F.L., Ramos, M, & Pelham, W.E, Jr. (2022). The effect of stimulant medication on the learning of academic curricula in children with ADHD: A randomized crossover study. *J. Consult, & Clin. Psychol.*, 90(5), 367-380.

Perez-Alvarez, M. (2017). The four causes of ADHD: Aristotle in the classroom. *Fron. Psychol.*, 8, 928.

Pies, R. (2019). Debunking the two chemical imbalance myths, Again. *Psychiat. Times,* https://www.psychiatrictimes.com/view/debunking-two-chemcical-imbalance-myths-ag

Pittelli, S.J. (2002). Meta0analysis and psychiatric genetics [letter to the editor]. *Am. J. Psychiatry,* 159, 496-497.

Raine, W. (2009, Sept.). *Western Australia Ministerial Implementation Committee for Attention Deficit Hyperactivity Disorder,* Raine Attention Deficit Hyperactivity Disorder Study, Perth, Australia: Telethon Institute for Child Health Research.

Raine, W. (2010, Jan.). *Attention Hyperactivity Disorder Study: Draft—Long-term outcomes associated with stimulant medication in the treatment of ADHD in children.* Perth, Australia: Telethon Institute for Child Health Research.

Rojo-Marticalla, M., Arija, V., Alda, J.A., Morales-Hidalgo, P., Esteban-Figuerola, O., & Canals, J. (2022). Do children with Attention-Deficit/ Hyperactivity Disorder follow a different dietary pattern than that of their control peers? (2022). *Nutrients,* 14(6), 1131—1156.

Seitler, B.N. (2006). On the implications and consequences of neurobiological etiology of Attention Deficit Hyperactivity Disorder. *Ethical Human Psychology and Psychiatry,* 8(3), 229-240.

Seitler, B.N. (2008). Successful child psychotherapy of Attention Deficit/ Hyperactive Disorder (ADHD): An agitated depression explanation. *Amer. J. Psychoanalysis.* 68, 276-294.

Seitler, B.N. (2011). Is ADHD a real neurological disorder or collection of psychosocial symptoms? Implications for treatment in the case of Randall E. *Journal of Infant, Child, and Adolescent Psychotherapy,* 10(1), 116-130.

Seitler, B.N. (2017). Sophistry and ADHD: The Dual Myths of Organicity and Biochemical Imbalance and the Ensuing Medication Tidal Wave. In, *From cradle to Couch: Essays in Honor of the Psychoanalytic Developmental Psychology of Sylvia Brody.* [Eds. Burton N. Seitler & Kim S. Kleinman]. NY: International Psychoanalysis Books.

Sonuga-Barke, E., Thompson, M., Abikoff, H., Klein, R. & Brotman, L.M. (2006). Nonpharmacological interventions for preschoolers with ADHD: The case for specialized parent training. *Infants & Young Children,* 19(2), 142-153.

Spencer, T., Abikoff, H.B., et al., (2006). Efficacy and safety of mixed amphetamine salts extended release (Adderall XR) in the management of oppositional defiant disorder with or without comorbid attention-deficit/ hyperactivity disorder in school-aged children and adolescents: A 4-week, multicenter, randomized, double-blind, parallel group, placebo-controlled forced-dose-escalation study. *Clinical Therapeutics,* 28(3), 402-418.

Spencer, T., Wilens, T., et al., (1995). A double-blind crossover comparison of methylphenidate and placebo in adults with childhood onset attention deficit hyperactivity disorder. Archives of General Psychiatry, 52(6), 434-443.

Stolzer, J. (2005). ADHD in America: A bioecological analysis. *Ethical Human Psychology and Psychiatry*, 7(1), 65-76.

Van Cleave, J. & Leslie, L.K. (2008). Approaching ADHD as a chronic condition: Implications for long-term adherence. *J. Psychosocial Nursing and Mental Health*, 46(8), 28-37.

Storebø, O.J. & Gluud, C. (2020). Methylphenidate for ADHD rejected from the WHO Essential Medicines List due to uncertainties in benefit-harm profile.

Storebø, O.J., Faltinen, E., Zwi, M. et al. (2018). The jury is still out on the benefits and hams of methylphenidate for children and adolescents with attention-deficit/hyperactivity disorder. *Clin. Pharmacol. Ther.*, 104(4), 606-609.

Storebø, O.J., Pedersen, N., Ramstad, E., et al. (202018). Methylphenidate for attention deficit hyperactivity disorder (ADHD) in children and adolescents-assessment of adverse events in non-randomized studies. *Cochrane Database Sys. Rev.* 5:cd012069. Doi: 10.1002/1651858.CD012069. pub2

Thapar, A. & Cooper, M. (2016). Attention deficit hyperactivity disorder. *Lancet.*, 387, 1240-1250.

Travell, C. & Visser, J. (2006). 'ADHD does bad stuff to you:' Young people's and parents experiences and perceptions of attention deficit hyperactivity disorder (ADHD). *Emot. Behav. Diffic.*, 11, 205-216.

Valenstein, E.S. (2002). *Blaming the Brain*. NY: Free Press.

Watson, G.I., Arcona, A.P. & Antonuccio, D. (2015). The ADHD drug abuse on American college campuses. *Ethical Human Psychology and Psychiatry*, 17(1) 5-21.

What's the "Deficit" in ADHD? A Wider View of an All-Too-Common Diagnosis

Ben Bernstein

Joshua, aged 13, was referred to me with a history of poor grades and being disruptive as the class clown. For the last forty years I have focused my psychology practice on how stress affects human performance. In addition to working with doctors, dentists, attorneys, athletes, stage performers, and many others in high stress occupations, my five decades of teaching at every level of the educational system informs my work with students, including those diagnosed with ADHD, who have performance issues in school.

Joshua (names are changed) was referred by his pediatrician, who had recommended to Josh's parents that he undergo a full battery of neuro-psych testing. According to the report, Josh "wasn't paying attention in class" and was "acting out." Based on testing, Josh was diagnosed with ADHD.

When Josh walked into my office he was immediately drawn to the bookshelves which are filled with a wide variety of objects. "Do you see something you like?" I asked him. Josh pointed to an unusually shaped quartz crystal and said, "That". I took down the crystal, handed it to him, and started to explain what it was. He cut me off, "Yeah, I know," and then he proceeded to talk in a very animated manner about the origin of crystals and about geology in general.

Ben Bernstein, Ph.D., is a psychologist and educator.

Taken by the scope of his knowledge and enthusiasm for the subject and—obvious to me, a teenage urge to impress—I followed up with some relevant questions. The conversation was lively, and ended with my saying how much I enjoyed talking with him. Then I asked, "Josh, do you know why your parents brought you here today?" He paused, and, staring at me in a hesitating, searching way, finally said, "School is so *boring*."

My career in education began in 1968 as a volunteer teacher in the first Head Start program in Maine. From there I landed in elementary schools in poverty-stricken Bedford-Stuyvesant, Brooklyn, where I was thoroughly disheartened by the near military conditions of enforced silence and strict discipline. I thought, *school has to be better than this,* and my search took me to London, England, where I was trained and then taught in one of the legendary "British infant schools" of the early 1970's. Classrooms there were organized into activity centers and each day the children chose to cook, or do carpentry, or sew, or dress up, or paint. As teachers, we honored and merged the two meanings of the word "interest"—we taught the children what was in their interest, in a way that was interesting to *them*.

Reading, writing and math were integrated into the kids' activities, central to their planning, problem solving and execution of ideas. When a child had difficulty understanding and learning something—fractions, for instance—it was never the child's "problem," it was always the teacher's challenge to find a way for the child to "get it." When a recipe called for a "quarter cup of flour" we took a full cup and divided and measured it into four equal parts. Then, the abstract "1/4" made sense and became operational once a child fully grasped what "one over four" symbolized.

The classrooms in London were lively, active *communities*. One of my principal teachers, Viola Spolin, in her landmark book *Improvisation for the Theater,* said, "Community is a phenomenon of the spirit that comes and goes and must be deliberately sought after." The classrooms in England were highly spirited.

Contrast this with the lifeless classrooms I observed in public schools in the U.S. In one, I charted the activities of the teacher and her students over a three-week period. My findings were grim: seventy-five percent of the teacher's actions were directed to getting the children to be quiet. Almost fifty percent of the children's activities had to do with spitting back "right answers." The other fifty percent was spent fooling around, sneaking food, writing, passing notes, and so on. The children were variously bored, agitated, minimally engaged, and noisy. The teacher had to keep quieting them down. The kids would stay hushed for a little while, then they would regurgitate more stuff, then become bored and rowdy, and then the teacher struggled to quiet them down again. And so, the cycle kept repeating. For most of these students, like for Josh, school was boring. Josh, and many others like him, were *dis-spirited.*

Over the years I have had numerous students like Josh referred to me. Kids who were chronically poor performers in their academic work, usually singled out by teachers as having "problems": unable to pay attention to the great frustration of their parents and teachers, with a tendency to act out and be disruptive. Then they were permanently stamped "ADHD."

Saraya, age 12, was brought to me because "she drifted off during classes." Saraya acted out by spacing out. Again, neuro-psych testing, again the diagnosis: ADHD.

One of the reports on Saraya stated, "She writes imaginative stories." Her stories—always about a twelve-year-old girl—contained a portal through which the girl would escape to fantastic worlds of color, light and adventure. When I met Saraya, I showed genuine interest in her stories, which led to an animated conversation about all kinds of things that interested her as a twelve-year-old: cool clothes, her own music playlists, drawing and her personal portal.

At Saraya's IEP meeting, her teachers all agreed, "Saraya isn't paying attention." When it was my turn to contribute I said, "But Saraya is paying attention to *something*." I proceeded to tell them about Saraya's portal and how she escaped through it to a world far more interesting and engaging than the one in the classroom.

As another example, Max's parents wanted Max, age 10, to attend a private middle school. Two of application requirements were a math proficiency test and an interview. The trouble was Max couldn't "do" math, and he didn't speak. In school, when the teacher taught math, Max withdrew into himself, looking down at his desk or, more usually, doodling. His pediatrician and teachers suspected ADHD.

In our first session Max seemed frightened. He had a hard time looking at me. All my attempts at conversation elicited only curt monosyllabic answers. In the second session, I took a different tack. From his parents, I knew that Max liked to draw, so I laid out different size sheets of paper on the floor of my office, along with an assortment of colored markers, crayons and pastels. When Max came in I said, "Let's not talk today, Max." Pointing to the floor, I said, "You can draw if you want to."

Though he gave me a slightly wary, *What are you up to?* look, Max began drawing. Over the next forty minutes he was thoroughly engaged drawing a collection of differently-sized dinosaurs. Before the end of the hour, I asked him if there was a story about the drawing. Without looking at me he said, "This is a family," and he pointed out the two parent dinos and the two kids— the girl and the boy. The girl was the older of the two.

From Max's parents, I had learned that his older sister, Julia, had the year before been accepted at a very exclusive private high school. To prepare her for that interview, the father—a recent refugee from a war-torn country—hid behind doors in their house and when Julia passed by he jumped out and surprised her with questions. If she didn't answer the questions to his satisfaction, Dad yelled at her.

When Max returned for the next two sessions he continued to draw and—keeping my focus on the drawings—we talked about the story as it evolved. Since Max was growing more comfortable talking with me (I wasn't jumping out from behind doorways), I gently asked him what was happening with math. He told me that he didn't understand what the teacher was talking about but was afraid to tell her. "Why?" I asked him. "They [his parents] will get angry."

I asked Max if it would be OK with him if I spoke with his parents and teacher to tell them that I instructed him to say "I don't understand" as soon as he couldn't follow what was going on, and that I'd get them to promise to be understanding and helpful. Max liked my suggestion and I engaged the parents and teacher in our plan.

In three weeks, Max's "problems" with math cleared up. He went on to have the interview, and was accepted to the school.

How was it that these three students—and almost countless others I've worked with over the last forty years—are diagnosed with ADHD when there are conditions in which they are calm and their attention is riveted?

Here's what I've come up with: The "attention deficit" these kids have been branded with is not *their* inability to pay attention—to be present to the task at hand—but in the deficit of attention they've *received*. They live in a vacuum— they're supposed to give their attention to things they don't care about or understand, but who's paying attention to *them*? Who is dialed into their interests and what motivates *them*?

When they didn't pay attention, they were labeled "inattentive" or they were shunned or punished. This often leads to aberrant behavior—hyperactivity—which is a backward, unproductive way of getting attention. The outcome: the diagnosis of ADHD.

To claim a child is not "paying attention" is to beg the question: what are we expecting children to attend to? While the answer seems fairly obvious—the required school curriculum—there is a deeper issue at work here which I would like to explore, and that is the subject of *focus*.

For the last fifty years my work has been centered on human performance: what are the conditions necessary for a person to perform at his or her best? Briefly put there are two: (1) an optimal relationship between arousal and performance; and (2) maintaining the optimal states for learning in body, mind and spirit.

In the early twentieth century two psychologists, Yerkes and Dodson, studied how arousal affects performance. The "Yerkes-Dodson" bell curve shows us that when arousal is too low [the left-hand tail of the curve] there is little motivation and performance suffers. On the right-hand tail, when arousal is too high, overstimulation and exhaustion compromise problem-solving and, again, performance suffers. At the apex of the curve there is just the right amount of arousal, which produces a state of optimal performance. Athletes call this "the Zone."

In the three case studies I cited earlier, we can see how this operates: Josh was bored (too little arousal; left side of the curve), Max was anxious and shut down (over arousal, right side), and Saraya,

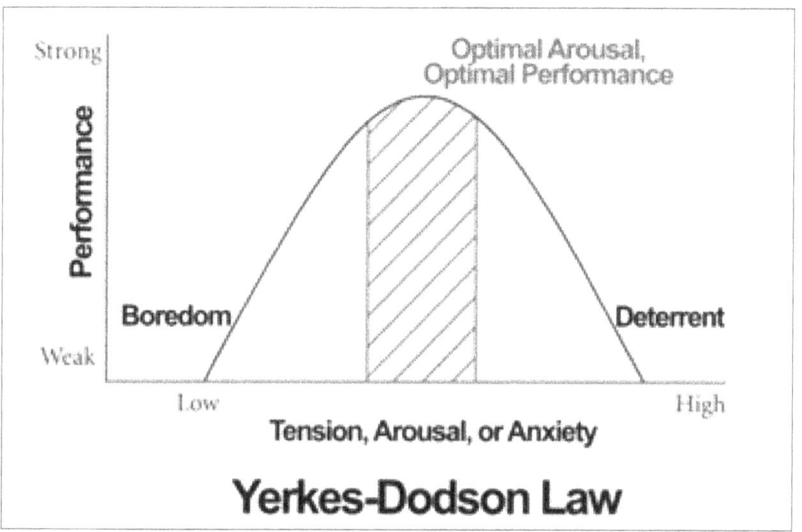

flipping between being under- and over-stimulated, found a way of checking out completely by escaping through her imaginary portal.

What actually creates the conditions for being in "the Zone"? Athletes talk about it in vaguely mystical tones: *Man ... last night I was in the Zone!* as if that state magically came upon them. Research and clinical experience demystify this: being in the Zone is a state that can be consciously attained.

In any performance situation (in any life situation) the body, mind and spirit are all involved. Optimal arousal and performance require a balance: the body needs to be calm, the mind confident and the spirit focused. Calm means you are in a state of relaxed readiness, not tense." "Confident" means that you are giving yourself positive, affirming messages ("I can do this," "I've got what it takes," etc.). And "focused" means you have a goal and you are consistently taking actions that move you to towards the goal.

I use the model of a three-legged stool to give a concrete, graphic representation of this:

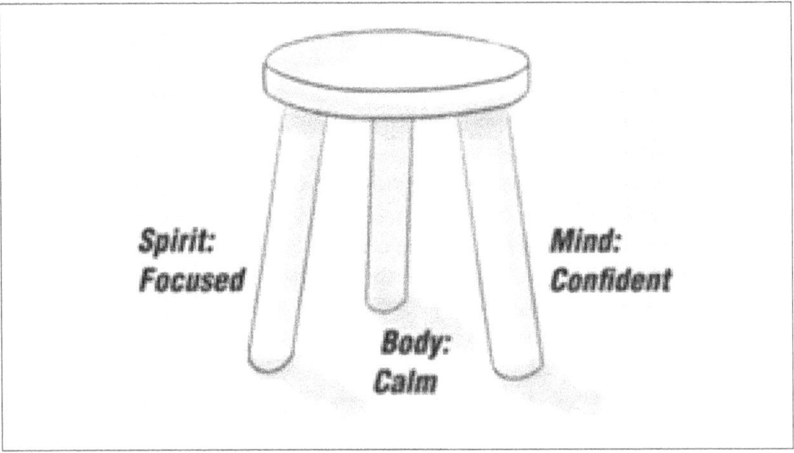

When all three legs are equally strong, the stool is a sturdy platform for optimal performance. When one (or more) of the legs is short or weak, the imbalance creates performance problems.

The diagnostic criteria for "inattention" in the DSM-V all point to a difficulty or failure in ability to attend. Children who don't or can't pay attention are slapped with the label of being "inattentive" and thus qualify for the diagnosis of ADHD.

The problem with this is two-fold: (1) an expectation that children should be able to attend to whatever we put in front of them; and (2) inattentive children have "a problem." Their inattention is considered the product of a "scattered mind" or an overactive nervous system rather than a lack of engagement of the spirit.

I have been most fortunate to have worked in vastly different educational environments—those in which children are actively engaged and those in which they are not. In the former (British infant schools, and select classrooms and schools in the US), the children, their teachers and the environment as a whole was highly *spirited*. In the latter, the spirit is squelched to the point of being asphyxiated.

Bringing "spirit" into a conversation about public education is fraught with controversy. We are conditioned to attach "spirit" to "religion" and become entangled in a hot-headed, irrelevant debate about whether the spirit has a place in the classroom. Also, "spirit" doesn't fit neatly into any quantifiable category. As per everything else in Western science, if we can't see it, we can't study it, and therefore, effectively, it doesn't exist.

As a performance psychologist, I consider spirit to have a distinct and essential function in learning and life: spirit informs our goals. While goals engage the body and mind, they originate in the spirit. Spirit directs us to what we want to accomplish. It supports us in taking actions that are aimed at accomplishing our goals. Think of spirit as the power generator. It produces the energy that sparks every one of our achievements. Throughout history, spirit has moved men and women to become great leaders, scientists, poets, musicians, and athletes.

In performance terms, the optimal state for the spirit is to be *focused*. According to the dictionary, "focus" has a two-pronged definition. As a noun, it is "the center of interest or activity." Think of the bullseye in the very center of a dartboard. As a verb, it is "to direct action toward a particular point or purpose." Think of throwing the dart directly to this point.

The word "focus" comes from the Latin root that means "hearth" or "fireplace." Traditionally, the hearth was the center of the home, a gathering place of warmth and light and sustenance. In my performance model, focus has these qualities. Our goals come from our center, the fireplace of our being, our spirit. When you stay focused, you are feeding and sustaining your fire, which generates energy and nourishment.

In the conventional classroom, the goal is what the teacher is mandated to accomplish, *ipso facto* the student's goal must be aligned with what the teacher must cover. If the student is not engaged, she or he is labeled as "having a problem" and subject to being diagnosed as ADHD.

I am making the case that inattention (difficulty focusing) is not necessarily a mind-body problem. It is very often the result of an unengaged spirit.

In the case of every student who has been sent to me with an ADHD diagnosis, I have been told "he can't concentrate" or "her mind wanders." The word "concentrate" conjures up a stern, gnarly schoolteacher straight out of a Dickens novel who will whack you on the knuckles when your attention wanders. The truth is that it is not in the mind's nature to concentrate. Typically, it jumps all over the place, from a fragment of a song, to what you had for breakfast, to criticism over some flimsy comeback in an argument, to a fantasy about the upcoming weekend. Keeping your mind on one track is like walking a pack of dogs that all want to run in different directions. The moment you pull one into line, another one runs off. Holding them together is hard work and eventually it wears you out. You can keep yelling at the dogs, of course, but after a while they'll stop listening to you.

Contrast concentrating, which is harsh, to focusing, which is nurturing. When you try to concentrate, you often feel as if you're being forced to do something somebody else expects of you. When you focus, however, your actions are self-directed. Your goal is coming from your spirit and is important to you. You are cooperating with your Self.

Children are naturally active, curious and engaged with the world: they need to have that fire—their spirit— nurtured. When a fire isn't tended it goes out. In each of the three case studies I've cited, their spirit as starved of attention. The fire had been reduced to embers. Once someone showed genuine interest in *them*, the fire was stoked and the "problems" cleared up.

This is as true for issues with "inattention" as it is for "hyperactivity." In too many cases I have observed that the child who can't "sit still" (what child was built to "sit still"?), is crying out for attention by being the class clown or running around the room. Both are ways that command attention, but in a very unproductive, soul-damaging manner.

Recently, I received a call from a 53-year-old man, I'll call "Bob." Bob had failed a professional licensing exam three times due to debilitating test anxiety. His internet search turned up my book *Crush Your Test Anxiety*, which he read. "I felt like you were talking to me," he said. He then went on to say, "I have ADHD," which he stated matter-of-factly, as if he was telling me his height or hair color.

In kindergarten Bob had trouble with reading (which, in those days, was actively taught in kindergarten classrooms) and he "couldn't do numbers." He was required to repeat kindergarten. By third grade, he couldn't concentrate in class. In the fourth grade, he was tested and diagnosed with ADHD. As the years progressed, and the school curricula became more complex and competition with peers intensified, Bob's academic problems grew worse. He made two attempts enrolling in college but dropped out. "It wasn't for me," he said. "I just couldn't do it."

Note, however, Bob's significant "back story": Starting at age 6, he was a very active athlete. By the time he reached high school he was ranked nationally as a track star. He was also the president of his class and the head of the student judiciary committee. Reaching further back, when Bob was in third grade his father had opened a fast food restaurant, and after school Bob was dropped off frequently at "the store" where he learned to make milkshakes, use the cash register, and help serve the clientele, who took a real shine to him. How much more engaging all of this was, as he said, "than being stuck at a school desk staring at the back of someone's head."

Bob admitted, "School tests were always a problem," but then told me an intriguing story. "On a math test in high school I got all the answers wrong. But then the teacher asked to look at my worksheet and saw, that in fact, I had solved all the problems correctly!"

I'm offering Bob's story as an example, common in my practice, of an adult who has, for years, lived and suffered from a childhood ADHD diagnosis. As a young child, Bob was lost from the get go, left back (in kindergarten!), but was much more engaged in the lively environment of his Dad's restaurant than in the boring, stagnant classroom environment, and he had a lot of success as an athlete.

What was revealing about the math test story is that Bob actually knew the math and had answered all the questions correctly, but when he crossed the threshold to the answer sheet he messed it all up. Now he was coming to me to help him pass a test that he had failed three times. My diagnosis: when Bob had to perform "academically" he was unsteady in all three "legs"— he became extremely jittery and nervous (body), he was feeding himself negative self-talk ("I can't do this, I'm going to get it wrong"—mind) and his focus (his goal—spirit) was to "get it all over with as fast as possible." All of this was a product of having suffered through a school system that failed *him.*

As with the three youngsters I cited earlier in this chapter, Bob's inner experience (curiosity, drive, taking on challenges) was mismatched with the messages he received in school: "You can't do this, you have a problem, you might as well give up."

How many kids are diagnosed with ADHD simply because no one has really spent the time and energy connecting with them? And how many kids get stuck with the diagnosis because it's an easy one to medicate, or to get extra time on tests, or just get more *attention*, however negative.

Over the years I've noticed that kids—particularly adolescents—are increasingly outspoken about how school is boring, how it's a waste of time and a pain in the butt, how they don't see the relevance to what they are learning, and how their teachers are uninspired and disconnected.

Granted, it's nearly impossible for a teacher to compete with dopamine-inducing video games, the riptide of social media, the attention-sucking universe of smart phones, and the horribly divisive political atmosphere about what should or should not be taught in American schools. Given the enormous challenges of teaching and learning during a global pandemic, it's a wonder that teachers even *continue teaching*. But they are caught up and trapped in a system that is historically oriented to outdated, irrelevant curricula, that breeds competition and out-scoring one another, and puts the premium on product rather than process.

"Education" has two Latin roots: *educere* and *educare*. Educere means "to bring forth, to lead out"; *educare* means "to shape." When we slap a child with a diagnosis of ADHD, we are shaping them for life, having forgone the absolutely vital first step of drawing forth the child for who he or she is.

But none of this—or maybe all of it—still does not change the basic fabric of human relationships and what we need from one another: nurturing, positive attention. We all need it, for who we *are*.

One way or the other children are going to get attention, even if they have to be "naughty" or "have problems". Why don't we upend that whole process and lovingly nurture kids for who they *are*?

ADHD as a Symptom of Attachment Insecurity: We Are Failing Our Children

Erica Komisar

There is enough research, statistical evidence, and case material from my own work and that of my colleagues to make a strong argument that as a society we are failing our children: there has been a dramatic increase in emotional, social, and behavioral difficulties like ADHD, anxiety, and depression in children from toddlerhood to adolescence.

The statistics for ADHD are frightening. According to the Centers for Disease Prevention and Control (CDC), 11 percent of children between the ages of four and seventeen years in the United States have been diagnosed with ADHD. This is a dramatic 16 percent increase since 2007. In addition, two-thirds of those children were treated with stimulant medications such as Ritalin and Adderall.[1] These stimulants are being prescribed to younger and younger children, and we don't yet know the long-term effects of changing the

---

Erica Komisar, LCSW, is a clinical social worker, psychoanalyst, and parent guidance expert based in New York City, USA.

[1] Division of Human Development and Disability, "Attention-Deficit/Hyperactivity Disorder (ADHD)," National Center on Birth Defects and Developmental Disabilities, Centers for Disease Control and Prevention, updated May 4, 2016, https://www.cdc.gov/ncbddd/adhd/data.html

brain's chemical balance and how it will affect a child's developing body and mind.[2]

ADHD is the brain's hypervigilant response to environmental stress. It is the "flight" part of the fight or flight response–the evolutionary response human beings possess for coping with stress. We medicate our children because we think it will help to relieve their pain, but in reality we are only silencing the symptoms of their pain.

There is a connection between high levels of cortisol, the stress hormone, and distractibility. Cortisol is an adaptive hormone and is produced by the HPA system when we are under stress. It activates the HPA system, or the "fight or flight" reaction. The hippocampus is the part of the brain that shuts down the cortisol response after the threat is gone. The problem is that since kids today are living in chronically stressful environments, the hippocampus does not shut off the stress response.

Consider the analogy of a lightbulb in the kitchen that you leave on overnight and that burns out the next day because it's been on too long. That's what happens to the stress-regulating part of the brain in kids when the stress response is chronic: when children are faced with intense frustration they cannot manage, or they are confronted with expectations they cannot meet. The distractibility, agitation, and difficulty sitting still that we see in children with ADHD is the flight response. Impulsivity and aggressive behavior is the fight response. These are protective responses of our bodies to a perceived threat.

---

[2] National Institute of Mental Health, "Prescribed Stimulant Use for ADHD Continues to Rise Steadily," September 18, 2011, https://www.nih.gov/news-events/news-releases/prescribed-stimulant-use-adhd-continues-rise-steadily#:~:text=The%20prescribed%20use%20of%20stimulant,Research%20and%20Quality%20(AHRQ).

Children are often identified as having ADHD starting as early as preschool, which is when many parents come to see me for guidance. The symptoms their children show include an inability to sit for long periods of time in the classroom; difficulty staying engaged in one activity for long; and the need to get up and move their bodies when they are in a social setting, often (but not always) accompanied by impulsive aggressive behavior like hitting or biting.

Why is this happening to our children? One key factor, I believe, is that because so many of us are ambitiously pursuing our own individual needs, we forget how we evolved as social creatures. Too often, mothers are putting their work and their own needs ahead of their children's. I know this issue is a very controversial one–so controversial, in fact, that few dare to address it.

Colleagues and researchers write about children and their primary caregivers and won't use the word *mother*. Clinicians are reluctant to make direct correlations publicly between an emotionally disengaged or physically absent mother and a child's personality, social functioning, and even mental illness, but it is what we discuss as clinicians amongst ourselves. A growing body of evidence from neuroscience, attachment, and epigenetic research supports the link between attachment insecurity and ADHD that we have seen in our clinical practices.

Sensitive nurturing and resilience to stress

The foundation for resilience to stress starts from ages 0 to 3, the first critical window of brain development. By the end of 3 years of age, 85% of the right brain, or the part of the brain that is responsible for emotional regulation and resilience to stress, is developed.

In the first three years of life, it is the interaction of child and mother or other primary attachment figure that establishes the child's patterns of response and trust in people and their environment, as well as his/her individual capacity to cope with environmental stress. A mother's sensitive nurturing and soothing presence in those years is a powerful influence on a child's ability to stabilize his or her emotions and the ability to cope with stressful events and feelings throughout life.

It is a mother's job to buffer her children from any moment-to-moment stress, and that buffering is internalized and helps the child to be resilient toward stress in the future. This early relationship creates the foundation for a lifetime of emotional health and stability. When a child does not get enough parental soothing and presence, he or she can lack the ability to regulate stress and strong emotions including sadness, anger, frustration, fear and excitement, leading to the symptoms we see in ADHD.

A mother's boredom with her nurturing role and/or her depression, disengagement, or absence can all lead to a disruption in a baby's development. According to Dr. Andrew Garner, co-author of the American Academy of Pediatrics' "Policy Statement and Technical Report on Toxic Stress," "Toxic stress reflects an inability to turn off the body's stress response. Toxic stress happens in the absence of resilience. Resilience is the ability to adapt to adversity in a healthy manner. The buffer for toxic stress is engaged nurturing."[3] Engaged nurturing requires a calm, reflective, and responsive mother.

Garner also noted that early adversity such as neglect, maternal depression, or lack of a secure attachment may produce a lasting and

[3] Andrew S. Garner, Jack P. Shonkoff, and the Committee on Psychosocial Aspects of Child and Family Health, Committee on Early Childhood, Adoption, and Dependent Care, Section on Developmental and Behavioral Pediatrics. "The Lifelong Effects of Early Childhood Adversity and Toxic Stress." *Pediatrics* 129, no. 1 (2012): e232-46.

chronic stress response, which alters the brain's ability to cope with stress in the future. It may also produce symptoms like ADHD. This kind of a stress response in young children can lead to less visible yet permanent changes in brain structure and function.[4]

The limbic system and stress regulation

Research has shown that a baby's developing limbic system–the part of the brain that controls the autonomic nervous system and regulates our stress response–is positively shaped by sensitive parenting and maternal presence and that early stressful experiences or social adversity can, as developmental neuroscientist Nim Tottenham explained, "increase the risk for psychopathology [mental or emotional illness]."[5]

According to research by Thomas Insel, former director of the National Institute of Mental Health, this is the result of a negative feedback loop in which stress promotes the production of a specific stress hormone, which in turn suppresses the release of oxytocin. However, the release of oxytocin in the baby's brain, which is promoted by nurturing, protects the brain from the negative effects of stressful events.[6]

The amygdala, an almond-shaped part of the limbic system that helps to regulate stress, is not meant to be activated during the first year of

---

[4] Ibid.

[5] Nim Tottenham and Margaret A. Sheridan, "A Review of Adversity, the Amygdala and the Hippocampus: A Consideration of Developmental Timing," *Frontiers in Neuroscience* 3, no. 68 (January 2010), doi:10.3389/neuro.09.068.2009.

[6] Thomas R. Insel, James T. Winslow, Zuoxin Wang, and Larry J. Young, "Oxytocin, Vasopressin, and the Neuroscience Basis of Pair Bond Formation," in *Vasopressin and Oxytocin*, ed. Hans H. Zingg, Charles W. Bourque, and Daniel G. Bichet, *Advances in Experimental Medicine and Biology* 449 (New York: Springer, 1998), link.springer.com/chapter/10.1007/978-1-4615-4871-3_28.

a child's life. But by not being physically or emotionally present for babies, we are exposing them to stress too early and activating the amygdala. Premature activation of the amygdala means that it will cease to function well in regulating stress throughout a child's life, leading to ADHD symptoms.[7, 8]

Attachment difficulties

John Bowlby, known as "the father of attachment," expressed the opinion that attachment security is the scaffolding on which we as humans determine whether we can trust our environment and the people in it. It is the key to mental health and emotional well-being long term.[9]

Mary Ainsworth, who is considered one of the matriarchs of attachment research, found there were three types of attachment: secure, insecure avoidant, and insecure ambivalent.[10] Mary Main, a prominent attachment researcher, later identified a fourth type, insecure disorganized, and also identified the attachment styles in infancy that correspond to emotional security or pathology in the future.[11]

Ainsworth created what is now known as the Strange Situation Experiment, a series of separations and reunions between mothers

---

[7] Dylan G. Gee, et al., "Early Developmental Emergence of Human Amygdala-Prefrontal Connectivity After Maternal Deprivation," *Psychological and Cognitive Sciences* 110, no. 39 (September 2013), doi: 10.1073/pnas.1307893110

[8] Elina Thomas, et al., "Newborn Amygdala Connectivity and Early Emerging Fear," *Developmental Cognitive Neuroscience* 39, (June 2019), doi: 10.1016/j.dcn.2018.12.002

[9] John Bowlby, *A Secure Base: Parent-Child Attachment and Healthy Human Development* (New York: Basic Books, 1988).

[10] Mary D. Salter Ainsworth, Mary C. Blehar, Everett Waters, and Sally N. Wall, *Patterns of Attachment: A Psychological Study of the Strange Situation* (New York: Psychology Press, 2015).

[11] Beatrice Beebe and Frank M. Lachmann, *The Origins of Attachment: Infant Research and Adult Treatment* (London: Routledge, 2014).

and one-year-old babies.[12] First, a mother and baby enter a room and the mother plays with her baby. Next, a stranger enters the room and engages the baby, and the mother leaves the room. The mother reenters the room and is reunited with the baby and the stranger exits, leaving the mother and baby alone. Then the mother leaves the room again, leaving the baby alone, and finally she returns and is reunited a second time with the baby.

This critical research highlighted the importance of secure attachment for the well-being and mental health of babies. How a child responds in the Strange Situation and how securely attached he is as twelve months old are related to his emotional health and emotional competence as an adult.

Ainsworth found that *securely attached* babies were upset when their mothers left the room but sought physical closeness, were easily comforted, and overall seemed happy to see their mother on her return. Between eight and eighteen months old, secure babies cycled between attachment and exploration: exploring the world using their body and newly found motor skills, and returning to the physical proximity of their mother, whom they used as a secure base from which to begin exploring again.

She found that babies who were *insecurely* attached to their mothers fell into one of two categories: They either had a consistent strategy to deal with their mother's attachment difficulties, as in the case of *insecure avoidant* babies or *insecure ambivalent* babies, or they had no clear strategy, as can be seen in insecure disorganized babies. Ainsworth, and later Beatrice Beebe, an attachment and infant-parent communication researcher, found that it was overall better

[12] Mary D. Salter Ainsworth, et al., *Patterns of Attachment.*

for the baby's mental health to be avoidant or ambivalent than disorganized.[13] However, each of these attachment disorders can be correlated to later specific mental health conditions.

Insecure ambivalent babies were emotionally volatile, clingy when their mother left, and hysterical when she returned. They suffered from intense separation anxiety and were unable to be easily comforted by their mother and were often angry at her. Their mothers were often anxious, and these babies absorbed their mother's fear and anxiety and rarely felt safe in the world or trusted those around them to comfort them. They clung to their mothers and rarely learned to regulate their own emotions. This led to anxiety later in development.

Babies who seemed uninterested or did not respond to their mother's departure with much emotion were classified as *insecure avoidant*. They did not seek much contact with their mothers before the separation and seemed to be able to occupy themselves with toys and objects in the room. They seemed interested in the stranger and could allow her to calm them when their mother left the room; they reacted only when they were left completely alone. These babies relied on their own resources to self-regulate rather than relying on their mother as a source of comfort. This attachment disorder is most strongly linked to depression.

Insecure avoidant babies adapt to their absent mothers by detaching emotionally and avoiding the pain of a relationship with their mother. Insecure avoidant children often lack empathy and show signs of uncontrolled aggression and anger at a young age; these children often come to the attention of parent guidance experts, therapists, and teachers when they go to preschool. They may be the bullies of

---

[13] Beatrice Beebe, et al., "On the Origins of Disorganized Attachment and Internal Working Models: Paper I. A Dyadic Systems Approach," *Psychoanalytic Dialogues* 22, no. 2 (April 2012), doi: 10.1080/10481885.2012.666147

the class or seek negative attention when they are in distress or hurt; they tend to withdraw rather than seek comfort from their mother. They may express their distress and anxiety physically, which is why many are labeled as having behavioral problems or ADHD.

Insecure disorganized babies alternated between different methods of coping: one moment ignoring their mother and pushing her away, the next moment clinging desperately. They were often very angry at the mother and unable to be comforted easily. Though their first impulse may be to seek comfort, when these babies are close to their mother, they feel frightened of precisely the person who should be comforting them with their fears. In the Strange Situation conditions, these babies may run up to their mother when she returns to the room, then pull away and curl up into a ball. Or they may become very aggressive and hit or throw things at the parent. They may alternate between crying and laughing. Disorganized attachment disorder is most strongly linked to Borderline Personality Disorder later in life.

Attachment security is passed down generationally from mother to child. In all of these cases of attachment disorders, the mother is absent in one way or another. Psychoanalyst and clinical psychologist Peter Fonagy proposed that the defensive strategy most available to the child is the one that their attachment figure–most often their mother–habitually uses in response to distress, which they then make their own.[14]

Anxiety: Attentional difficulties

We are not born with the ability to sustain our focus; babies learn how to focus and increase their attention span from interacting with

[14] Peter Fonagy and Mary Target, "Attachment and Reflective Function: Their Role in Self-Organization," *Development and Psychopathology* 9 (1997): 679-700.

their mothers. This requires a mother to be interested in her child and what he or she is doing and to be able to focus her own attention on her baby without being constantly distracted. Mothers showing an active interest in their child, both verbally and nonverbally, are all simple forms of right brain to right brain interaction that have a profound effect on a child's development.

Of course, it's not possible to play with a baby every minute. When an alert baby doesn't have his mother's attention, he will turn to objects or his own hand or foot to occupy him. Girls are better at waiting for their mothers' attention than boys. Boys are more neurologically fragile, sensitive and will often become fractious or cry when their mothers are occupied. Boys' brains are also more susceptible to the effects of cortisol and anxiety, and a boy who is left to deal with his own distress or discomfort, unable to soothe himself, is more likely to be diagnosed with ADHD than a girl. According to Child Mind Institute, there are twice as many boys (12.1 percent) as girls (5.5 percent) diagnosed with ADHD.[15]

Anxiety: Increased aggression and behavioral problems

Children used to start preschool at four and daycare with large ratios of children to caregivers did not exist in great numbers. Until then, children stayed with their mother, who acted as their constant emotional regulator, especially for fear and aggression.

Today many preschool programs take children as young as eighteen months and daycare is rampant taking children as young as 6 weeks of age. That's a big difference in terms of emotional and physical development, as well as his impulse control. Changes in

[15] Child Mind Institute, "Children's Mental Health Report." https://childmind.org/awareness-campaigns/childrens-mental-health-report/

routine and environment, even small changes, can also trigger what we call regressive behavior–a child who's been successfully toilet trained begins to wet his pants, or one who has been relatively even-tempered hits or bites a classmate.

It's unrealistic to expect a two-and-a-half-year-old–especially a boy–to be able to sit quietly or contain his boundless physical energy in circle time. What some people see as misbehavior, "acting out," or symptoms of ADHD, I see as a normal reaction to being separated prematurely from a mother's safe and soothing presence before a child is developmentally ready.

Building attachment during the first three years

In other parts of the world, parents sleep with their newborn babies. Mothers breastfeed and do not separate from their infants or return to work prematurely and if they do, they take their babies with them. These cultural differences from what we have in the U.S. give babies the safety during their first year to build a foundation for emotional security. The early presence of the mother provides the stress buffering and emotional regulation which is the foundation of mental health. This sense of security over time allows the child to internalize that even if their mother is not immediately present, they can experience the same feelings of safety and soothing that they have when their mother is present.[16]

Overdiagnosis of ADHD

ADHD is too frequently misdiagnosed in the United States. Other countries, like France, consider ADHD as a psychosocial disorder

---

[16] Nim Tottenham. "Social Scaffolding of Human Amygdala-mPFCcircuit Development," *Social Neuroscience* 10, no. 5 (2015): 489-499.

and treat the condition by focusing on the underlying cause with psychotherapy and family counseling, an approach with which I strongly agree. This approach takes time and effort on the part of the parents. Far too often, pediatricians, teachers, and parents are too quick to medicate away the symptoms rather than deal with the underlying emotional issues.

Some children may need medication if their symptoms are extreme but only as a bridge until a child therapist who is psychodynamically oriented can pinpoint the underlying emotional stressors causing the symptoms. Medication is not a long-term or permanent solution. Many children and adolescents are quickly medicated to silence their emotional pain and to alleviate their symptoms because it's easier for the adults in their lives.

There are cases where medication can be useful in conjunction with psychotherapy for a limited time, particularly if the symptoms are intense or disruptive.[17] I see talk therapy as a long-term sustainable form of treatment with no unwanted physical side effects; temporary medication can give kids the ability to slow down and absorb the lessons of therapy. I do not believe that medication should ever be used as the sole treatment for these disorders.

What parents can do

It is important to seek help for children and adolescents as soon they begin showing ADHD symptoms. When children first show signs of stress, there is a window of opportunity to help them. Many parents who suspect their child has ADHD will first take them to a

---

[17] Mayo Clinic, "Attention-Deficit/Hyperactivity Disorder (ADHD) in Children." https://www.mayoclinic.org/diseases-conditions/adhd/symptoms-causes/syc-20350889

psychiatrist. What parents need to know is that many psychiatrists are trained to treat mental health issues with medication alone. The first stop for parents when they see symptoms in their child should be an adolescent or child talk psychotherapist or play psychotherapist. If children and adolescents do not receive help quickly enough, they develop defenses and their symptoms may submerge only to come back later with a vengeance. In addition, kids can become entrenched in behaviors that are even harder to treat.

Parents are in a rush for their children to become independent and grow up. However, as a society we need to remember how fragile and sensitive they are to stress and to losses and adversity of any kind no matter how nuanced. Social emotional development and forming healthy attachment at a young age builds the foundation for mentally healthy and resilient children. Being there as much as possible for the first three years of a child's life is critical to the foundation of their mental and emotional health so that they can build strong and healthy attachment.

For older children, parental presence is also important. If we replace judgment of children's limited ability to tolerate frustration, disconnection, and social isolation with understanding, empathy, and adaptation to their needs, then we can prevent these acute stress responses from becoming chronic mental illness. It is not a foregone conclusion that temporary symptoms of acute stress will lead to developing ADHD, but if parents misunderstand and mishandle or ignore the signs, as a result symptoms may become chronic and harder to treat.

As I have emphasized, medication should be a last resort for children and adolescents, not a first step, except in extreme crises. And even then, it should be a bridge to understanding our children, not the solution. Exercising sensitivity and empathy toward children, while trying to understand their limitations, can prevent distress and foster emotional and mental health in a country where ADHD diagnoses continue to increase.[18] If we can work to understand and alleviate children's underlying pain from loss, trauma, family/relational issues and attachment disorders rather than masking it with medication, we can build emotionally resilient and mentally healthy children who are heard, seen and understood rather than labeled and silenced.

[18] Centers for Disease Control and Prevention. "ADHD Throughout the Years," September 23, 2021, https://www.cdc.gov/ncbddd/adhd/timeline.html

ADHD: A bioecological assessment

Jeanne Stolzer

This chapter was penned a while ago, but it is more prophetic than dated. The epidemic of ADHD labeling has continued unabated and only increased over time, both in the United States and worldwide. The misguided, unscientific, and profit-motive-driven "diagnosing" of the so-called "mental disorder" of ADHD, while under scrutiny in some quarters (including in this volume and in this series), still reigns supreme. I hope that the following strikes you as a more accurate way to understand how the behaviors of childhood can be viewed than the one provided by the pseudo-medical model view.

The mass labeling and drugging of American children has reached epidemic proportions. Currently, Americans are immersed in a linear medical model which promotes the widespread use of psychotropic medications in child populations in order to control undesirable behaviors.

While no one has any idea of the long-term results of this giant proxy experiment, many academicians, researchers, and medical professionals are actively questioning the reliability and validity of this reductionistic and deterministic model. This chapter will explore

---

Dr. Jeanne Stolzer is professor of Family Science at the University of Nebraska-Kearney.

This chapter is an updated, adapted version of the article Stolzer, J. (2005) ADHD in America: A bioecological analysis. Ethical Human Psychology and Psychiatry, 7, 65-75.

the ADHD phenomenon using Urie Bronfenbrenner's bioecological theory.

Familial, political, economic, biological, medical, contextual, cultural, and historical system alterations will be explored in depth in order to gain new insights into the myth of ADHD. Particular attention will be given to the interactive nature of the various systems proposed by Bronfenbrenner, and integral linkages will be discussed. The goal of this chapter is to offer a theoretically sound alternative to the current medical model and to challenge the existing ADHD paradigm that pathologizes normal-range child behaviors.

Bronfenbrenner (1999) theorized that development is shaped by various interacting systems, which include the microsystem, the mesosystem, the exosystem, and the macrosystem. The core theoretical premise of the bioecological model is that human development is a function of the forces from all of the various systems, and the relationships that exist between the systems.

Bronfenbrenner (1989) has postulated that the various systems are bi-directional in nature as they are continually influencing us, and we in tum are continually influencing them. According to the corollaries contained within Bronfenbrenner's theory, the systems are intrinsically intertwined; alterations occurring on one level have the potential to affect the entire system (1989). Employing Bronfenbrenner's theory, the following sections will address the linkages that exist between the bioecological corollaries and the epidemic of attention deficit hyperactivity disorder (ADHD) in America.

The microsystem

The microsystem is defined as "a pattern of activities, roles, and interpersonal relations experienced by the developing person in a given face-to-face setting with particular physical and material features" (Bronfenbrenner, 1989, p. 67).

The microsystem is characterized by direct, intimate, interactional processes as familial relationships and close friendships are the cornerstone of this system. Bronfenbrenner has hypothesized that significant others continually influence individual development by altering and/or maintaining particular environments that either encourage optimal developmental processes, or suppress the probability of optimal developmental trajectories (1999).

Over the course of the last century, Americans have dramatically altered their parenting practices. For 99.9% of our time on earth, humans have practiced what I shall refer to in this chapter as "attachment parenting" (Dettwyler, 1995). Attachment parenting is characterized by long-term breast-feeding, child-led weaning, co-sleeping, and staying in close physical proximity to one's offspring throughout early childhood (Stuart-Macadam & Dettwyler, 1995).

Humans, along with other warm-blooded vertebrates, have been categorized as mammals because they sustain their young with milk secreted from their breasts (Ben Shaul, 1962). Humans, while typed as mammals according to specific and measurable biologic characteristics, are also social creatures who construct and maintain particular cultural customs (Stuart-Macadam & Dettwyler, 1995). For millions of years, breast-feeding human young was considered a fundamental component of the maternal experience; conception, pregnancy, birth, and lactation were perceived as intrinsically intertwined. Until the early 1900s, the collective human culture dictated that breast-feeding was an integral and natural component of the birthing process (Dettwyler, 1995).

In 1900, 98% of all children in the United States of America were breast-fed; weaning at the tum of the century in America occurred between 2 and 4 years of age (Stuart Macadam & Dettwyler, 1995). Currently, less than half of American infants are fed human milk, and more than 80% of these children are weaned by 6 months of age (U.S. Department of Health and Human Services, 2000). These statistics clearly indicate that a significant biocultural shift has occurred within the perimeters of the microsystem over the last 100 years.

Researchers have analyzed weaning rates in traditional hunter-gatherer societies and have concluded that the majority of children currently living in these societies are weaned between 2 and 5 years of age (Dettwyler, 1995; Wickes, 1953). Prevailing ideologies in the West dictate that long-term nursing is pathological, yet when analyzing worldwide weaning rates (where the norm is 2.9 years), it appears that it is the West that is atypical in comparison to the majority of the earth's inhabitants (Wray, 1990).

It is a possibility that biological changes within the microsystem have led to alterations in the mother-child relationship. Strictly controlled studies have concluded that lactating females differ significantly from their non-lactating cohorts. Lactating females present an altered physiological state as lactation stimulates the pituitary gland to activate the secretion of oxytocin and prolactin (Lawrence, 1994). These specific hormones are elevated in lactating women, and prolonged elevation of these hormones is due to the frequency, intensity, and duration with which a child nurses (Jelliffe & Jelliffe, 1986; Lawrence, 1994).

Researchers have documented that elevated oxytocin levels are highly correlated with maternal nurturance (Stuart-Macadam & Dettwyler, 1995); the desire to stay in close physical proximity to one's offspring (Insel & Shapiro, 1992); and a significant decrease in maternal anxiety levels (Uvnas-Moberg, Widstrom, Nissen, & Bjorvell, 1990). Research has also indicated that elevated oxytocin levels are associated with an overall sense of maternal well-being and feelings of calmness and serenity (McCarthy, Kow, & Pfaff, 1992). Although it cannot be assumed that maternal behavior is entirely hormonally regulated, there are indications that hormones such as oxytocin do have the potential to affect the mother-child relationship, thus affecting the long-term developmental trajectory of the individual child (Silber, Larsson, & Uvnas-Moberg, 1991).

Research indicates that oxytocin and prolactin alter not only maternal behaviors, but perhaps more importantly, these hormones have been found to alter maternal perceptions (Dettwyler, 1995; McCarthy et al., 1992). It has been hypothesized that lactation facilitates the ancient mother-child "dance"; an evolutionary partnership that has been perfected over millions of years to ensure optimal physiological and psychological interdependence (Stuart-Macadam & Dettwyler, 1995). It is a possibility that when disruptions in the "dance" occur, psychological, biological, cognitive, and social processes may be altered for both mother and child, thus opening the door for the unprecedented parental acceptance of the myth of ADHD in America.

Seminal research indicates that breast-feeding decreases the incidence of problematic child behaviors. Maslow's 1946 study concluded that breast-fed children, when compared to their artificially-fed cohorts, displayed significantly fewer behavioral problems (Maslow & Szilagy-Kessler, 1946). Holloway (1949) demonstrated that children who were breast-fed were significantly more likely to display pro-social behaviors and to engage in self-regulation. From an evolutionary standpoint, it would appear that breastfeeding ensures optimal developmental trajectories in child populations, and may also positively influence maternal perceptions and behaviors (Stuart-Macadam & Dettwyler, 1995). However, in order to fully understand what role breast-feeding plays in the prevention of childhood behavioral disorders, more research is needed in order to establish the magnitude and direction of this hypothesized relationship.

Breast-feeding is not the only ancient mammalian practice that has been altered by modem-day Americans. Palmer (1991) has stated, "The practice of co-sleeping has been the norm since the dawn of human civilization" (p. 107) and that this ancient practice continued unabated until the 1900s. Quandt (1985) has asserted that along with the advent of unisleeping practices came the manufacturing of products that were intended to keep mother and child separated (i.e., playpens, strollers, cribs, bottles, formula, pacifiers, etc.). McKenna and his colleagues (1993) demonstrated that traditional child-rearing practices (which include keeping the child in close physical proximity during the day and night) encourages optimal dyadic cue reading and lead to a distinct type of mother and child synchronicity, a synchronicity that has been perfected over 5-7 million years of hominid evolution.

In American culture, co-sleeping is viewed as atypical. However, co-sleeping can be seen across cultures, across historical time, and across mammalian species. Currently, 80% of the world co-sleeps (Fogel, 2001), yet the majority of Americans eschew this ancient mammalian practice (Palmer, 1991). Americans have become quite adept at keeping parent and child separated (particularly during the nighttime hours). We give pacifiers, blankets, bears with human heartbeats—things intended to suffice in lieu of parental comfort. We teach our children very early on to depend on these things to comfort them. From an evolutionary standpoint, the ancient practice of co-sleeping increased the child's rate of survival and ensured optimal parent-child attachment (Dettwyler, 1995). Data confirm that until approximately 100 years ago, parent-child co-sleeping was practiced throughout the world (Lancaster & Lancaster, 1982).

Dettwyler (1995) has postulated that the ascent of the formula industry in tandem with the American practice of unisleeping illustrates specific cultural practices which infringe upon our mammalian heritage, a heritage that was framed by natural selection over millions of years to ensure the optimal development of women and children. It has been hypothesized that disruptions within the microsystem (i.e., attachment disruption) can lead to a myriad of problems in the mother-child dyad (Bowlby, 1988). Furthermore, disruptions occurring within the microsystem have the potential to negatively impact broad-based systemic functioning, thus altering the course of humankind (Bronfenbrenner, 1989, 1999).

At the present time, we have no way of knowing how alterations in ancient mammalian parenting practices impact ADHD traits. What is certain is that those who have a vested interest in promoting the myth of ADHD have completely ignored the enormous complexities surrounding this issue, and have refused to take into account evolutionary processes. Instead of employing a bioecological model when analyzing ADHD traits, we have chosen instead a reductionistic and deterministic model that promotes the mass labeling and drugging of children. The medical model promotes the theory of the "neuro logically disordered brain," and in doing so, neglects to take into account other possible explanations for ADHD-typed behaviors.

Perhaps relationship changes occurring within the microsystem have made parents more willing to accept the myth of ADHD. When ancient maternal behaviors are modified, it is a distinct possibility that psychological, biological, cognitive, and social processes may be altered in both the parent and the child. Couple these evolutionary alterations with the rise of the pharmaceutical industry and the widespread acceptance of mainstream psychiatry, and it is no surprise that the myth of ADHD has been unconditionally accepted by the masses.

The mesosystem

The mesosystem is defined as the "linkages and processes taking place between two or more settings containing the developing person" (Bronfenbrenner, 1989, p. 227). The mesosystem includes daycare settings, the educational system, and the workforce. Children are affected in various ways by the functioning of the mesosystem, and alterations within this system may in fact be correlated with the increasing rates of ADHD in America.

Perhaps because we are moving away from our mammalian heritage (i.e., ancient attachment parenting practices), we have come to believe that parents are dispensable. Americans have recently constructed an ideology that assumes that children can be away from their parents during the vast majority of their formative years and attachment processes will proceed unaltered. Seventy-five percent of all children under 12 months of age are currently in full-time non-parental care in the US (Fogel, 2001).

Daycare workers in this country have the highest turnover rates of any profession. They are paid extremely low salaries, receive little if any benefits, and report high levels of stress (Fogel). Currently, there are no federal regulations regarding training or education for daycare workers, nor are there uniform laws regarding teacher-child ratios (Fogel). The fact of the matter is we are involved in one giant proxy experiment; never in the history of humankind have we relegated our parental responsibilities to uninvested, unrelated strangers.

Do we really assume there will be no consequences associated with this experiment? Ethologists have known for decades that if you try this "daycare experiment" with any other mammal, catastrophic disruptions in the attachment process will result. Yet, we, the most advanced nation on earth, have convinced ourselves that we are different from other mammals. We have conned ourselves into accepting the myth of "quality time" and in doing so, have successfully assuaged our collective parental guilt.

There is a common misconception that the "era of the working mother" has made attachment parenting impossible. However, historical data indicates that women have worked for thousands of years while practicing attachment parenting (Stuart-Macadam & Dettwyler, 1995). It is the modern era that has decreed that parenting and working cannot occur simultaneously. "Working" is not inherently incompatible with parenting; it is our particular culture that has drawn this line. The dichotomy that prevails in the West between the public and private spheres is essential to this debate.

Parenting has been defined in the West as a private-sphere practice, while working is defined as a public activity (Carballo & Pelto, 1991; Stuart-Macadam & Dettwyler, 1995). According to this dichotomous worldview, attachment parenting is forbidden within the boundaries of the public sphere, thus perpetuating our cultural acceptance of paying someone other than a parent to care for our children.

Baumslag and Michels (1995) have asserted that specific, national policies would help to promote attachment parenting in America. They propose a federally mandated maternal health policy which includes guaranteed job reinstatement; flexible work schedules; flextime; part-time work; job sharing; option to work from home; and guaranteed parental leave options. The fact is, we value the worker above the parent. Currently in America, a woman's worth is based on her economic earning power and not on her competence and commitment in the maternal arena. Until we can collectively face these facts, any proposed change in policy that would benefit our children seems remote at best. It is more likely that we will continue to label our children with mythical diseases such as ADHD rather than address those policies and ideologies which perpetuate the mass labeling and drugging of American children.

Van Esterik (1994) has acknowledged that scholars who advocate for children may be accused of subscribing to an "anti-woman sentiment." Van Esterik has called for a paradigm shift that would honor women for their contributions to the public sphere and for their provision of optimal care for their children. The dichotomy of the public and private spheres may prohibit women from excelling in the workplace, and it clearly diminishes a woman's inimitable, biosocial capacity as a unique and irreplaceable force in the life of her child (Stuart-Macadam & Dettwyler, 1995; Van Esterik, 1994).

Compulsory schooling is yet another example of how mesosystemic processes have been altered over the last 100 years. Recess is no longer deemed a necessary part of the curriculum and cuts in physical education have become widespread. Research has confirmed that children who are given the opportunity to engage in large motor outdoor activities during the course of the school day exhibit significantly fewer behavioral problems (Pellegrini, 1988). In spite of this fact, teachers across this country continue to use "staying in for recess" as punishment for inappropriate behavior, a practice which may in fact increase the probability of behavioral problems at school.

American classrooms are overcrowded, and teacher-child ratio is an ongoing problem. Furthermore, teachers are now assuming the role of psychologist, psychiatrist, and/or neurologist. Let us not forget that teachers are not trained as psychologists, psychiatrists, or neurologists. Teachers have a teaching certificate as they are trained in curriculum and instruction, not in diagnosing "neo neurological" disorders (Cohen, 2004). The majority of teachers' colleges in the US do not require teachers to take classes in development. How is it that teachers can accurately implement an appropriate curriculum when they have no training in child development? How is a teacher to identify normal-range, age-appropriate behaviors when the teacher has little if any training in this area? Furthermore, teachers have swallowed the myth that disruptive behavior indicates some type of brain abnormality, yet research clearly indicates that "ADHD traits" have been highly adaptive throughout human history (Jensen et al., 1997).

It appears that the study of child development has gone by the wayside when it comes to defining atypical behavior in the classroom. Children by their very nature are inattentive, spontaneous, active, and messy (Breggin, 1995). These attributes do not indicate an underlying neurological pathology; they are instead innate behaviors that have been documented across cultures, across historical time, and across mammalian species.

There is clearly an economic incentive to label children with a myriad of mythical diseases in this country. Children who have been diagnosed with ADHD (as well as other "brain disorders") are covered under the Americans with Disabilities Act (ADA), and as such, schools receive federal monies in order to accommodate such students (Cohen, 2004). ADHD rates in child populations vary considerably from school to school; private schools that do not benefit economically from labeling students tend to have much lower rates of ADHD in their populations (Cohen, 1994). In this current climate where children are forced to sell magazine subscriptions in order to supplement their school budget, it is not surprising that ADHD rates in public schools across this country are skyrocketing. Somehow, the schools must meet their budgetary expenses, but it cannot, and must not, be at the expense of our children.

Daycare, the dichotomy of the public and private spheres, and compulsory schooling were covered under mesosystemic functioning.

We have, in the course of one generation, altered attachment processes, the mother-child relationship, and perceptions regarding normal-range child behaviors within the educational system. All of these alterations can be seminally linked with the advent of ADHD in America. Now, let us focus our attention on the exosystem.

The exosystem

The exosystem is defined as "the linkages and processes taking place between two or more settings, at least one of which does not ordinarily contain the developing person, but in which events occur that influence processes within the immediate setting that does contain that person" (Bronfenbrenner, 1989, p. 227).

A review of the literature indicates that the pharmaceutical industry has a vested economic interest in promoting the myth of ADHD. Parenting magazines, television, and doctors' offices routinely advertise psychotropic drugs for use in child populations. This unprecedented flood of advertising has strengthened our collective acceptance of the myth of ADHD in America. The pharmaceutical industry openly promotes the "disease model" and it is clear that this promotion is motivated by economic gain (Jureidini & Mansfield, 2001). The pharmaceutical industry has helped much in assuaging parental guilt as claims from the industry assure the American parent that the cause of their child's behavior is "brain related" and has nothing whatsoever to do with parenting, institutionalized schooling, national policies, or cultural ideologies. The pharmaceutical industry also promotes the belief that "brain disorders" (i.e., ADHD) in children require the use of psychotropic medications in order to control undesirable child behaviors (Breggin, 2001).

Perhaps most disturbing is the economic alliance that exists between the pharmaceutical industry and the medical community.

The pharmaceutical industry methodically promotes ADHD as a neurological disorder; routinely funds major medical conferences; dominates research funding in the area of ADHD; provides financial incentives for physicians who prescribe specific drugs; and funds groups such as Children and Adults with Attention-Deficit Hyperactivity Disorder [CHADD] who openly promote psychotropic medications in child populations (Breggin, 2001; Jureidini & Mansfield, 2001). Do we really believe that the biochemistry of the human brain is responsible for the epidemic of ADHD in America? How is it possible that in the course of one generation, child brains have been altered to such an extent that they cannot function properly unless they are mutated with psychotropic medications (Levine, 2004)? This is the myth that the medical community and the pharmaceutical industry have perpetuated in America and we have been willing to accept this myth without question (Breggin, 2001).

In the 1950s, ADHD did not exist. In 1970, 2000 American children were diagnosed as "hyperactive." By 2003, 6 million American children had been diagnosed with a "brain disorder" called ADHD and the vast majority of these children have been prescribed dangerous and addictive psychotropic medications in order to control their disruptive behavior (Levine, 2004). Why is this "brain disorder" not found in other cultures? Why is this "brain disorder" not found in other species? Why is this "brain disorder" not documented across history? The answer to these questions is because this "brain disorder" does not exist (Baughman, 2004).

Forces emanating from within the exosystem that have a vested economic interest in promoting the myth of ADHD include the United States Government, the medical community, and the pharmaceutical industry. The economic alliance that exists between the medical community, the pharmaceutical industry, and the government will continue to thrive if left unchecked. As Americans, we must demand that this economic alliance be severed, and that authentic research (i.e., research that is not funded by the pharmaceutical industry) is used as the "gold standard" when implementing national policies that affect American children and their families.

The macrosystem

The macrosystem consists of overarching patterns that can be found in a given culture. These patterns include ideologies, activities, world views, and belief systems which are hypothesized by Bronfenbrenner (1989) to be the societal blueprint for a particular culture.

Macrosystemic functioning has been greatly altered over the last generation. Our collective perceptions of childhood have changed, and what were once regarded as normal-range child behaviors are now defined as "disorders of the brain." Do millions of American children actually suffer from unprecedented brain disorders? What could have altered the developing brains of our children to such an extent that millions of American children are diagnosed with "disorders of the brain" when only a generation ago this epidemic was unheard of?

ADHD traits may in fact be the result of millions of years of adaptation. It would stand to reason that the most active of the species would be the genetic line that survived throughout the course of evolutionary time (Jensen et al., 1997). ADHD traits may also be linked to disruptions in the attachment process, which may lead to parental acceptance of the theory of the "neurologically disordered brain." What is certain is that children's brains have not been altered neurologically in the course of one generation (Baughman, 2004). Breggin (2004) has stated that perhaps we prefer the chemically-altered brain over the non-chemically-altered brain as normal-range child behaviors do not fit in with the frenzied world we have created for ourselves and for our children. While physicians, pharmaceutical companies, parents, and school personnel insist that children who display ADHD traits are neurologically abnormal, no scientific evidence exists to support this supposition (Baughman; Breggin, 2002; Cohen, 2004).

Childhood itself has been greatly altered. It is common in 21st century America for children to sit for hours at a computer, TV, or video game. They are continually immersed in artificial light, and surrounded by four walls with no exposure to the earth or to the sun-elements which they have been immersed in for millions of years (Wilson, 1993). Our children are largely sedentary as the "roaming" of the past has been replaced with strict and unalterable schedules. Children are inundated with unhealthy diets as parents are under intense pressure to climb the corporate ladder. Preservatives, dyes, antibiotics, and hormones are ingested on a daily basis with no end in sight. These are significant biocultural changes and these changes must be addressed if we are to legitimately challenge the myth of ADHD.

Our collective perception of "boyhood" has also been altered dramatically. Males across species, across cultures, and across historical time have displayed ADHD traits (Breggin, 2001; DeGrandpre, 1999). The behavior of boys has remained constant, but our collective perceptions of these unique and ancient male attributes have been recalibrated in order to accommodate the medical model of development. How have we successfully convinced academicians, physicians, teachers, and parents across this country that what was once considered typical, normal, and desirable boy behavior is now the result of an atypical brain?

Employing an evolutionary perspective, males were designed to be extremely active, combative, physical, and protective in order to ensure the survival of their species (Breggin, 1995). While some theoreticians may argue that environment is the sole cause of ADHD traits, the fact remains that male-typed behaviors have been documented for thousands of years, across diverse geographical locations, and across mammalian species. We have lost the wisdom of our ancestors who knew unequivocally that boys and girls were very, very different. We cannot now, nor have we ever been able to, dictate that males will follow female developmental trajectories.

It appears that we are left with two choices; either we can reassume our historical theoretical stance which supports the notion that developing males and females follow divergent developmental pathways, or we can continue to insist that young males develop according to the criterion set forth by their female cohorts. Since it seems highly unlikely that we will ever successfully force young males to develop according to traditional female norms, we can expect to see more and more of our male children diagnosed as "brain disordered," when in actuality, they are following typical, historically documented male developmental patterns.

Bowlby (1988) hypothesized that culture was so potent a force that it could actually override biological predispositions. For millions of years, males have been perfecting the art of "maleness," and this "maleness" was considered to be extremely valuable to the functioning of society. What are we to do now that these ancient and unique male traits are currently defined as pathological? The answer is that we construct a mythical brain disorder and use psychotropic medications to alter the structure of the male brain so that males will behave according to our newly acquired cultural scripts.

Conclusion

Bronfenbrenner (1989) postulated that an alteration within one system had the potential to affect every level of systemic functioning.

For the first time in recorded history, modern-day Americans have successfully altered every one of the above-described various systems. Parenting, lifestyle, schooling, medicine, policy, and cultural ideologies have all been profoundly altered in a relatively short time. These historical alterations unquestionably affect child development, yet we continue to label individual children as "disordered" when the fact is that it is the system alterations that are negatively affecting our nation's children.

By applying simplistic "band-aid" solutions such as labeling children with mythical neurological disorders, we do not have to work to change those familial, societal, political, and cultural forces which are at the root of the myth of ADHD in America. It is much easier to buy into the myth of ADHD. By accepting this scientifically illegitimate disease, we as American adults can continue to live exactly as we are living, deluding ourselves into believing that the problem lies within the individual child. The time has come for us to take a collective stand and to demand change on every level. Our children are counting on us.

References

Baughman, F. (2004). Understanding attention deficit hyperactivity disorder (ADHD): An early diagnosis is a key factor for treatment. Retrieved October 29, 2004, from www.adhdfraud.com.

Baumslag, N., & Michels, D. L. (1995). Milk, money and madness: The culture and politics of breast feeding. London: Bergin and Garvey.

Ben Shaul, D. M. (1962) The composition of the milk of wild animals. *Zoological Yearbook*, 4, 333- 342.

Bowlby, J. (1988). *A secure base: Parent-child attachment and healthy human development*. New York: Basic Books.

Breggin, P. (1995). Are behavior-modifying drugs over-prescribed for America's school children. *Insight on the News*, 11(31), 18.

Breggin, P. (2001). *Talking back to ritalin: What doctors aren't telling you about stimulants for children.* (Rev. ed.). Cambridge, MA: Perseus Publishing.

Breggin, P. (2002). *The ritalin fact book.* Cambridge, MA: Perseus Publishing.

Breggin, P. (2004). *ICSPP Conference.* New York: American Psychological Association.

Bronfenbrenner, U. (1999). Environments in developmental perspective: Theoretical and operational models. In S. Friedman & T. Wachs (Eds.), *Measuring environment across the lifespan* (pp. 3-28). Washington, DC: American Psychological Association.

Bronfenbrenner, U. (1989). Ecological systems theory. *Annals of Child Development*, 6, 187-249.

Carballo, M., & Pelto, G. H. (1991). Social and psychological factors in breastfeeding. In F. Falkher (Ed.), *Infant and child nutrition worldwide.* Boca Raton, FL: CRC Press.

Cohen, D. (2004). *Contesting ADHD: Dissenting views on psychiatric diagnosis and treatment of children.* Paper presented at the University of Nebraska-Kearney, Kearney, NE.

DeGrandpre, R. (1999). *Ritalin nation.* New York: Norton.

Dettwyler, K. (1995). The cultural context of breastfeeding in the United States. In P. Stuart Macadam & K. Dettwyler (Eds.), *Breastfeeding: Biocultural perspectives.* New York: Aldine De Gruyter.

Fogel, A. (2001). *Infancy: Infant, family and society.* Belmont, CA: Wadsworth Publishing.

Holloway, A. R. (1949). Early self-regulation of infants and later behavior in play interviews. *American Journal of Orthopsychiatry*, 19, 612-613.

Insel, T., & Shapiro, S. (1992). Oxytocin receptors and maternal behavior. *Annals of the New York Academy of Sciences*, 652, 122-140.

Jelliffe, D. B., & Jelliffe, E. F. P. (1986). The uniqueness of human milk updated: Ranges of evidence and emphases in interpretation. *Advances in International Maternal and Child Health*, 6, 129-147.

Jelliffe, D. B., & Jelliffe, E. F. P. (1978). *Human milk in the modem world*. Oxford, England: Oxford University Press.

Jensen, P. S., Mrazek, D., Knapp, P. K., Steinberg, L., Pfeffer, C., Schowalter, J., et al. (1997). Evolution and revolution in child psychiatry: ADHD as a disorder of adaptation. *Journal of the American Academy of Child and Adolescent Psychiatry*, 36(12), 1572-1679.

Jureidini, J., & Mansfield (2001). Does drug promotion adversely influence doctors' abilities to make the best decisions for patients. *Australasian Psychiatry*, 9, 95-100.

Lancaster, J. B., & Lancaster, C. S. (1982). Parental investment: The hominid adaptation. In D. Ortner (Ed.), *How humans adapt; A biocultural odyssey* (pp. 35-50). Washington, DC: Smithsonian Institution Press.

Lawrence, R. A. (1994). *Breastfeeding: A guide for the medical profession* (4th ed.). St. Louis, MO: C.V. Mosby.

Levine, B. (2004). *Mental illness or rebellion: How biopsychiatry diverts us from examining a society toxic to well-being*. Paper presentation; ICSPP Conference, New York, New York.

Maslow, A., & Szilagy-Kessler, I. (1946) Security and breastfeeding. *Journal of Abnormal and Social Psychology*, 41, 83-85.

McCarthy, M., Kow, L., & Pfaff, D. W. (1992). Speculations concerning the physiological significance of central oxytocin in maternal behavior. In C. A. Pederson, J. Caldwell, G. Jirikowski, and T. R. Insel (Eds.), *Oxytocin in maternal, sexual, and social behaviors: Annals of the New York Academy of Sciences, Vol. 65* (pp. 70-80). New York: The New York Academy of Sciences.

McKenna, J. J., Thomas, E. B., Anders, T. F., Sadeh, A., & Schechtman, V. L. (1993) Infant-parent co-sleeping in evolutionary perspective: Imperatives for understanding sleep development and SIDS. *Sleep*, 16(3), 263-282.

Palmer, G. (1991). *The politics of breastfeeding*. London: Harper Collins.

Pellegrini, A. D. (1988). Elementary school children's rough-and-tumble play. *Early Childhood Re search Quarterly*, 4, 245-260.

Quandt, S. A. (1985). Biological and behavioral predictors of exclusive breastfeeding duration. *Medical Anthropology*, 9, 139-150.

Sharav, V. (2004, October). *Screening for mental illness: The merger of eugenics and the drug industry*. Paper presented at the ICSPP Conference, New York, NY.

Silber, M., Larsson, B., & Uvnas-Moberg, K. (1991). Oxytocin, somatostatin, insulin, and gastrin concentrations vis-a-vis late pregnancy, breastfeeding, and oral contraceptives. *Acta Obstetricia et Gynecologica Scandinavica*, 70, 283-289.

Stuart-Macadam, P., & Dettwyler, K. (1995) Breastfeeding: *Biocultural perspectives*. New York: Aldine DeGruyter.

U.S. Department of Health and Human Services. (2000). *Blueprint for action on breastfeeding*. Washington, DC: Author.

Uvnas-Moberg, K., Widstrom, A., Nissen, E., & Bjorvell, H. (1990). Personality traits in women 4 days postpartum and their correlation with plasma levels of oxytocin and prolactin. *Journal of Psychosomatic Obstetrics and Gynecology*, 11, 261-273.

Van Esterik, P. (1994). Breastfeeding in feminism. *International Journal of Gynecology and Obstetrics*, 47(Suppl.), 41-54.

Wickes, I. G. (1953). A history of infant feeding. *Archives of Diseases in Childhood*, 128, 151. Wilson, E. 0. (1993). Biophilia and the conservation ethic. In S. R. Kellert & E. 0. Wilson (Eds.),

The biophilia hypothesis. Washington, DC: Island Press/Shearwater.

Wray, J. D. (1990). Breastfeeding: An international and historical review. In F. Falkher (Ed.), *Infant and child nutrition worldwide: Issues and perspectives* (pp. 61-99). Boca Raton, FL: CRC Press.

Medicating Preschoolers: How "Evidence-Based" Psychiatry has Led to a Tragic End

Robert Whitaker

In its May 25, 2021 issue, JAMA published a report on the comparative efficacy of two medications for treating preschoolers diagnosed with ADHD.[1] Both methylphenidate and guanfacine were deemed to be beneficial, and in an accompanying editorial, JAMA told of how this retrospective review of patient charts added to the evidence base for this practice.[2]

The editorial's first paragraph, which was written by Tanya Froehlich, a professor at the University of Cincinnati College of Medicine, set forth a medical context for the study:

"Recognition of attention-deficit/hyperactivity disorder (ADHD) in the preschool age group is on the rise, with an increase in preschool ADHD rates in US nationally representative samples from 1.0% in 2007 to 2008 to 2.4% in 2016. Having a preschool-age child (i.e., 3-5 years) with ADHD is associated with numerous negative

---

Robert Whitaker is an author, former journalist, and founder of the madinamerica.com website.

First published on madinamerica.com.

[1] E. Harstand, et al. (2021). α2-Adrenergic Agonists or Stimulants for Preschool-Age Children With Attention-Deficit/Hyperactivity Disorder. *JAMA* 325(20):2067-2075. doi:10.1001/jama.2021.6118

[2] T. Froehlich (2021). Comparison of Medication Treatments for Preschool Children With ADHD: A First Step Toward Addressing a Critical Gap. *JAMA* 325(20):2049-2050. doi:10.1001/jama.2021.5603

outcomes in the home (e.g., disordered parent-child relationships, elevated family stress), as well as out-of-home settings (e.g., impaired preacademic skills, peer interaction difficulties, expulsion from preschool and childcare settings), underscoring the importance of identification and treatment. Guidelines from the American Academy of Pediatrics and the Society for Developmental-Behavioral Pediatrics (SDBP) recommend behavioral interventions as first-line treatment for preschool-age children with ADHD. However, behavioral interventions alone do not sufficiently improve ADHD-related symptoms and impairment in a large percentage (>80%) of children."

That opening paragraph makes a number of "evidence-based" assertions: that ADHD is a valid disorder; that it can be reliably diagnosed in preschoolers; that there is progress being made in recognizing this disorder in this age group; that untreated ADHD in preschoolers leads to bad outcomes in home and childcare settings; and that behavioral treatment fails to resolve ADHD symptoms in most preschoolers. Therefore, according to this argument, there is scientific reason to conclude that there is a pressing need to study drugs being prescribed to preschoolers so diagnosed.

The editorial's second paragraph asserts that clinical trials have already shown methylphenidate to be an effective treatment. The American Academy of Pediatrics guideline, Froehlich writes, recommends "stimulant methylphenidate as initial pharmacotherapy for preschool-age children with ADHD because it is the medication with the most evidence of efficacy and safety in this age group."

The need for this effective drug to be compared to guanfacine is that "alternative medication options are sometimes needed given the diminished efficacy and higher rates of adverse effects associated with methylphenidate in preschool-age children compared with school-age children." Organizations such as SDBP and the

American Academy of Child and Adolescent Psychiatry's Preschool Psychopharmacology Working Group recommend a2-adrenergic agonists such as guanfacine when a preschooler doesn't tolerate methylphenidate well, even though the "evidence base is remarkably limited regarding management of ADHD" with these drugs in this age group.

In short, the editorial is promoting the notion that prescribing methylphenidate to preschoolers diagnosed with ADHD is an evidence-based practice, and now, with this retrospective review of charts for toddlers treated either with methylphenidate or guanfacine, there is evidence being gathered to support guanfacine's use in this age group as well.

Yet, imagine this thought experiment. If the "evidence-based" assertions were removed from the discussion, what would most people think about giving a three-year-old who "talks excessively" or "who is easily distracted" a 5-mg dose of methylphenidate three times a day, which is a dosage deemed "optimal" in toddlers?

They would likely think it was a form of child abuse. Indeed, an adult who gives methylphenidate to a two-year old without a prescription is understood to have committed a federal crime.[3]

That's the power of an assertion that a practice is "evidence-based." It flips that instinctual thinking. An act that seems to be a form of child abuse, doing evident harm to the child, is understood to be a helpful medical treatment.

---

[3] National Drug Intelligence Center, "Ritalin fact facts," archived January 1, 2006. Accessed on August 27, 2022 at: https://www.justice.gov/archive/ndic/pubs6/6444/index.htm

Psychiatry's evidence base for preschool ADHD

Turn the clock back to 1979, and there would have been very few pediatricians or child psychiatrists who would have prescribed stimulants to preschool children. Psychiatry's construction of an evidence-base for this practice, which began to take off in the 1990s, consists of three claims:

- ADHD is a neurological disorder characterized by genetic and brain volume abnormalities.
- ADHD can be reliably diagnosed.
- Methylphenidate is a safe and effective treatment for preschoolers "with ADHD."

If there is good science behind these claims, then it could be argued that medicating preschoolers diagnosed with ADHD is a helpful treatment. If the claims are based on biased and misleading interpretations of research findings, then this is a practice without a scientific justification, and the specter of child abuse comes into view.

Genetic and brain volume abnormalities in ADHD

The diagnosis of "attention deficit disorder" was created in 1980, when the American Psychiatric Association (APA) published the third edition of its *Diagnostic and Statistical Manual* (DSM-III). There was no such diagnosis in the two prior editions of the DSM, and when the APA published DSM-III, it adopted a disease model for diagnosing and treating mental disorders. In her 1984 book *The Broken Brain*, Nancy Andreasen—the long-time editor in chief of the *American Psychiatric Journal*—set forth this new conception: "The major psychiatric illnesses are diseases. They should be considered medical illnesses just as diabetes, heart disease and cancer are." The thought was that "each different illness has a different specific cause."[4]

This conception of psychiatric disorders meant that "attention deficit disorder," from the outset, would be conceptualized—and treated—as a medical/biological problem, with the thought that a line could be drawn that separated the ADD child from the normal child. That diagnosis soon morphed into attention deficit hyperactivity disorder (ADHD).

However, with the APA having adopted this disease model, research into the biology of ADHD was tainted from the start. Psychiatric researchers did not design their studies to assess *whether* those diagnosed with ADHD suffered from a brain illness (or abnormality). They sought to *find* such abnormalities to validate the disorder the APA had created. Researchers have focused on three such possibilities: chemical imbalances, genetic associations, and abnormalities in brain structures (or size).

In the 1980s and 1990s, the chemical imbalance theory of mental disorders was all the rage, a theory born from discoveries of how psychiatric drugs acted on the brain. Antipsychotics block dopamine receptors in the brain, and so researchers hypothesized that schizophrenia was due to too much dopamine in the brain. Antidepressants up serotonergic activity, and so researchers hypothesized depression was due to too little serotonin. Ritalin (methylphenidate) increases dopamine activity and so ADHD was hypothesized to be due to too little dopamine.

---

[4] N. Andreasen. *The Broken Brain.* (New York: Harper & Row, 1984): 29-30, 133.)

Today, the chemical imbalance theory of mental disorders has been mostly discarded. As Kenneth Kendler, co-editor in chief of *Psychological Medicine* wrote in 2005, "We have hunted for big simple neurochemical explanations for psychiatric disorders and not found them."[5] While advocacy organizations, such as CHADD, may still inform the public that "people with attention deficit hyperactivity disorder may have different levels of dopamine than neurotypical people," this pathology is no longer posited as a primary feature of ADHD in the medical literature.[6]

Although no specific gene (or genes) for ADHD have been found, ADHD experts now regularly tell of how there is a genetic element that contributes to its "heritability." The World Federation of ADHD International Consensus Statement, which was published in September 2021, asserted that there is a "polygenic cause for most cases of ADHD, meaning that many genetic variants, each having a very small effect, combine to increase risk for the disorder. The polygenic risk for ADHD is associated with general psychopathology and several psychiatric disorders."[7]

A 2010 study published in *The Lancet* is often cited as proof of this "polygenic" component.[8] The study compared whole genome scans of 366 children diagnosed with ADHD with those of 1047 non-ADHD children. In a press release, the authors of the study stated

---

[5] K. Kendler (2005). Toward a more philosophical structure for psychiatry. *Am J Psychiatry* 162:433-440. https://doi.org/10.1176/appi.ajp.162.3.433

[6] CHADD: "What to know about ADHD and dopamine." Accessed on August 27, 2022 at: https://chadd.org/adhd-in-the-news/what-to-know-about-adhd-and-dopamine/.

[7] S. Faraone, et al (2021). The World Federation of ADHD International Consensus Statement: 208 Evidence-based conclusions about the disorder. Neuroscience & Biobehavioral Reviews 128, 789-818. https://doi.org/10.1016/j.neubiorev.2021.01.022

[8] N. Williams, et al (2010). Rare chromosomal deletions and duplications in attention-defi cit hyperactivity disorder: a genome-wide analysis. Lancet 376, 1401-1408. DOI: https://doi.org/10.1016/S0140-6736(10)61109-9

"now we can say with confidence that ADHD is a genetic disease and the brains of children with this condition develop differently to those of other children."[9]

ADHD children, if the press release were to be believed, had been found to have genetic abnormalities that weren't present in "normal" children. But as UK psychiatrist Sami Timimi wrote in his book *Insane Medicine,* which was serialized on Mad in America, the actual data didn't support that conclusion.[10]

The researchers reported that 15.7% of the ADHD group had "copy number variants"— abnormal bits of genetic code known as CNVs—in their genomes, compared to 7.5% of the control group. This meant that 84% of the ADHD group did not have this polygenic abnormality, which means that this abnormality, in fact, was *not* characteristic of those so diagnosed.

A 2017 article in Genome Medicine is an example of research that has led to the second part of the genetics claim, which is that there is a polygenic abnormality common to neuropsychiatric disorders.[11] In the study, an international group of investigators reported that they had found CNVs on two genes (DOCK8/KANK1) significantly more often in those diagnosed with ADHD and four other psychiatric disorders than in healthy controls. This was evidence, they wrote, of a "common genetic component involved in the pathogenesis of neuropsychiatric disorders."

---

[9] Wellcome Trust, September 30, 2010 press release. First direct evidence that ADHD is a genetic disorder: Children with ADHD more likely to have missing or duplicated segments of DNA. Accessed on August 27, 2022 at: https://www.sciencedaily.com/releases/2010/09/100929191312.htm

[10] Serialized at: madinamerica.com/insane-medicine/

[11] J. Glessner et al (2017). Copy number variation meta-analysis reveals a novel duplication at 9p24 associated with multiple neurodevelopmental disorders. *Genome Med* 9, 106. https://doi.org/10.1186/s13073-017-0494-1

Here is the data for the ADHD group. Of the 1,241 youth in the ADHD cohort, four—0.32%—had CNVs in these two genes. That meant that 99.7% of the ADHD group didn't have this genetic abnormality. However, since only 0.1% of the control group had this abnormality, the authors concluded that the ADHD patients were three times more likely to have it than healthy controls.

The data was similar for the other four psychiatric disorders. In total, only 32 of the 7,849 people with a psychiatric diagnosis had a CNV abnormality in their DOCK8/KANK1 genes (0.4%). There was an increased "odds ratio" that this abnormality occurred in those diagnosed with psychiatric disorders, but it occurred so rarely that this difference was meaningless. The "odds ratio" calculations were an example of science employed to mislead, rather than to inform.

The flaws with the brain volume research are much the same. The studies involve averaging volumes in an ADHD group compared to non-ADHD controls, and while the effect size differences in these composite comparisons are quite small, meaning that there is a great overlap in the distribution curves of volumes for both groups, the research is cited as evidence of brain differences in individuals with ADHD.

In 2017, *Lancet Psychiatry* published a "mega-analysis" of such studies.[12] The 82 authors declared that theirs was the largest dataset of its kind. It was composed of MRI scans measuring brain volumes in 1,713 people diagnosed with ADHD and 1,529 controls, with this research having been conducted at 23 sites around the world. Theirs was a definitive study, and they declared it showed that *individuals* with ADHD had smaller brains than normal.

---

[12] M. Hoogman, et al (2017). Subcortical brain volume differences in participants with attention deficit hyperactivity disorder in children and adults: a cross-sectional mega-analysis. *Lancet Psychiatry* 4, 310-319. https://doi.org/10.1016/S2215-0366(17)30049-4

"The data from our highly powered analysis confirm that patients with ADHD do have altered brains and therefore that ADHD is a disorder of the brain," they wrote. "This message is clear for clinicians to convey to parents and patients, which can help to reduce the stigma that ADHD is just a label for difficult children and caused by incompetent parenting."

Headlines in CNN, Newsweek, WebMD, and other media all echoed this claim. "Study finds brains of ADHD sufferers are smaller," Newsweek wrote.

However, this conclusion was belied by the effect sizes that the researchers reported for the various brain volume comparisons. The Cohen's D effect sizes ranged from 0.01 to 0.19, meaning that the distribution of brain volumes in the two groups, in comparison after comparison, were nearly identical. The effect size for "intracranial volume" was 0.1, which is depicted in the graphic below:

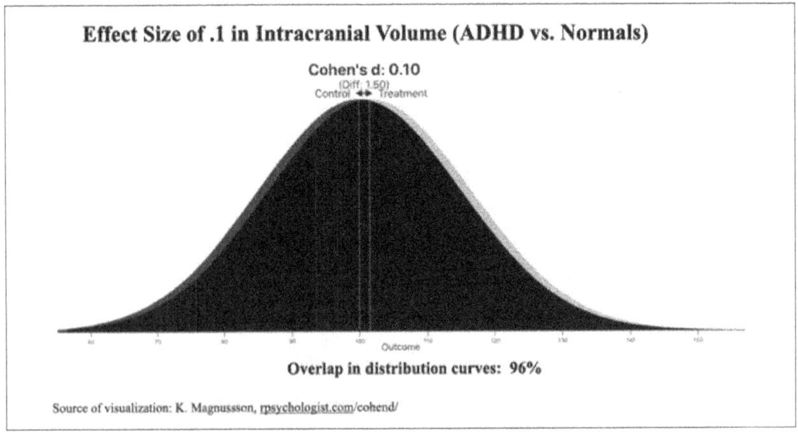

With an effect size of 0.1, there is a 96% overlap between the two groups. Pick a random individual diagnosed with ADHD in the study, and there would be a 47% chance that he or she would have a *bigger brain* than the median of the control group (and a 53% chance to have a smaller brain than the median.)

While such research is easily deconstructed, it is the conclusion drawn by the authors that gets entered into the ADHD evidence base. These findings are then incorporated into consensus statements, medical textbooks, clinical guidelines, and information provided to the lay public.

Here is a sampling of this process:

The World Federation of ADHD International Consensus Statement: "Findings from genetics or brain imaging . . . indicate a consistent set of causes for the disorder."

The American Academy of Child and Adolescent Psychiatry: "ADHD is a brain disorder. Scientists have shown that there are differences in the brains of children with ADHD . . . Research has shown that some structures in the brain in children with ADHD can be smaller than those areas of the brain in children without ADHD."[13]

The Centers for Disease Control and Prevention: "Although the exact causes of ADHD are not known, research shows that genes play a role."[14]

WebMD: "Experts aren't sure what causes ADHD. Several things may lead to it, including . . . genes, chemicals, brain changes" (and more).[15]

---

[13] American Academy of Child and Adolescent Psychiatry. "ADHD and the Brain." Accessed on August 27, 2022, at: https://www.aacap.org/AACAP/Families_and_Youth/Facts_for_Families/FFF-Guide/ADHD_and_the_Brain-121.aspx.

[14] Centers for Disease Control and Prevention. "Research on ADHD." Accessed on August 27, 2022 at: https://www.cdc.gov/ncbddd/adhd/research.html

[15] WebMD. "Attention-Deficit Hyperactivity Disorder (ADHD). Accessed on August 27, 2022 at: https://www.webmd.com/add-adhd/childhood-adhd/attention-deficit-hyperactivity-disorder-adhd

The root cause of this misinformation is that ever since DSM-III was published, psychiatric researchers have been searching to identify biological causes for ADHD, and with that impulse in play, they have regularly misrepresented their own data. Very small group differences compared to controls are represented as abnormalities found in *individuals* diagnosed with ADHD, even though the study data, when properly parsed, show that not to be true.

Indeed, once the data are reviewed, here is the finding that comes clear: Decades of research into the "biology" of ADHD failed to find any pathology that was characteristic of *individual* children so diagnosed. The search for chemical imbalances, ADHD genes, and brain volume abnormalities all turned up negative. Any reported group differences in the genetic and brain volume studies were quite small and showed that most ADHD children fell within "normal" limits.

ADHD can be reliably diagnosed

Psychiatry's declaration that ADHD has genetic and biological underpinnings leads to the conclusion that it is a discrete disorder that can exist in preschool children (or is a disorder present at birth that will become manifest as the child develops.) However, for the prescribing of methylphenidate to be considered "evidence-based," a second conclusion must be drawn, which is that this discrete illness can be reliably diagnosed in preschoolers. Otherwise, such prescribing practices would lack a medical justification and treating toddlers who might not have this condition with a stimulant could be seen as doing great harm.

The National Drug Intelligence Center even makes this point: methylphenidate is safe only when prescribed "for a legitimate medical condition."[16] Otherwise, it should be considered a drug

[16] National Drug Intelligence, ibid.

of abuse, one that can cause "psychotic episodes, cardiovascular complications, and severe psychological addiction."

As is well known, there is no biological marker for diagnosing ADHD. From its inception, the diagnosis has been made on an assessment of behaviors—inattention, impulsivity, and hyperactivity—said to be symptoms of the disorder. The specific criteria for the diagnosis have changed with each iteration of the DSM, with each updated volume making it easier to make the diagnosis. Prevalence studies reflect this expansion, with the percentage of youth said to have ADHD increasing from 3% in the early 1980s to 5% after DSM-IV was published in 1994, and to 10% in the DSM-5 era.[17]

While the changing criteria and prevalence studies tell of a diagnosis that is a construct, as opposed to an illness found in nature, the ADHD professional community has steadfastly maintained that it is a "real" disorder that can be reliably diagnosed. The field has created an evidence base for this belief, in large part through its use of rating scales to measure the symptoms set forth in the DSM.

Psychiatry, of course, has created rating scales for all of its major disorders, which quantify symptom scores and thus lend an aura of scientific objectivity to the diagnoses. The rating scales may also be used to draw a theoretical line separating those who meet the criteria for the disorder and those who do not, which is how the ADHD rating scales are used.

One such tool is the SNAP-IV Teacher and Parent Rating Scale, which was created after DSM-IV was published.[18] The ADHD questionnaire

---

[17] Centers for Disease Control and Prevention. "ADHD Throughout the Years." Accessed on August 27, 2022 at: https://www.cdc.gov/ncbddd/adhd/timeline.html.

[18] SNAP-IV 26-Item Teacher and Parent Rating Scale. Accessed on August 22, 2022 at: http://www.shared-care.ca/files/Scoring_for_SNAP_IV_Guide_26-item.pdf.

lists nine behaviors related to the "inattention" domain and nine behaviors related to the "hyperactivity impulsive" domain, with the parent or teacher rating the presence of the behavior on a scale of 0 to 3 (0 = not at all, 1 = just a little, 2 = quite a bit, 3 = very much).

Sample Questions on SNAP-IV Rating Scale

Scale: 0 to 3 for each question	Not at all	Just a little	Quite a bit	Very much
13. Often has difficulty playing or engaging in leisure activities quietly				
14. Often is "on the go" or often acts as if "driven by a motor"				
15. Often talks excessively				
16. Often blurts out answers before questions have been completed				

The possible range of scores is 0 to 27 for each of the two subtypes. SNAP guidelines define scores less than 13 as "not clinically significant," and scores above that line of demarcation are categorized as mild, moderate, or severe symptoms of ADHD. Here is the SNAP scoring table:

Not clinically significant: < 13
Mild symptoms: 13 – 17
Moderate symptoms: 18 - 22
Severe symptoms: 23 - 27

Another such tool is the Vanderbilt assessment scale. Today, a parent or teacher can go online, answer questions related to the frequency of a child's symptoms and performance in school, push the "calculate" button, and immediately learn whether the child "meets criteria" for the disorder and its various subtypes.[19] It's a yes or no bottom line.

When SNAP, the Vanderbilt, and other ADHD rating scales were introduced, other researchers then assessed their "reliability" and "validity." These assessments are difficult to understand, but methodologies are discussed, numbers are crunched, tables of statistics are published, and a conclusion is drawn about the scales' merits. A 2003 review published in the *Journal of the American Academy of Child and Adolescent Psychiatry* gave them all excellent grades: ADHD "rating scales can reliably, validly, and efficiently measure DSM-IV-based ADHD symptoms in youths," the authors wrote. "They have great utility in research and clinical work."[20]

The rating scales developed after DSM-IV was published in 1994 were deemed useful for measuring symptoms in school-age children. The thought at that time—the late 1990s, early 2000s—was that ADHD couldn't be reliably diagnosed in preschool children, as even "normal" three-year-olds were often inattentive, impulsive, and ran about like they had motors inside them. But then physicians began prescribing stimulant medications to toddlers with behavioral problems, and that led to the release of the ADHD Rating Scale IV, Preschool Version.[21]

This scale is similar in kind to the SNAP-IV, with 18 questions scored on a scale of 0 to 3. Scores are tallied compiled for inattention subtype,

---

[19] NICHQ Vanderbilt Assessment Scale. Accessed on August 22, 2022 at: https://www.mdapp.co/nichq-vanderbilt-assessment-scale-calculator-519/.

[20] B. Collett, et al (2003). Ten-year review of rating scales. V: scales assessing attention-deficit/hyperactivity disorder. *Journal of American Academy of Child & Adolescent Psychiatry* 42:1015-37. doi: 10.1097/01.CHI.0000070245.24125.B6.

[21] ADHD Rating Scale IV – Preschool Version. Accessed on August 27, 2022 at: https://fliphtml5.com/xibq/ekgw.

hyperactivity/impulsivity subtype, and composite type. The cutoff for symptoms "suggestive" of ADHD is the 93% percentile mark, i.e., scores in the top 7% are seen as meeting criteria for a diagnosis.

Sample Questions on ADHD Rating Scale IV - Preschool Version

Scale: 0 to 3 for each question	Rarely or never	Some-times	Often	Very often
9. Has difficulty organizing tasks and activities (i.e. choosing an activity, getting materials, doing steps in order)				
10. Is "on the go" or acts as if "driven by a motor"				
11. Avoids tasks that require sustained mental effort (i.e. puzzles, learning ABC's, writing name)				
12. Talks excessively				

Although the rating scales are not supposed to be used to make a diagnosis, they are said to identify children who need to be referred to a psychiatrist for a diagnostic evaluation. The numerical scores promote an understanding, which permeates the medical literature, that there are children "with ADHD," and children "without ADHD," a description that signals there is no in-between space. A child either has the "neurological" disorder or doesn't.

In 2002, Russell Barkley and other prominent figures in the ADHD world published an "International Consensus Statement on ADHD" that made this point clear.[22] Evidence that ADHD was a "real medical condition," they wrote, was so abundant that to question its validity

[22] R. Barkley, et al (2002). International Consensus Statement on ADHD. *Clinical Child and Family Psychology Review* 5: 89 – 111.

was "tantamount to declaring the earth flat, the laws of gravity debatable, and the periodic table in chemistry a fraud."

The recently published World Federation International Consensus Statement made a similar claim, albeit in more moderate language.[23] ADHD was a "valid disorder" and the fact that it could be reliably diagnosed was an essential part of the evidence establishing its validity. "Well-trained professionals in a variety of settings and cultures agree on its presence or absence using well-defined criteria," they wrote. However, just as the genetics and brain volume research can be easily deconstructed, so too can this assertion that ADHD is a distinct disease that can be reliably diagnosed. The pretense is self-evident.

While scales may spit out a bottom-line score, the assessing of symptoms is a subjective exercise. When does a toddler's "difficulty organizing tasks and activities" fall into the "often" category, as opposed to the "very often" category? When does "talks excessively" move from the "sometimes" category into the "often" category? The scores change depending on which box the parent or teacher checks. Even more to the point, the scores fall on a *spectrum*, and then cutoff numbers are arbitrarily drawn to distinguish those who "have" symptoms suggestive of ADHD and those who do not.

Should the cutoff be one standard deviation above the mean? If so, this will mean that 16% of all children will have scores at the far end of the spectrum, and thus have symptoms suggestive of ADHD. Or should the cutoff be 1.5 standard deviations above the mean? If so, this will result in 6.5% of all children "meeting the criteria" for ADHD. The cutoff lines used in ADHD rating scales vary, with most drawing a cutoff within this range of 1 to 1.5 standard deviations above the mean.

---

[23] Faraone, ibid.

None of this tells of a disease found in nature. The assessing of symptoms is a subjective exercise, symptom scores fall on distribution curve, and then a line—somewhere along that distribution curve—is arbitrarily set to identify those who meet criteria for the disorder. Yet, it is the pretense—that ADHD is a discrete neurological disorder that can be reliably diagnosed—that rules in the medical literature and in the public mind. Articles in medical journals regularly tell of "children with ADHD" and children "without ADHD."

This mindset is on display in the *JAMA* editorial. The title is "Comparison of Medication Treatments for Preschool Children With ADHD." The first word in the editorial then reifies that understanding. The writer does not tell of an increase in the *diagnosis* of ADHD in preschoolers, but rather of how *recognition* of ADHD in preschoolers has increased.

That is a difference in word choice that reveals all. And it sets the table for the field to declare that prescribing stimulants to preschool children is a helpful thing to do.

The preschool ADHD treatment study (PATS)

The science reviewed above, if interpreted in an unbiased manner, tells of how ADHD is a diagnostic construct that groups together children with certain behaviors that impair their ability to function in certain environments (at least in the eyes of teachers and parents). The biology that may be associated with such behaviors is unknown, and no specific biology—genetic or brain abnormality—has been found that is common to all those so diagnosed. There is a distribution curve in the ratings of behaviors said to be characteristic of ADHD, and those so diagnosed fall at the far end of that curve.

[xx] Mayo Clinic, "Attention-Deficit/Hyperactivity Disorder (ADHD) in Children." https://www.mayoclinic.org/diseases-conditions/adhd/symptoms-causes/syc-20350889

With that conception, arising from forty years of research, one possible societal response would be to see if changing the child's environment could be helpful, which could include society creating more nurturing environments *for all children*. The problem doesn't necessarily lie *within* the child, but rather arises from the child's response to his or her *environment*. Society could see the "prevalence" of the disorder as a marker of distress in society. However, the understanding that ADHD is a distinct disorder, characterized by genetic and brain abnormalities, and that this disorder can be reliably diagnosed, leads to the conclusion that a medical intervention is warranted.

While behavioral treatment may be the initial intervention offered to preschoolers, when a disorder is said to lie within the individual, drug treatment quickly becomes a go-to intervention, particularly once a drug has been deemed to be "safe and effective." The NIMH's Preschool ADHD Treatment Study (PATS), which was conducted in the early 2000s, is cited as providing evidence for prescribing methylphenidate to this age group.

The inclusion criteria required the toddlers to score above the 93rd percentile on the Conners Parent and Teaching rating scales for ADHD (1.5 standard deviations above the mean). There were 303 preschoolers enrolled into the study, which had a complicated multi-phase design.[24]

Here are the results from each phase of the study:[25]

---

[24] S. Kollins, et al (2006). Rationale, design, and methods of the Preschool ADHD Treatment Study (PATS). *Journal of American Academy of Child & Adolescent Psychiatry* 45:1275-1283. doi: 10.1097/01.chi.0000235074.86919.dc.

[25] L. Greenhill, et al (2006). Efficacy and safety of immediate-release methylphenidate treatment for preschoolers with ADHD. *Journal of American Academy of Child & Adolescent Psychiatry* 45:1284-1293. doi:10.1097/01.chi.0000235077.32661.61.

1. *Parent-training:* Before the 303 children were exposed to methylphenidate, the parents were given a 10-week parent training course, and if a child significantly improved during this period, the child did not continue to the next step of the study. Many parents also dropped out during this period. This left 183 preschoolers who entered the drug-testing phases of the study.

2. *Tolerability test:* The 183 children went through four weeks of open-label treatment to see if they could tolerate the drug, and those who could not, as evidenced by their experiencing adverse effects, were removed from the study. Fourteen children were discontinued during this phase.

3. *Assessment of a "best dose" response:* 165 children entered into a five-week "titration" study. Each week, a child would be prescribed a different dose of methylphenidate administered three times a day (1.25 mg, 2.5 mg, 5 mg, and 7.5 mg), with the fifth week a placebo dose. At the end of each week, parents and teachers assessed the children's symptoms on two rating scales to ascertain how they had fared during the seven days on that particular treatment.

   The researchers reported that there were significant decreases in ADHD symptoms during the weeks the toddlers were on a 2.5 mg, 5 mg, or 7.5 mg dose of methylphenidate compared to their week on placebo. Only the 1.25 dose failed to provide this benefit. The effect sizes for the three "effective" doses were small, with an effect size of 0.43 for the 15-mg daily dose, deemed the "optimal dose" of methylphenidate for this age group.

   During the five weeks, the top five adverse events spontaneously reported by parents were decreased appetite, emotional outbursts, difficulty falling asleep, irritability, and repetitive behaviors or thoughts.[26] These adverse events occurred more frequently during the weeks they were on methylphenidate than during their week on placebo.

4. *Randomization phase:* After the titration trial, the blind was broken to identify the specific dose of methylphenidate the child had done best on (or whether a child had markedly improved during the week of placebo treatment). Then, following a 24-hour washout, the 114 toddlers still in the trial were randomized to their "best dose" of methylphenidate or to placebo. The primary outcome was "excellent response" at the end of four weeks as measured on the SNAP scale.

   Twenty-one percent of the methylphenidate cohort achieved that response compared to 13% of the placebo group, a difference that was not statistically significant. Only 77 of the 114 finished the four weeks of treatment.

5. *Open label maintenance:* All of the children enrolled into the methylphenidate phases of the study were eligible for 10 months of open-label treatment, with this phase designed to assess the longer term "safety and tolerability" of methylphenidate. One hundred forty children entered this study, with the percentage suffering various adverse events charted at the start of the 10 months and again at the end, with the thought that the percentage would decline as the preschoolers became more accustomed to the drug. The table below details the findings:

[26] T. Wigal, et al (2006). Safety and tolerability of methylphenidate in preschool children with ADHD. *Journal of American Academy of Child & Adolescent Psychiatry* 45:1294-1303. doi: 10.1097/01.chi.0000235082.63156.27

Adverse Effects in Maintenance Phase of PATS Study

Adverse effect	Change over ten months
Crabby/irritable	44% to 24%
Appetite loss	42% to 41%
Prone to crying	37% to 27%
Skin-picking	37% to 34%
Trouble sleeping	29% to 20%
Worried/anxious	28% to 24%
Tearful/sad/depressed	24% to 9%
Stomachaches	17% to 8%
Social withdrawal	16% to 8%
Listless/tired	12% to 3%

Source: T. Wigal (2006): Safety and tolerability of methylphenidate in preschool children with ADHD. *J Am Acad Child Adolesc Psychiatry* 45:1294-1303.

In addition, of the 95 children who remained on methylphenidate for the 10 months, annual growth rates were 20% less than expected, and weight gain was 52% less than expected.

Deconstructing PATS

Once the PATS trial is detailed in this way, what conclusions can be drawn? The first is that parents of 120 of the 303 preschoolers enrolled into the trial decided—after the parent training phase—not to expose their child to methylphenidate. That's 40% of all parents.

The second is that the efficacy of methylphenidate, on a primary outcome measure, only appears during the five-week titration trial, which involved comparing reduction of ADHD symptoms during the weeks they were on methylphenidate to the week they were switched to placebo.

The third is that the titration trial was biased by design against placebo. The placebo period began with the toddlers being abruptly withdrawn from whatever dose of methylphenidate they had been on, and given that discontinuation studies of methylphenidate have found that behavioral symptoms often rapidly worsen following abrupt withdrawal, it could be expected that the behavior of many of the toddlers would deteriorate during their seven days on placebo.

Yet, even with this biased design, at the 15-mg daily dose that was deemed optimal, the "effect size" was only 0.43. With this effect size, the number needed to treat is 7. You would need to treat seven preschoolers with methylphenidate to produce one additional favorable outcome (in terms of reduction of symptoms.) The other six are exposed to the hazards of the drug without any benefit beyond placebo.

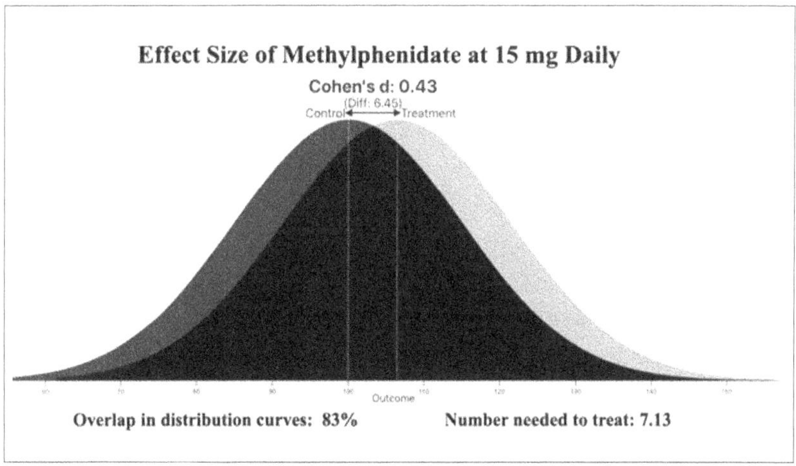

The fourth is that there is no evidence anywhere in this trial of the preschoolers treated with methylphenidate functioning better. In the parallel phase study, the primary outcome was achieving an "excellent response," which presumably would lead to better functioning, but there was no statistically significant difference between "best dose" of the drug and placebo. Indeed, of the 183 toddlers who were exposed to methylphenidate, there were only 13 ever described as having an "excellent response" while on the drug.

Meanwhile, the toddlers put on methylphenidate frequently suffered moderate to severe adverse events, and the 10-month maintenance phase told of toddlers that, while being treated with methylphenidate, were often crabby, prone to crying, picking at their skin, having trouble sleeping, worried, and without much of an appetite. At the end of 10 months, they were notably shorter and lighter in weight than they normally would have been.

The flaw in evidence-based medicine

The bottom line-conclusion drawn from this study—that methylphenidate is a safe and effective treatment for preschoolers diagnosed with ADHD—reveals a flaw that is baked into "evidence-based" prescribing of medications. If a trial finds that a drug produces a greater reduction of symptoms than placebo, with the difference "statistically significant," then it is deemed to be an effective treatment for the related disease, and regularly prescribed to all those so diagnosed. But that endpoint—reduction of symptoms better than placebo—is just one data point among many produced in a trial of a drug, and an examination of this broader collection of data is needed to assess its likely *overall* impact on a diagnostic group.

What you find in the PATS trial is the following:

- Many toddlers apparently got better with parent training as a first intervention.

- Of the 183 children exposed to methylphenidate at some point during the study, 21 "discontinued treatment because of intolerable methylphenidate adverse events."

- The effect size in reduction of symptoms during the titration phase was small, such that at an optimal daily dose of 15 mg, six of seven toddlers treated with methylphenidate will suffer the adverse effects of the drug without any additional benefit beyond placebo in reduction of ADHD symptoms.

- In the randomized four-week trial, only 21% had an excellent response to the drug, compared to 13% in the placebo group. This means that if you medicated 100 preschoolers with methylphenidate, there would only be eight additional "excellent responders" than there would have been otherwise.

- Adverse effects on methylphenidate were frequent and told of behavioral deterioration, particularly in the 10-month maintenance phase.

- At the end of 10 months, the toddlers were shorter and weighed less than normal.

That is the picture that emerges from a recap of all the data. If you do the math, there is only a small percentage of preschoolers—10% to 15%—that could be said to enjoy a benefit from the treatment in terms of reduction of symptoms over the short term. That means that 85% or so of all toddlers treated with methylphenidate will experience the adverse effects of that drug without receiving any additional benefit, a net result that tells of harm done.

Yet, in evidence-based medicine, there is a hyper focus on symptom reduction, with even a small effect size deemed proof of efficacy, and that is how the PATS trial led to a conclusion that methylphenidate is a safe and effective treatment for toddlers diagnosed "with ADHD." As the *JAMA* editorial states, the American Academy of Pediatrics recommends methylphenidate as "initial pharmacotherapy for preschool-age children because it is the medication with the most evidence of efficacy and safety in this age group."

One final note on the PATS trial: in the published report of the safety and efficacy results, the authors collectively disclosed 72 "relationships" with pharmaceutical companies, with the manufacturers of ADHD drugs prominent on the list of disclosures.

The PATS follow-up: A childhood on drugs

Even with the 10-month maintenance phase, the PATS trial didn't provide insight into how the lives of these toddlers unfolded over the longer term once they had been diagnosed as "having ADHD." However, PATS investigators did conduct two follow-up assessments of their ongoing medication use, at three and six years, and the results are heartbreaking.[27]

Here are the results:

Medication Use Three and Six Years Later

Medication Use	At Three Years N=206	At Six Years N= 179
No medication	34%	27%
Stimulant monotherapy	41%	40%
Atomoxetine, alone or with stimulant	9%	5%
Antipsychotic, usually with a stimulant	8%	13%
Other pharmacotherapy	7%	15%
Total on a psychiatric drug	66%	73%

Source: B. Vitiello (2015): Pharmacotherapy of the Preschool ADHD Treatment Study (PATS) Children Growing Up. *J Am Acad Child Adolesc Psychiatry* 54:550-556

[27] B. Vitiello, et al (2015). Pharmacotherapy of the Preschool ADHD Treatment Study (PATS) Children Growing Up. *Journal of American Academy of Child & Adolescent Psychiatry* 54: 550–556. doi:10.1016/j.jaac.2015.04.004.

The findings tell of stolen childhoods. These children were diagnosed with ADHD as preschoolers and that turned two-thirds of them into persistent mental patients who grew up constantly on psychiatric drugs. At their tenth birthdays, this group would have no memory of being alive without the mind-altering effects of psychiatric drugs. Which begs the next question: What fate awaits them as they move into their teenage years and into adulthood? While there are long lists of adverse effects associated with longer-term use of stimulants and other psychiatric drugs, which collectively tell of impaired physical health and social development, there is an absence of good research on how such drugs may fundamentally alter brain development over time. However, there have been animal studies studying the effects and those studies have sounded an alarm.

For example, repeated exposure to stimulants was found to cause rhesus monkeys to exhibit "aberrant behaviors" long after the drug exposure had stopped.[28] Preadolescent rats treated with stimulants moved around less as adults, were less responsive to novel environments, and showed a "deficit in sexual behavior"."[29] Such findings have led at least a few investigators to conclude that stimulants may damage the brain's "reward system," and thus to a concern that medicating a child may produce an adult with a "reduced ability to experience pleasure."[30]

Aberrant behaviors, a deficit in sexual behavior, a reduced ability to experience pleasure . . . if these animal studies are any guide,

---

[28] S. Castner, et al (1999). Long-lasting psychotomimetic consequences of repeated low-dose amphetamine exposure in rhesus monkeys. *Neuropsychopharmacology* 20:10-28. doi: 10.1016/S0893-133X(98)00050-5.

[29] C. Bolanos, et al (2003). Methylphenidate treatment during pre- and periadolescence alters behavioral responses to emotional stimuli at adulthood. Biological Psychiatry 15: 1317-29. doi: 10.1016/s0006-3223(03)00570-5.

[30] W. Carlezon, Jr. (2003). Enduring behavioral effects of early exposure to methylphenidate in rats. *Biological Psychiatry* 15: 1330-7. doi: 10.1016/j.biopsych.2003.08.020.

preschoolers prescribed stimulants for ADHD, who then stay on this medication as they grow up, will have sharply diminished lives as adults because of this "medical intervention."

The bottom line

The *JAMA* editorial was occasioned by a report, based on a retrospective review of pediatric health records, that compared the risks and benefits of guanfacine to methylphenidate when prescribed to preschoolers diagnosed with ADHD. The authors reported that both drugs led to improvements in the majority of children "with differing adverse effect profiles."

The accompanying editorial told of how this was a "first step toward addressing a critical gap" in the evidence base for treating preschool ADHD. Both drugs are now being routinely prescribed to toddlers, and, the editorial argued, it was important to ascertain which class of drugs should be the preferred drug treatment for this age group. Randomized clinical trials comparing guanfacine to methylphenidate would be a vital next step in the evidence base supporting such prescribing.

The editorial stirred a different question investigated in this Mad in America report: How is it that the medical community came to think that prescribing stimulants to preschoolers on a daily basis was a helpful thing to do? What was the makeup of the "evidence base" that could lead to such a practice? While one can be skeptical of the motivations of those who construct the evidence base, the motivation of pediatricians who follow it, prescribing methylphenidate in ways recommended by clinical care guidelines, is not subject to such skepticism. Pediatricians pick that specialty because they want to be promoters of health in newborns and the young.

Thus, the focus of this MIA report is how "evidence-based" medicine, particularly when constructed in the squishy scientific realm of psychiatry, can do harm. In this case, you find a story of researchers seeking to find evidence of a disease, which could then be used to validate a diagnostic construction drawn up by a medical guild, drawing conclusions that weren't supported by the data. Pretense snuck into the "evidence base," and then came the fatal flaw regularly cooked into conclusions drawn from clinical trials, which is that a slight reduction of symptoms translates into evidence of a "safe and effective" drug, even though most patients may be receiving no benefit. In that way, you end up with an "evidence base" for prescribing stimulants daily to a three-year-old.

There is one other way that "evidence-based" medicine fails in this instance. There is never any consideration of a fundamental question: What rights does the child have? Preschoolers are in the first stage of their journey into the mysterious world of life, and if there is a core existential aspect to growing up, it is the experience of struggling to know one's own mind, of one's own essential makeup, and as part of that struggle, of gaining some control over one's behavior. As the saying goes, you want to see what you can make of yourself. The medicating of preschoolers, with that medicating becoming a constant and often evolving into polypharmacy by the time they are in elementary school, robs them of that future.

That is a story of a great tragedy, of existential loss, and yet in American medicine today, it is recommended as an evidence-based treatment for the 2.6% of preschoolers—that's one in every 38—said to "have ADHD." Readers can decide whether this is a story of "evidence-based" medicine enabling a practice that, without that sheen of science, could rightfully be described as child abuse.

Psychopharmacology and the Treatment of ADHD: What Role Should Clinical Psychologists Play?

Robert Foltz, Judy Kupchan, and Alexandra Pope

Attention-Deficit/Hyperactivity Disorder (ADHD), one of the most commonly diagnosed psychiatric disorders among children and adolescents (Song et al., 2021), is characterized by symptoms of inattention, hyperactivity, and/or impulsivity which impair daily functioning in more than one environment (American Psychiatric Association [APA], 2022).

Inattention can manifest in a variety of behaviors including difficulty focusing, inability to stay on task, and disorganization unrelated to lack of understanding, while hyperactivity is typically exhibited through excessive motor activity such as fidgeting, tapping, or talking when deemed inappropriate (APA, 2022). These symptoms are typically chronic (Visser et al., 2014) and impair children's development and functioning in social, academic, and/or occupational domains (APA, 2022).

Of the 18 DSM-5-TR criteria for this condition, only six are required to secure a diagnosis of ADHD. This translates to thousands of potential

---

Robert Foltz, Psych.D., is associate professor of clinical psychology at the Chicago School of Professional Psychology, USA.

Judy Kupchan and Alexandra Pope are clinical psychology doctoral students at the Chicago School of Professional Psychology.

symptom configurations, all representing ADHD. Moreover, the word "often" begins each criterion, leaving one to wonder, how often is often enough to identify this "neurodevelopmental disorder?" Moreover, to what degree does context influence how 'often' these behaviors emerge?

As ADHD is classified as a *neuro*developmental disorder, it is important to note the neurological foundation, or lack thereof. Of course, the brain is involved in everything we do, but the American Psychiatric Association (2022) highlights:

- No biological marker is diagnostic for ADHD. Although ADHD has been associated with elevated power of slow waves (4-7 Hz 'theta') as well as decreased power of fast waves (14-30 Hz 'beta'), a later review found no differences in theta or beta power in either children or adults with ADHD relative to control subjects.

- Although some neuroimaging studies have shown differences in children with ADHD compared with control subjects, meta-analysis of *all* neuroimaging studies do not show differences between individuals with ADHD and control subjects ... No form of neuroimaging can be used for diagnosis of ADHD (p. 72).

It is fair to assume that if reliable data existed to identify the pathognomonic neurological foundation for this disorder, it would have been presented in the most recent edition of the DSM-5-TR. In its absence, and with the acknowledgement that our current neuroimaging cannot be used to diagnose the condition, clinicians should be cautious about making such claims.

In 2017, the Lancet Psychiatry published an article purporting to identify specific neurological differences between ADHD and "normal" youth (Hoogman et al., 2017). Upon further scrutiny, the neurological differences were dubious, and the ADHD children had higher IQ scores than controls at 16 of 20 sites in the study (Corrigan & Whitaker, 2017). Many efforts have been made to determine reliably identified differences in the brains of those with – and without – ADHD, yet these differences remain elusive.

Over the past 10 years, the age range of individuals diagnosed with ADHD has expanded significantly to include preschool-aged children as well as adults. A recent global meta-analysis indicated that 7.2% of children around the world have a diagnosis of ADHD (Thomas et al., 2015), six years being the median age of diagnosis (Visser et al., 2014).

In the United States, 8.4% of children from ages 2 to 17 have been diagnosed with ADHD, with about two-thirds receiving pharmacological treatment and about half engaged in behavioral treatment, totaling approximately 6.2 million youth (Danielson et al., 2018). Further, the CDC reported that over 10,000 toddlers between the ages of 2 and 3 years old are being medicated for the treatment of ADHD, despite the FDA's lack of approval of the use of stimulants in this age group (Leo & Lacasse, 2015). Meanwhile, about one-quarter of children in the U.S. have not received any sort of treatment for ADHD at all (Danielson et al., 2018).

Treatment recommendations

Following a rigorous review of the treatment literature between 2011 and 2016, the American Academy of Pediatrics (AAP) released the most recent clinical practice guidelines for evaluating, diagnosing, and treating children and adolescents with ADHD in 2019 (Wolraich et al., 2019). In instances where the intervention was found to be, at minimum, supported by "trials or diagnostic studies with minor limitations" and "consistent findings from multiple observational studies" and demonstrative of a preponderance of benefits over harm to the individual being treated, the committee made a strong recommendation for the treatment in question (Wolraich et al., 2019, p. 4). Clinicians are urged to accept strong recommendations unless a "clear and compelling rationale for an alternative approach is present" (Wolraich et al., 2019, p. 4).

Table 1. Recommendation Overview based on AAP ADHD Practice Guidelines (2019)

Age	Primary Recommendation	Secondary Recommendation
4 – 6	Parent Training in Behavior Management (PTBM)	Methylphenidate if PTBM does not yield sufficient improvement, or if behavioral strategies are unavailable.
6 – 12	FDA approved ADHD medications	Behavioral interventions should be offered in conjunction with medication
12 – 18	FDA approved ADHD medications	Consider the use of behavioral strategies

A comment on preschool children

It should be noted that methylphenidate has not yet been approved by the Food and Drug Administration (FDA) to be prescribed to preschool-aged children due to a paucity of research surrounding its use in this age group, thus it is currently being prescribed on an "off-label" basis (Wolraich et al., 2019).

Evidence to support the efficacy and safety of methylphenidate in preschool-aged children is limited to one multisite study and ten other smaller, single-site studies for a total sample size of 269 children (Greenhill et al., 2006; Greenhill et al., 2008). More recently, Harstad et al., (2021) completed a retrospective analysis of 497 preschool-aged children, examining alpha-adrenergic agonists and stimulant medication. Their report of improvement (noted in 78% of those taking stimulants) is based on retrospective chart reviews scored with the Clinical Global Improvement Scale. However, it is noteworthy that "moodiness/irritability" occurred in 50% of these stimulant-treated children, among other side-effects.

Absent from the AAP Guidelines were findings from "the most comprehensive available evidence base to inform patients, families, clinicians, guideline developers, and policymakers on the choice of ADHD medications across age groups" (Cortese et al., 2018, p. 1). This meta-analysis of efficacy and tolerability included over 10,000 children and adolescents across published and unpublished randomized controlled trials.

Remarkably, this exhaustive review determined that evidence to support the use of medications to effectively treat ADHD could not be recommended beyond 12 weeks of intervention. Beyond that, the research is insufficient to recommend any stimulant medications for the treatment of ADHD (Cortese et al., 2018). Indeed, the longest study conducted to understand the effects of medication treatment (the Multimodal Treatment of ADHD – MTA study) also notes the diminished benefits of stimulant treatment over time (Jensen et al., 2007).

In contrast to the conviction in the committee's recommendations for medication treatment of ADHD in children and adolescents, the committee is less definite in its guidelines surrounding psychosocial treatments for children and adolescents with ADHD. Specifically, they maintain that the long-term effects of psychosocial treatments have yet to be determined and that some non-medication treatments including mindfulness, cognitive training, supportive counseling, and social skills training have either insufficient evidence to support them or have been found to yield little to no change in ADHD symptoms.

Moreover, the committee reports that cognitive-behavioral approaches have not been found to produce meaningful improvements in daily functioning (Wolraich et al., 2019). With respect to behavioral approaches to therapy, the committee reports that although psychopharmacological treatment with stimulants has been found to have a stronger and more immediate effect on the core symptoms of ADHD, parents tend to be more satisfied with behavioral approaches which address both the symptoms and the functions of ADHD behaviors (Wolraich et al., 2019). Furthermore, the positive effects of behavioral treatments tend to persist post-treatment, whereas the positive effects of medication stop as soon as the medication is no longer being taken (Wolraich et al., 2019). Finally, the guidelines concede that skills-based and school-based training interventions have been found to be beneficial for children and adolescents with ADHD (Evans et al., 2018; Evans et al., 2014; Evans et al., 2016; Langberg et al., 2018; Schultz et al., 2017).

Despite the AAP's acknowledgment that certain psychosocial approaches to therapy may be beneficial for the treatment of ADHD in children and adolescents, stimulants are still strongly recommended as the first line of treatment in almost every age group. Even for children under six who cannot be prescribed stimulants with FDA approval, the guidelines encourage clinicians to weigh the potential risks of initiating medication treatment on an off-label basis against the harm that delaying medication treatment may bring.

Of note, the clinical guidelines for the treatment of adult ADHD recommend stimulants and the non-stimulant atomoxetine as first-line interventions as well, followed by the prescription of antidepressants (Post & Kurlansik, 2012; Mészáros et al., 2009). Given that ADHD is one of the most common psychiatric disorders of childhood currently affecting 8.4% of children from two to 17 years of age, almost two-thirds of whom are taking medication to address their symptoms, it is critical for clinical psychologists to be trained in psychopharmacology to be informed and knowledgeable participants in the multidisciplinary care of their child and adolescent clients (Danielson et al., 2018).

In view of psychopharmacology being the primary method of treatment for ADHD in children, and authoritative organizations such as the American Academy of Pediatrics recommending their use, establishing an understanding of the risks that come with taking these medications is vital for both non-prescribing clinicians as well as parents. As with most medications, psychopharmacological treatments for ADHD have a variety of side effects that vary with the class of medication and the individual patient.

Let us begin with the "mechanism of action" – how they work. Stimulant medications' action is to dramatically increase the availability of dopamine and norepinephrine (catecholamines) within the central nervous system. One process for this is blocking "catecholamine transporters." Once dopamine is released into the synapse (space between neurons) to send its signal, the unused neurochemical would be reabsorbed into the presynaptic neuron. This normal reuptake process is enabled through the catecholamine transporters. When the transporter is inhibited (blocked), dopamine and norepinephrine would remain available within the synaptic space longer. For example, Ritalin, as a potent dopamine transporter inhibitor, has been identified to be twice as potent as cocaine (Jackson, 2005). Another process to increase the availability of dopamine is by stimulating the release. Promoting the release of catecholamine further enhances the availability of dopamine and norepinephrine.

Understanding how they "work" also requires an understanding of the potential negative impact, or side-effects, of medication use. The potential adverse effects of ADHD medications should not be taken lightly and must be closely monitored by all members of the ADHD client's care team, including clinical psychologists, as they are likely to be meeting with the client on a more frequent basis compared to the medication-prescribing colleague. Side-effects from stimulant medications are wide-ranging and can impact a variety of systems in a child's developing body.

Table 2. A partial list of adverse effects includes (Elbe, Black, McGrane and Procyshyn, 2019):		
Restlessness	Tics	Dysphoria / sadness
Irritability	Stomach Aches	Cause / worsen psychotic symptoms
Anxiety	Headaches	Obsessive Compulsive Symptoms
Insomnia	Cardiac complications	Weight loss
Anorexia	Growth impact	May cause suicidal ideation
Aggression/hostility	Gastrointestinal distress	
May precipitate manic / hypomanic symptoms	May lower seizure threshold	

While we think of stimulants to be "short-acting" (that is, their effect occurs in a short period of time), discontinuing these medications can indeed create more clinical challenges. For instance:

"Abrupt discontinuation after prolonged use may result in dysphoria, irritability or a rebound in symptoms of ADHD; increase in sleep and appetite ... and if taken in conjunction with an antipsychotic agent, sudden discontinuation of the stimulant may result in the emergence of extra-pyramidal side effects previously masked by the stimulant's anticholinergic properties and competition at the D2 receptors" (Elbe, Black, McGrane & Procyshyn, 2019, p. 30).

Prolonged use is not the only concern. In addition to the effects noted above, animal research has revealed concerning impact on the developing central nervous system in children that are already struggling to function in academic, social, and home settings. For example, research using Adderall in monkeys resulted in "long-lasting behavioral oddities, such as hallucinations, and cognitive impairment" in just six- and twelve-week trials (Higgins, 2009, p. 42).

Research on mice – when comparing methylphenidate versus cocaine exposure over two weeks – demonstrated "cocainelike structural and chemical alterations in the brains of mice given methylphenidate" (Higgins, 2009, 41). Cognitive problems included deficits in working memory, which persisted for years. Another study involving monkeys demonstrated amphetamine-induced brain damage with dosing that mimicked dosing in humans (Higgins, 2009).

It is particularly important for clinical psychologists to be aware of the side effects that these medications may induce because psychologists typically see their patients with greater frequency than psychiatrists and other clinical care providers with prescription privileges. Thus, clinical psychologists have a greater opportunity to monitor, identify, and report potential side effects to other members of the client's care team, who may then choose to titrate the medication dose to achieve maximum benefits with more tolerable side effects.

Moreover, ignorance of potential ADHD medication side effects might lead clinical psychologists to misattribute side-effects in their patients to comorbid diagnoses that the patients may not actually have. Thus, clinical psychologists must be trained in the side effects of psychopharmacological interventions for ADHD to be able to serve their clients ethically and competently.

Given the prevalence and strong recommendations for the use of medications in ADHD, there must be compelling evidence, right? As mentioned above, the largest study examining treatments for ADHD was the MTA Study (Pelham, 1999). Researchers compared behavior modification, to methylphenidate, to combined treatment, to a community control group. While medication continued for the first 14-month period, behavior modification was discontinued after 6 to 9 months. In the short-term, combined treatment, and stimulants alone, outperformed behavior modification, but all groups significantly improved.

As Jackson (2005) details, MTA researchers continued to evaluate treatment trajectory between 14 and 24 months. They examined scores for ADHD symptoms, Oppositional Defiant Disorder symptoms, and Social Skills (all rated by parents and teachers), as well as Wechsler Individual Achievement test of reading, and Negative Parental Discipline score. "On three of the five outcome measures (ADHD symptoms, social skills, and negative parental discipline), *the groups receiving medication demonstrated a deterioration in their condition. In contrast, patients in the behavioral therapy or community comparison groups of the study remained stable*" (Jackson, 2005, p. 276).

Long-term MTA outcomes point to an even more disappointing picture. Six to eight years following the enrollment in the study, "despite initial symptom improvement ... children with combined-type ADHD exhibit significant impairment in adolescence" (Molina et al., 2009, p. 484). Further, "the MTA group as a whole was functioning significantly less well than the non-ADHD classmate sample" (Molina et al., 2009, p. 494) and "children still taking medication by 6 and 8 years fared no better than their nonmedicated counterparts, despite a 41% increase in the average daily dose" (Molina et al., 2009, p. 496).

As ADHD symptoms are often first identified in the school setting, it is likely that stimulant use is driven by the effort to improve functioning in this setting. However, a recent study refutes the overall benefit of medication related to academic outcomes. In a study of 173 children diagnosed with ADHD, medication was seen to have an improvement in "seatwork productivity and classroom behavior" but "there was no detectable effect of medication on learning the material taught during instruction" (Pelham et al., 2022, p. 367).

The urgency for clinical psychologists to be informed on the use and implications of psychopharmacological treatments of ADHD is amplified by the fact that ADHD is a chronic condition (Wolraich et al., 2019). Although the manifestation of symptoms may change as children move into adolescence and adulthood, children diagnosed with ADHD at a young age will typically continue to experience ADHD-related symptoms and impairment into adulthood (Wolraich et al., 2019). As such, it is important to consider which modalities of treatment are most sustainable for long-term use and most effective in addressing the underlying functions of ADHD behaviors. In general, the positive effects of behavioral therapies have been found to persist after treatment, but the positive effects of medication on ADHD symptoms have been found to cease when medications are no longer being taken (Wolraich et al., 2019).

Moreover, the MTA studies were pivotal in exposing the long-term effects of stimulant treatment on ADHD symptoms in children

(Pelham, 1999). They revealed that combined treatments were most effective in reducing symptoms and that pharmacological treatment alone should only be recommended when the provider is "not concerned with their patient's long-term outcomes, which will be unaffected by medication" (Pelham, 1999, p. 989). In other words, long-term benefits related to the reduction of ADHD symptomatology were absent, and long-term, ongoing symptoms persisted for those treated with stimulants and those left untreated (Swanson et al., 2017). One possible explanation for the lack of lasting effects of stimulant treatment is that stimulants may serve to reduce ADHD symptoms but fail to address issues that may be underlying or causing those symptoms.

Moreover, a recent comprehensive review of the literature on the association between ADHD and trauma found that deficits in affect modulation linked to trauma exposure in childhood may exacerbate symptoms typically associated with ADHD (for example, restlessness, poor concentration, inattention, irritability, and functional impairments) and/or create a vulnerability for the development of this disorder (Szymanski et al., 2011). In the context of this obvious lack of empirical clarity regarding the true etiological nature of ADHD, being able to differentiate the impact of trauma from ADHD symptoms is critical as this diagnostic clarification differentially impacts treatment efforts.

Viewed in this light, stimulant treatment may fail to produce lasting effects on ADHD symptoms because it may not address deep-seated issues underlying ADHD symptoms, such as early exposure to trauma (APA, 2022). Given the persistence of ADHD over the lifespan (Wolraich et al., 2019) and the fact that psychopharmacological treatments have not been found to yield long-term effects (Schweren et al., 2019), selecting an exclusively psychopharmacological line of treatment for a chronic case of ADHD may require taking medications for the rest of one's life.

However, such a course of treatment may be complicated by the multitude of contraindications of stimulant use which cause 30% of adult ADHD clients to discontinue taking their medications (Faraone et al., 2004), all the while potentially failing to address underlying issues at the root of clients' symptomology and distress. As part of clinical psychologists' ethical obligation to take reasonable steps to avoid harming their clients, clinicians must be informed enough to consider such factors when referring their clients out for psychopharmacological consultations or working with clients who are also receiving a psychopharmacological course of treatment (APA, 2017).

The important role for psychologists

Optimal outcomes for children with ADHD are lacking. While medications are recommended as the first line of intervention for these 6.2 million children and adolescents diagnosed with ADHD, the American Academy of Pediatrics (AAP) also recommends psychotherapeutic interventions as an additional service that clients with ADHD should receive (Wolraich et al., 2019).

Because psychologists experience significantly more client-contact than other members of the client care team – particularly in comparison to providers with prescription privileges, like psychiatrists and pediatricians – psychologists play a critical role in being able to closely monitor symptom progress or deterioration. In the context of the significant and growing prevalence of ADHD in the United States, the complex and largely unknown nature of this disorder's etiology, and the fact that psychopharmacological interventions are the treatment of choice for ADHD, it is vital that clinical psychologists receive comprehensive education and training in the use and implications of these medications to be best prepared to serve their clients.

A survey of APA Accredited Clinical Psychology doctoral programs in the United States

How prepared are clinical psychologists to serve children with ADHD?

It is clear that clinical psychologists must be educated in psychopharmacology as part of their clinical training to be best prepared to serve children with ADHD. A recent study (Foltz et al., 2022) aimed to quantify how many APA accredited clinical psychology doctoral training programs require coursework in psychopharmacology, with the intention of shedding light on the preparedness of psychologists entering the field.

To address this question, 254 doctoral-level Clinical Psychology programs accredited by the American Psychological Association (APA) in the United States were studied. 70% of the programs were Ph.D. programs and 30% of the programs were Psy.D programs. A confident assessment of the available psychopharmacology classes was acquired of approximately 90% of the sampled programs.

The survey revealed that only 26% of the 254 APA accredited clinical psychology doctoral programs in the United States (or 66 programs) *require* coursework in psychopharmacology. Assuming the first-year cohorts reported remain intact, this translates to 1443 students entering the field from these programs with a foundational education in psychopharmacology.

In the context of the prevalence of ADHD, its persistence across the lifespan, and the practice guidelines for the treatment of children and adolescents with ADHD which prioritize psychopharmacological treatment interventions, the paucity of future clinical psychologists with formal training in psychopharmacology is alarming.

Although it would seem imperative for clinical psychologists to be educated and trained on the various implications surrounding the psychopharmacological treatment of children and adolescents with ADHD, including the risks of medication use in certain age groups, the multitude of side effects of ADHD medications, and their limited effect on long-term outcomes, the reality is that less than half of doctoral students in the United States will graduate with adequate preparation to serve as informed care providers of children and adolescents with ADHD.

Licensed clinical psychologists play a critical role in (1) assessing for and diagnosing ADHD, (2) providing treatment recommendations and referrals, and (3) monitoring client progress through their frequent and consistent psychotherapy sessions. In this way, clinical psychologists are in the best position to monitor side-effects of prescribed stimulants in conjunction with symptom improvement or deterioration, given that they see their clients more frequently and consistently than psychiatrists and pediatricians.

Moreover, as the only party in the clinical care provider team who lacks a financial stake in the prescription of medications, clinical psychologists have a professional and ethical obligation to consider the implications around the psychopharmacological treatment of ADHD prior to recommending that their clients engage in a medication consultation with a prescribing treatment provider.

In the context of the 2.5-fold increase of amphetamine use in the United States from 2006 to 2016 (Piper et al., 2018), the need for impartial treatment providers to make informed and unbiased recommendations is becoming increasingly urgent. It is deeply troubling how few of our future clinical psychologists will be entering the field in a few short years without adequate preparation to serve clients with ADHD, one of the most diagnosed psychiatric disorders among children and adolescents (Song et al., 2021).

The responsibility to address this gaping hole in the training of clinical psychology doctoral students falls on the American Psychological Association. We call upon the APA to include psychopharmacology coursework in the required curriculum of APA accredited clinical psychology doctoral programs to ensure that our future psychologists are best prepared to serve children and adolescents with ADHD effectively, competently, and ethically.

For too long, parents and providers have been overly confident in the medication treatments of ADHD. Claims about the neurobiology of ADHD, while commonly touted as fact, have yet to be established. Medication treatments, while considered the frontline approach, can only sustain short-term gains. And while many have seen the initial response to medication as "proof" of this neurodevelopmental condition, the subsequent deterioration in treatment response is too often attributed to "difficult to treat" or "non-responder" patients to our best treatments. Clearly, our best treatments are not good enough. Our children and families deserve better. Psychologists should take an active role in re-evaluating what works, and what doesn't, and strive toward innovative modifications to our 'best practices.

References

American Psychological Association. (2017). Ethical principles of psychologists and code of conduct (2002, amended effective June 1, 2010, and January 1, 2017). Retrieved from: http://www.apa.org/ethics/code/index.html

APA-Accredited Programs, Clinical Psychology. American Psychological Association. (2021). Retrieved from https://accreditation.apa.org/

Corrigan, M. and Whitaker, R. (2017). Lancet Psychiatry Needs to Retract the ADHD-Enigma Study. MIA Report: Authors' conclusion that individuals with ADHD have smaller brains is belied by their own data. Retrieved from: https://www.madinamerica.com/2017/04/lancet-psychiatry-needs-to-retract-the-adhd-enigma-study/

Cortese, S., Adamo, N., Giovane, C., Mohr-Jensen, C., Hayes, A., Carucci, S. et al. (2018). Comparative efficacy and tolerability of medications for attention-deficit hyperactivity disorder in children, adolescents, and adults: a systematic review and network meta-analysis. *Lancet Psychiatry, August.* Published online. doi: 10.1016/S2215-0366(18)30269-4

Danielson, Bitsko, R. H., Ghandour, R. M., Holbrook, J. R., Kogan, M. D., & Blumberg, S. J. (2018). Prevalence of parent-reported ADHD diagnosis and associated treatment among U.S. children and adolescents, 2016. *Journal of Clinical Child and Adolescent Psychology,* 47(2), 199–212. https://doi.org/10.1080/15374416.2017.1417860

Diagnostic and statistical manual of mental disorders: DSM-5-TR (5th edition, text revision.). (2022). Washington, DC: American Psychiatric Association Publishing.

Diagnostic and statistical manual of mental disorders: DSM-5. (5th ed.). (2013). American Psychiatric Association.

Diagnostic and statistical manual of mental disorders: DSM-IV-TR. (4th ed., text revision.). (2000). American Psychiatric Association.

Elbe, D., Black, T., McGrane, I., and Procyshyn, R. (Eds). (2019). Clinical Handbook of Psychotropic Drugs for Children and Adolescents. Boston MA: Hogrefe Publishing.

Evans, S. W., Langberg, J. M., Egan T., & Molitor, S. J. (2014). Middle school-based and high school-based interventions for adolescents with ADHD. *Child and Adolescent Psychiatric Clinics of North America,* 24(4), 699-715. https://doi.org/10.1016/j.c.hc.2014.05.004

Evans, Langberg, J. M., Schultz, B. K., Vaughn, A., Altaye, M., Marshall, S. A., & Zoromski, A. K. (2016). Evaluation of a school-based treatment program for young adolescents with ADHD. *Journal of Consulting and Clinical Psychology, 84*(1), 15–30. https://doi.org/10.1037/ccp0000057

Evans, S.W., Owens, J. S., Wymbs, B. T., & Ray, A. R. (2018). Evidence-based psychosocial treatments for children and adolescents with attention-deficit/hyperactivity disorder. *Journal of Clinical Child and Adolescent Psychology, 47*(2), 157–198. https://doi.org/10.1080/15374416.2017.1390757

Faraone, Spencer, T. J., Montano, C. B., & Biederman, J. (2004). Attention-deficit/hyperactivity disorder in adults: A survey of current practice in psychiatry and primary care. *Archives of Internal Medicine (1960), 164*(11), 1221–1226. https://doi.org/10.1001/archinte.164.11.1221

Foltz, R., Fogel, K., Kaeley, A., Kupchan, J., Mills, A., Murray, K., Pope, A., Rahman, H., and Rubright, C. (2022). Addressing the Psychopharmacology Training Gap in Accredited Clinical Psychology Programs. [Manuscript submitted for publication]. Department of Clinical Psychology, The Chicago School of Professional Psychology, Chicago Campus.

Greenhill, Kollins, S., Abikoff, H., McCracken, J., Riddle, M., Swanson, J., McGough, J., Wigal, S., Wigal, T., Vitiello, B., Skrobala, A., Posner, K., Ghuman, J., Cunningham, C., Davies, M., Chuang, S., & Cooper, T. (2006). Efficacy and safety of immediate-release methylphenidate treatment for preschoolers with ADHD. *Journal of the American Academy of Child and Adolescent Psychiatry, 45*(11), 1284–1293. https://doi.org/10.1097/01.chi.0000235077.326613.61

Greenhill, L. L., Posner, K., Vaughan, B. S., & Kratochvil. (2008). Attention deficit hyperactivity disorder in preschool children. *Child and Adolescent Psychiatric Clinics of North America, 17*(2), 347-366. https://doi.org/10.1016/j.chc.2007.11.004

Higgins, E. (2009). Do ADHD drugs take a toll on the brain? *Scientific American Mind,* July/August.

Hoogman, M., Bralten, J., Hibar, D., Mennes, M., Zwiers, M., Schweren, L., et al. (2017). Subcortical brain volume differences in participants with attention deficit hyperactivity disorder in children and adults: a cross-sectional mega-analysis. *Lancet Psychiatry*, 4(4). 310-319.

Harstad, E., Shults, J., Barbaresi, W., Bax, A., Cacia, J. et al. (2021) a2-Adrenergic Agonists or Stimulants for Preschool-age Children with Attention-Deficit / Hyperactivity Disorder. *JAMA*, 325(20). 2067-2075. doi:10.1001/jama.2021.6118

Jackson, G. (2005). Rethinking Psychiatric Drugs: A guide for informed consent. Bloomington, Indiana: Authorhouse.

Jensen, P., Arnold, L., Swanson, J., Vitiello, B., Abikoff, H., et al. (2007). 3-year follow-up of the NIMH MTA study. *Journal of the American Academy of Child and Adolescent Psychiatry, 46*(8). 989-1002.

Langberg, J. M., Dvorsky, M. R., Molitor, S. J., Bourchtein, E., Eddy, L. D., Smith, Z. R., Oddo, L. E., & Eadeh, H. M. (2018). Overcoming the research-to-practice gap: A randomized trial with two brief homework and organization interventions for students with ADHD as implemented by school mental health providers. *Journal of Consulting and Clinical Psychology, 86*(1), 39–55. https://doi.org/10.1037/ccp0000265

Leo, J., Lacasse, J. R. (2015). *The New York Times* and the ADHD epidemic. *Society (New Brunswick)*, 52(1), 3–8. https://doi.org/10.1007/s12115-014-9851-5

Mészáros, Czobor, P., Bálint, S., Komlósi, S., Simon, V., & Bitter, I. (2009). Pharmacotherapy of adult attention deficit hyperactivity disorder (ADHD): A meta-analysis. *The International Journal of Neuropsychopharmacology, 12*(8), 1137–1147. https://doi.org/10.1017/S1461145709990198

Molina, B., Hinshaw, S., Swanson, J., Arnold, L., Vitiello, B., et al. (2009). The MTA at 8 Years: Prospective follow-up of children treated for combined-type ADHD in a multisite study. *Journal of the American Academy of Child & Adolescent Psychiatry, 48*(5). 484-500. doi: 10.1097/chil.obo13e31819c23d0

Pelham. (1999). The NIMH multimodal treatment study for attention-deficit hyperactivity disorder: Just say yes to drugs alone? *Canadian Journal of Psychiatry, 44*(10), 981–990. https://doi.org/10.1177/070674379904401004

Pelham, W., Altszuler, A., Merrill, B., Raiker, J., Macphee, F. et al. (2022). The effect of stimulant medication on the learning of academic curricula in children with ADHD: A randomized crossover study. *Journal of Consulting Psychology, 90*(5). 367-380. doi: 10.1037/ccp0000725

Piper, Ogden, C. L., Simoyan, O. M., Chung, D. Y., Caggiano, J. F., Nichols, S. D., & McCall, K. L. (2018). Trends in use of prescription stimulants in the United States and Territories, 2006 to 2016. PloS One, 13(11), e0206100–e0206100. https://doi.org/10.1371/journal.pone.0206100

Post, & Kurlansik, S. L. (2012). Diagnosis and management of attention-deficit/hyperactivity disorder in adults. *American Family Physician, 85*(9), 890–896.

Schultz, B. K., Evans, S. W., Langberg, J. M., & Schoemann, A. M. (2017). Outcomes for adolescents who comply with long-term psychosocial treatment for ADHD. *Journal of Consulting and Clinical Psychology, 85*(3), 250–261. https://doi.org/10.1037/ccp0000172

Schweren, L., Hoekstra, P., Marloes, v. L., Oosterlaan, J., Nanda Lambregts-Rommelse, Buitelaar, J., Franke, B., & Hartman, C. (2019). Long-term effects of stimulant treatment on ADHD symptoms, social–emotional functioning, and cognition. *Psychological Medicine, 49*(2), 217-223. https://doi.org/10.1017/S0033291718000545

Song, Zha, M., Yang, Q., Zhang, Y., Li, X., & Rudan, I. (2021). The prevalence of adult attention-deficit hyperactivity disorder: A global systematic review and meta-analysis. *Journal of Global Health, 11*, 04009–04009. https://doi.org/10.7189/jogh.11.04009

Swanson, Arnold, L. E., Molina, B. S., Sibley, M. H., Hechtman, L. T., Hinshaw, S. P., Abikoff, H. B., Stehli, A., Owens, E. B., Mitchell, J. T., Nichols, Q., Howard, A., Greenhill, L. L., Hoza, B., Newcorn, J. H., Jensen,

P. S., Vitiello, B., Wigal, T., Epstein, J. N., ... Stern, K. (2017). Young adult outcomes in the follow-up of the multimodal treatment study of attention-deficit/hyperactivity disorder: Symptom persistence, source discrepancy, and height suppression. *Journal of Child Psychology and Psychiatry, 58*(6), 663–678. https://doi.org/10.1111/jcpp.12684

Szymanski, Sapanski, L., & Conway, F. (2011). Trauma and ADHD - association or diagnostic confusion? A clinical perspective. *Journal of Infant, Child, and Adolescent Psychotherapy, 10*(1), 51–59. https://doi.org/10.1080/15289168.2011.575704

Thomas, R., Sanders, S., Doust, J., Beller, E., & Glasziou, P. (2015). Prevalence of attention-deficit/hyperactivity disorder: A systematic review and meta-analysis. Pediatrics, 135(4), 994-1001

Visser, S. N., Danielson, M. L., Bitsko, R. H., Holbrook, J. R., Kogan, M. D., Ghandour, R. M., Perou, R., & Blumberg, S. J. (2014). Trends in the parent-report of health care provider-diagnosed and medicated attention-deficit/hyperactivity disorder: United States, 2003-2011. *Journal of the American Academy of Child and Adolescent Psychiatry, 53*(1), 34–46. e2. https://doi.org/10.1016/j.jaac.2013.09.001

Wolraich, Hagan, J. F., Allan, C., Chan, E., Davison, D., Earls, M., Evans, S. W., Flinn, S. K., Froehlich, T., Frost, J., Holbrook, J. R., Lehmann, C. U., Lessin, H. R., Okechukwu, K., Pierce, K. L., Winner, J. D., Zurhellen, W., & Hagan, J. F. (2019). Clinical practice guideline for the diagnosis, evaluation, and treatment of attention-deficit/hyperactivity disorder in children and adolescents. Pediatrics (Evanston), 144(4). https://doi.org/10.1542/peds.2019-2528

Medicalization's Opportunity Costs: A Critique of the Societal Acceptance of ADHD

Anne Zimmerman

Attention spans vary widely. So does energy – the high-octane kid looks a bit different from the book worm. The psych industries have pathologized attention span, with increasingly broad criteria for ADHD.

Critiques of ADHD and the psych industries vary considerably in their identification of what has gone wrong and why it is wrong. I focus here on opportunity costs: the ways in which pathologizing behavior and treating it in the psych and medical arena is a distraction from societal solutions to behavioral issues.

ADHD is a product of the psych industries and the pharmaceutical industry that was spurred on by social constructs including social support for the diagnosed. To clarify, I do not find behavioral problems to be a hoax. Parents and teachers experience great difficulty with the behavioral problems of their children or students. But ADHD is classic disease creep, or perhaps, more accurately "disorder" creep.

The DSM-5 describes behavior that is subjective and quite mainstream. I shy away from the word normal here, as so many kids fidget and fail to complete tasks and engage in many of the items

---

Anne Zimmerman, JD, MS is an author, editor, and the founder of *Modern Bioethics*.

on the ADHD checklist that it would be a mere judgment to draw a line between normal and abnormal. The psych industries are more comfortable with line drawing than I am. If a line is to be drawn, and a legitimate disability recognized, the criteria should be stricter and limited to severe cases. As is, the DSM-5 definition is too broad, based only on judgments, and not grounded in science.

There is buy-in from a complex web of institutions that follow the psych and pharmaceutical industries. General practitioners buy in, and they prescribe ADHD medications. Insurance buys in and covers the medicines using diagnosis codes. Schools buy in and teachers refer children through the counseling or nurses' office. Testing organizations like the College Board and the Educational Testing Bureau buy in by allotting extra time for test-taking; and many parents buy in, with expectations of anything from better grades or test scores to an easier, more manageable parenting job, or merely because they follow doctors' recommendations.

The buy-in is happening at a personal level, case-by-case, in a clinical, educational, or social setting. But in the larger landscape of society, medicalization is changing how problems are approached, affecting the whole population. There is societal good in decreasing medicalization and taking on the societal deficits that are environmental, socioeconomic, and ecological that influence how society reacts to children's behaviors and supports children. But the clinical practice of pathologizing and prescribing as a first-line treatment, sometimes accompanied by some classroom accommodations or parental training, is problematic and diverts attention from much-needed change.

Taking a pill, the simplistic approach, has placed behavioral blame on the child exclusively and imposed a remedy on only the child. Properly contextualized, highly active children require patient parents, teachers, and doctors, strategies for coping and improving behaviors, and personal accountability for behavior as children mature. Societal patience is waning and being replaced by a drug, preventing parents from allowing children time to outgrow or resolve childish behavior. The many public policy and institutional strategies like more time outdoors, longer recess, healthier diets, smaller class sizes, and, in some cases, more individual attention, are more difficult to achieve. They require hard work, tax dollars, hands-on parents, and a shift in priorities. But a simple pill—that is tempting. And the pill affects the child, physically, mentally, socially, etc. but it does not change the environment, the ecosystem that makes it more difficult to let kids be kids.

Medicalization, looking at social problems through the lens of medicine (Lantz, Lichtenstein, and Pollack), leads to over-diagnosing, overprescribing, and over-assisting. In the United States, it threatens to change the fabric of classrooms and the development of social skills, and it creates demands on public services. Medicalization jeopardizes the role of science in society and the public's inclination to trust science. Yet somehow much of the public is accepting of (and complicit in) defining ADHD as an illness (or disorder) in need of medication.

"...[M]edicine transformed into a dominant form of regulation of social life (Zola 1972): it defines, normalizes, disciplines and controls people's lives. It is a source of power and is strictly related to the policy of the government and becomes a basis for biopolitics." (Domaradzki, 2013) Perhaps accepting medicine's influence even when it is outside the bounds of the accepted scientific method, as with the ADHD checklist, has begun to feel mandatory, and medicine has permeated society so much that it has many missionaries for its cause.

A look at how science earns public trust reveals that the trust may be in the scientific method as well as in the scientist (Shapin, 1995). But with ADHD there is not scientific precision "verified in a medical laboratory" (Macht, 2017, p. 91), and the definitions are subject to change, as seen from the time of Frederick Sill in 1902, through the designation "hyperkinetic reaction to childhood" noted in the 1960s, to the DSM-5, based on opinions and judgments rather than biological features or scientific discoveries.

The lens of medicine is simply the wrong approach to much of the behavior deemed symptoms of ADHD.

Conflict of interest and the numbers

Almost ten percent of children have been diagnosed with ADHD, including 15 percent of high school students. Data differs slightly by source, but about 62 to 65 percent of those diagnosed take medicine for their ADHD (CDC, 2022). The global ADHD therapeutics market was $29.56 billion in 2022. The market forecasters note that the COVID-19 pandemic is expected to increase the demand for ADHD drugs (Market Data Forecast, 2022). The American Psychiatric Association receives almost 30 percent of its funding from the pharmaceutical industry. ADHD advocacy groups including CHADD receive significant pharma money as well (Wired, 2015). It has long been common for patient advocacy groups to be funded by pharma (Rose, 2013). The psychiatrists contributing to the DSM-5 had financial ties to industry (Cosgrove and Krimsky, 2012).

During the COVID-19 pandemic, psychiatric appointments held virtually led to a new business: platforms designed to dispense psychiatry and stimulants. Cerebral is an example of an online platform for those seeking mental health treatment. One former employee disclosed that the company encouraged its employees to prescribe stimulants to 100 percent of the clients (Mosendz and Melby, 2022). Their advertising practices bait customers and dangle drugs as easily accessible.

In the case of Cerebral, a customer thought her care coordinator, Eileen Davis, was an actual person working on coordinating her care. Really Eileen Davis was a made-up name assigned to hundreds of care coordinators so that they could interchangeably handle customer concerns and coordinate online visits designed to propel sales. Customers who had the sense that, like in some medical offices, a care coordinator had been assigned to their case and understood their symptoms and medical history were wrong. (Mosendz and Melby.)

Many ADHD-diagnosed children take stimulants. The side effects of Adderall and Ritalin include trouble sleeping, loss of appetite, dry mouth, anxiety, increased heart rate, irritability, headache, and dizziness. Some severe side effects of Ritalin are cardiovascular reactions, including sudden death, stroke, and heart attack, increased blood pressure, increased heart rate (tachycardia), psychiatric adverse reactions, including worsening of a pre-existing psychiatric condition, development of new psychotic or manic symptoms, sustained and sometimes painful erections in males, poor circulation, including Raynaud's phenomenon, long-term suppression of growth and weight loss in pediatric patients, and potential for abuse and dependence (Eagle, 2020). It is clear that the harms may outweigh the benefits (Kazda, et al., 2021).

Diagnosis and treatment: The DSM-5 and professional recommendations

This section provides background on the status quo, i.e., treating the person rather than altering the society to accommodate typical and atypical behaviors of childhood. This individualistic approach to ADHD benefits pediatricians, the psych industries, and the pharmaceutical industry financially, to the tune of billions, although certainly there is not consensus in the medical community and some doctors are hesitant to prescribe.

The DSM-5 defines three types of ADHD:

- Combined Presentation: if enough symptoms of both criteria inattention and hyperactivity-impulsivity were present for the past 6 months

- Predominantly Inattentive Presentation: if enough symptoms of inattention, but not hyperactivity-impulsivity, were present for the past six months

- Predominantly Hyperactive-Impulsive Presentation: if enough symptoms of hyperactivity-impulsivity, but not inattention, were present for the past six months. (American Psychiatric Association: Diagnostic and Statistical Manual of Mental Disorders (DSM-5))

The DSM-5 lists a host of subjective attributes like getting out of one's seat when one is expected to remain seated, trouble waiting their turn, failing to finish tasks, and often loses things. These do not sound medical to me. Five or six of the circumstances listed would lead to a positive diagnosis, depending on the child's age. For the diagnosis, the behaviors are meant to be persistent and interfere with schoolwork or social functioning and not be explained by other mental or psychiatric disorders. Even the word "diagnosis" sounds misplaced as subjective observers would merely use their personal judgment (Cooper, 2004).

The American Association of Pediatrics (AAP) recommends evaluating anyone with "academic or behavioral problems" and showing "inattention, hyperactivity, or impulsivity." (CDC, 2022). That is so broad as to be unhelpful. The recommendation for those ages four to six is parent training or classroom interventions prior to trying medication, but for ages six to 18, the AAP guidelines, repeated by the CDC, recommend stimulants as a first-line treatment along with parent training and classroom intervention. There is evidence that medicines are prescribed to many children as young as three despite the recommendation to try other interventions first. (Schwartz, 2016; Cha, May 3, 2016).

Environmental causes for behavior patterns are missing completely from the DSM-5 and the American Association of Pediatrics' recommendations (and the CDC website, which simply sets forth the AAP recommendations and the DSM-5 criteria). There are known relationships between environmental toxins and impulsivity, mood, and behavior. Philip Landrigan was a pioneer in the field of children's environmental medicine and noted the effect of many pollutants, notably lead, on children's ability to focus and learn. He theorized and showed the link between exposure to chemicals and attention span and behavior (Landrigan, et al., 2002; See also Landrigan, 2011.)

Manuel Vallée asserts that environmental medicine is absent in clinical recommendations for two reasons: first, a turf war over medical jurisdiction that led psychiatry to emphasize pharmaceuticals and led pediatrics to move into psychiatric care; and second, ideological devotion to the paradigm of biomedicine that identifies disease and uses medicine to treat over the old-school public health paradigm that spoke to poverty and other social ills that result in poor health (Vallée, 2013.)

Additionally, the guidelines do not include the nonpharmaceutical solutions to undesirable behavior like diet and exercise that improve behavior, ability to learn, and overall health. A biomedical approach to prevention, wellness, and to resolving problematic behaviors found on the ADHD checklist includes addressing nutritional deficiencies, boosting the immune system and addressing chronic unwanted immune responses, developing healthy gut flora, and addressing high levels of toxic metals like mercury and lead (Hyman, 2015).

The teachers and school employees recommending evaluation and the professionals making ADHD diagnoses use peer groups for comparisons. People who are the youngest in their grades have more diagnoses (Macht, 2017, 172; Chen, et al., 2016; and Cha, March 14, 2016). The expectation should be that they are less mature, for example, than someone in their class who is nearly one year older, especially in younger years. Some diseases do make age-based comparisons, an important early detection tool, but in ADHD the comparison to others rises in importance in the absence of biological markers.

Most importantly, the clinical protocols ignore the causes and remedies rooted in society. ""While the physician may be 'doing good,' on an individual basis, they note, by enhancing the child's performance with medication, he or she may unwittingly be contributing to a 'social bad.' It's a well-known conundrum of child psychiatry that even an effective psychopharmacological intervention may permit a poor environment to continue or worsen. When American doctors distribute fifteen tons of Ritalin to children in just one year, are they accepting and abetting the fact of overcrowded classrooms, overwhelmed parents and teachers, and unreasonable standards?"" (Macht, p. 179, quoting Diller, L.H. (1998), p. 330, referring to Carol Whalen and Barbara Hencker.)

Logical fallacy: If medicine works, then the problem for which it works is of a medical nature

The definition of ADHD encompasses the normal. As stimulants improve attention span, their effect on the checklist in the behavioral questionnaire that determines ADHD is positive. It can and does address the behavior albeit for a short time as people develop tolerance and need higher doses and eventually effectiveness wanes. Similarly, stimulants would improve attention span and motivate those without an ADHD diagnosis. Stimulants stimulate. It is simply what they do in the short run regardless of who takes them.

Stimulants are in many respects an enhancement. The language of allowing people to fulfill their intellectual potential is highly misleading. It has the connotation of leveling a playing field or repairing a deficit. But at any level of natural academic achievement, any person may feel entitled to stimulants to unlock their potential: potential to accomplish more increases with the drug. Bringing a C student to a B or an A student to an A+ can be cloaked as helping the student meet their potential. Being a C student is not a sickness! (In the case of an F student who cannot function in classroom or social settings at all, there is likely a better case for some type of intervention.)

Stimulants may make people do more in a short time, or hyper-concentrate, but they would do that for anyone, not just those deemed to have ADHD. It is difficult to argue that they are an enhancement for some people and not for others. ADHD is distinctly different from strep throat or cancer where the remedy would likely be quite detrimental to someone without the disease. Here, the so-called remedy would have the same pros and cons for anyone. Allowing the mild and moderate cases access to stimulants is a slippery slope. As the line is pushed toward including more and more people in the ADHD sphere, more drugs are prescribed under the cloak of validity.

Society's willingness to tolerate or embrace enhancement and expand the definition of a disorder should be critically explored as the neurotechnology frontier will bring more questions about the blurred line between treatment and enhancement. Many bioethicists argue for equal access to drugs and technologies and for insurance coverage (for example, Yuste, et al., 2021). To me, their argument is stronger for treatments than enhancements.

Stimulants and extra time: Two sides of the same coin

Part of the diagnosis is that the behavior affects performance in school. Some parents feel justified in giving their children stimulants because of the DSM-5, the advice of their pediatrician or child psychiatrist, and the many other families approaching ADHD with the same medicine. It has been normalized. The more popular ADHD treatment is, the fewer people question its purpose and validity. They have normalized something akin to an athlete taking steroids. The kids take stimulants daily to help them study and take tests, especially college entrance exams like the SAT and ACT, and, in wealthy areas, even prep school entrance exams like the SSAT and the ISEE.

The U.S. News and World Report college rankings system (the rankings) designed in 1982 has influenced college admissions to the detriment of colleges and students. Rankings stigmatize low-ranked colleges leading some parents and students to overemphasize the importance of a high-ranked college and to lose sight of which characteristics feed the rankings. College rankings have changed how colleges recruit and operate. They play to the rankings criteria. An algorithm that is highly dependent on SAT scores for deciding a school's ranking has led students to hyper focus on SAT scores.

Colleges have kowtowed to rankings criteria, and students followed suit. But the rankings do not measure how much students learn at any given college (O'Neil, 2016). Rankings have led colleges to exaggerate SAT scores, to supply false data, and to have students retake the test after being admitted (O'Neil, 2016). While colleges collectively tried to improve the criteria that they had control over to move up in the rankings, they juggled the factors, leading to even more pressure on some people to score well to outweigh those accepted with lower scores.

Being selective is itself a rankings criterion. That makes colleges reject highly qualified students so that their ratio of how many accepted students choose to attend is higher. That interferes with the ability to predict reliable safety schools. The rankings fail to account for college tuition costs and measures of personal success (O'Neil, 2016). I do not challenge grades and scores as admissions factors; I find them very important. Learning at an appropriate pace with a cohort of students is imperative, but the rankings do not measure how well matched any candidate is to the teaching style or rigor, other than to technically note the graduation rate. I question the idea that a few elite colleges provide the best learning experiences for everyone. Struggling to keep up with college curricula that are too intense leads to the continuation of stimulant use at the college level, and fuels anxiety.

The nature of the rat race of college admissions has changed. Parents and students are more focused on status arguably than ever before. Stimulants, extra time on the test, and cheating, as evidenced by the college admissions scandals revealed in recent years, are proof that it is status rather than love of learning and the hope of academic rigor that attracts many students. It is credentialism over substance. ADHD enables parents in the cutthroat environment. The ethical difference between bribing a coach, having an imposter take an SAT, and drugging a child for the sake of bringing out the child's "true intellect" is difficult to pinpoint.

Without doctors, the diagnoses and stimulants would take on a different ethical appearance and might appear more like cheating and bribing. Furthermore, if the parents provided Red Bull, caffeine pills, or cocaine to achieve the focus and alertness, they would be criticized, and in the case of cocaine, arrested. The distinction is that doctors prescribe the stimulants, thereby validating their use and absolving parents of accountability. And it is not just parents.

Students themselves buy "smart drugs" on the internet (Cadwalladr, 2015) or get Adderall and Ritalin through friends with prescriptions (Talbot, M. 2009; Woods, 2009).

That diagnosis provides relief from "mother-blaming culture" is an example of a critical explanation for the rise of ADHD diagnoses (see Sammi Timimi, p. 97), and explains the willingness of mothers to go along. The theory is that the psychiatric industry essentially relieves the feelings of guilt and failure that mothers experience when their children are not meeting societal behavior standards. Mothers may also feel responsible for their child's inability to reach educational aspirations.

People generally want opportunity for themselves and their children. Striving for academic perfection can come at too high a cost. The ways in which society supports opportunity influence outcomes. Improving resilience may be better than treating people like machines meant to take in and relay information. The Americans with Disabilities Act (ADA) also validates the ADHD diagnosis. Formalities like diagnosis, prescription, and ADA accommodations make ADHD sound distinctly medical. Under the ADA, accommodations are mandatory, all under the guise of a level playing field. That creates incentives to get the label, take advantage of extra time, and then apply to schools without disclosure that extra time was taken on a standardized test.

From an ethics perspective, the use of extra time on tests for other societal reasons would be distinctly different. Some of the test optional schools place SAT testing in the realm of social justice and want to be sure that those without tutors and prep schools have equal access to the college. In some cases, extra time could arguably level a difference in access to high quality early education if it could be achieved without a diagnosis. Test optional approaches eliminate that need and make sense for schools that do not believe test scores should limit admissions opportunity.

Medical cultural authority: How can so many professionals and parents buy into widespread ADHD?

Speculation about the increase in ADHD is wide-ranging. The DSM-5 criteria are much broader; society is arguably more stressful, although medicalizing behavior serves to divert attention from relieving stress. None of the cultural explanations add up or seem more plausible than the general medicalized ideology, financial motivations of pharma, and the broad definition that includes so many normal childhood behaviors.

Industries that disrupt attention

In addition to the education, pharmaceutical, and psych sectors, the tech, gaming, social media, and advertising industries work against attention span. ADHD is linked to digital media use (Ra, et al. 2018). Endless scroll is an ethical problem, as it will offer blips that children quickly skim or click through. Concerned organizations have proposed limiting infinite scrolling as a recommended public policy. For example, see the Policy Reforms page on the Center for Humane Technology website (https://www.humanetech.com/policy-reforms). And compulsive behavior draws people to screens (Marvin, 2018). That compulsiveness can be misinterpreted as ADHD. Scholars note the negative impact of constantly shifting attention (Rosen and Gazzaley, 2016). The tech industry has significantly affected attention span and attention choice, making it difficult to interrupt people engaged in scrolling their social media.

Ads for ADHD medications on TikTok purposely blur the line between enhancement and treatment. The ads highlight improved focus rather than suggesting only those with deficits would need the drugs. Some of the ads even offer a very simple approach to obtaining the medicines: an online form and online appointment. (Wayt, 2022).

Opportunity costs: Neglecting the social causes, personal benefits, and realities of an array of behaviors

Pathologizing and medicalization pose two distinct sets of ethical dilemmas: first, potential and demonstrated harm from the diagnosis and intervention (for example, the side effects of stimulants); and second, the harm caused by forgoing a different path. Here, I am focusing on the second. Opportunity cost is "the loss of potential gain from other alternatives when one alternative is chosen." (Oxford Languages). To set opportunity cost into the language of ethics, doctors have obligations to do good and avoid harm and there are standards by which they achieve that, for example, the demand that they consider the best interests of the child.

Additionally, societal considerations look at what is lost or compromised when the medicalized path is taken. But the deeper issue is not just what these opportunity costs are, it is the ethical significance of forgoing them. It is arguable that forgoing a societal benefit to help an individual case is justified, and that a doctor's duty is to the patient, not the public. But the clash between the social sciences and medicine goes largely unresolved. Outside the doctor-patient relationship, medicalization leads to the neglect of policies, actions, and solutions that exist outside of the typical diagnose-and-treat paradigm.

The personal opportunity costs

Resilience. Improving each child's resilience, while not a medical problem, is important to success. Within the doctor-patient relationship, if a recommendation or treatment plan might interfere with resilience, that must be included in any analysis of the harms and benefits of medication. If the ADHD label absolves a child or parents of accountability, that itself might undermine resilience.

One way to develop resilience is allowing the child to outgrow behavioral patterns, learn new ones, and mature without medical intervention. Problem solving and emotional intelligence come with experiences and life lessons. There are risks associated with not problem solving independently in social settings. By leaning on medications and stressing the importance of classroom time, schools may be aggravating behavioral problems. The cognitive immaturity hypothesis suggests that some traits, like overconfidence, that lead to poor judgments, have a developmental benefit (Pellegrini and Bohn, 14). Rather than cuing a child to change behavior, allowing children to play independently leads children to develop confidence.

ADHD medicines meant to improve focus negatively impact free and creative time. Children return from breaks from organized learning more attentive (Pellegrini and Bohn, 2005, p. 15). Many organizations and the American Association of Pediatrics oppose denying recess as a form of punishment and some states prohibit denying recess as punishment (Jarrett, 2019) yet the practice persists, leaving those whose behavior and attention span would benefit from recess worse off.

Social cues. Another sacrificed benefit is the social cues a child learns from adults. Adults teach children to expand their attention span little by little, to sit a few minutes longer each day, and that they inevitably will have times in life where their behavior must conform to some degree with societal expectations. Adults can model the behavior they wish to instill.

When adults blame the ADHD, they react in various ways. They often become accepting of almost all the behavior rather than correcting behavior that is not appropriate. They also may give the child special treatment, which has pros and cons, and can result in the child being removed from the classroom. When adults ask whether the child remembered to take his medication, they teach the child that the behavioral situations are completely out of the child's control — they are not availing the ADHD child of the same adult reactions, punishments, and recommendations that the non-diagnosed children get. They are perhaps learning that they are helpless and need medicine to concentrate.

Creativity. There is a noted trade-off between focus and creativity. Martha Farah, a University of Pennsylvania cognitive neuroscientist, said, "I'm a little concerned that we could be raising a generation of very focused accountants." (Talbot, 2009). There are not enough studies that quantify what lost creativity might look like to society in the long run. The ability to focus and take in more information may leave less time for creating new thoughts and solving problems creatively. Stimulants may dampen the best traits of a highly creative problem solver. In the long run, they may limit opportunity as people develop more sameness in their thinking and in deciding which tasks are important to concentrate on.

Diet and exercise. Failure to address environmental factors like diet and exercise is an ethical lapse. Healthy diets and exercise contribute to whole body health. Mental and emotional health are tied to healthy gut flora, for example. Do we owe children the functional medicine approach to ADHD symptoms? I argue there is an ethical responsibility to address behavioral problems with diet before medicines. And if a biological cause is identified, it can be approached using diet and lifestyle first (Hyman, 2008). Diet and exercise have the added benefits of long-term disease prevention. There is a correlation between obesity and ADHD. Resolving the obesity through a healthy whole foods diet could be a key to relieving the behaviors deemed ADHD.

The child's home environment. In one vignette, Sammi Timimi describes a case of a child whose teacher's first response to a bad day was to ask the child whether he had taken his medication. The child had been on Ritalin for years and the effects were wearing off, so his dose was higher than the maximum approved dose. Once alternative theories about the child's behavior emerged, new ways to help him were proposed. An important factor in the child's life was that his father had been incarcerated. As a result of his incarceration, he withdrew himself whenever he felt angry so that he would not lose his temper in public, and perhaps risk another arrest. Similarly, the parents kept the child home on days when the child seemed most rambunctious so that the child would not be put in the position to be punished or to disrupt classes. The father's need to manage his own behavior informed how the parents dealt with the child (Timimi, 2002, 116-120). In this example, the child was somewhat a victim of the father's past trauma and fears, which led the parents to limit the child and cater to the ADHD diagnosis.

Societal opportunity costs

Across society, public policy and public health policy have the power to improve societal conditions, benefiting children. The failure to improve public policy once children are directed toward the psych industries and, often, medication has opportunity costs. Here are some of the missed opportunities:

Investment in play and free time. Nonacademic time during the school day—more recess—is imperative to childhood development. More parks, more time outside, and safer neighborhoods to enjoy walking and experiencing society are key lifestyle improvements for adults and children (Cecil, 2018).

When ADHD is over-diagnosed and medicines prescribed, the glaring lack of access to fields and playgrounds continues unresolved. The medication can make the dire need to play outside look less pressing. But there are organizations drawing attention to the significance of recess. Playing in a green space is very valuable and affects children's behavior positively. "Findings suggest that everyday play settings make a difference in overall symptom severity in children with ADHD. Specifically, children with ADHD who play regularly in green play settings have milder symptoms than children who play in built outdoor and indoor settings. This is true for all income groups and for both boys and girls." (Taylor and Kuo, M., 2011; Kuo, F.E., and Taylor, 2004).

Additionally, obesity correlates with ADHD (see Cortese, 2019). Recess plays a positive role in cognitive performance (Pellegrini and Bohn, 2005). Children fidget less and pay attention more after recess compared to before it (Ridgway, et al., 2003). Schools in the United States have decreased recess time (Pellegrini and Bohn, 2005). Poor performance in school is one of the issues that tempts parents and teachers to evaluate and then medicate children. Recess in a green space can negate some of the behavioral impediments to learning by improving attention span and focus.

The No Child Left Behind Act undermined recess. But sacrificing recess for more time learning was counterproductive: limiting recess leaves students worse off and does not correlate with improved scores. Also, countries with better performance on standardized tests tend to have more recess (Jarrett, 2019).

There is a social justice component to recess. Studies have shown that Black and poorer children have significantly less access to recess. One study showed that 85 percent of white children in the United States had access to recess while only 61 percent of African American and only 56 percent of those living below the poverty line had it (Jarrett, 2019, p. 3). "Large, urban, Southeastern schools with high poverty and high minority populations had the least recess, sometimes none at all." (Jarrett, 2019, p. 3 citing Fenton Communications report for the Robert Wood Johnson Foundation, 2007). The area of the country with the most ADHD is the Southeast. Among the six states with the most ADHD diagnoses (measured by whether a child had ever had an ADHD diagnosis), five are in the South. Kentucky, Arkansas, and Louisiana top the list with 16.6, 15.1, and 14.2 percent, respectively (CDC, 2020).

Class size. Inner city schools also have large class sizes. Those diagnosed with ADHD stay on task more in small group instruction than in larger (whole) groups (Hart, et al., 2011). There is an ongoing social movement striving for small class size (Walker, 2019). Relating behavioral traits that are difficult for teachers to teach around to the broader system of public-school education can benefit everyone. Teacher shortages may be partially caused by the need to oversee a large group of children. That is, teachers and students both benefit from smaller class sizes.

Teaching quality. "If the idea of giving a pill as a substitute for better teaching seems repellent—like substituting an I.V. drip of synthetic nutrition for actual food—it may nevertheless be preferable to a scenario in which only wealthy kids receive a frequent mental boost." (Talbot, 2009). That idea is repellent. High quality teaching is an important goal of any education system.

Repairing the cutthroat nature of academics and college admissions. ADHD is a side effect of the push for super-achievement. Parent persistence in wanting name brand educational opportunities for children who would not otherwise be admitted fuels the desire for a diagnosis. Without the dog-eat-dog nature of admissions, the temptation of extra time or the validation of medicine that comes with prescriptions would decrease. But as early as pre-school, the desire to get students ahead, seems to correlate with more rigor or intensity and more need to have them behave more like the mean behavior than the outlying behavior. Again, rankings do students a disservice.

Conflicts of interest. There is an ongoing opportunity to improve trust in pharma. Pathologizing and prescribing is a missed opportunity. Doctors and drug companies could prove they are not motivated by sales and profits by changing the broad definition in the DSM-5. The doctors, psychiatrists, and psychologists contributing to the DSM-5 had insurmountable financial conflicts of interest (Cosgrove and Krimsky, 2012). The pro-medication bias is suspect, and it undermines everything else pharma does from vaccines to cures for diseases.

Focus on the mild at the expense of the severely mentally challenged. Beeker, et al. argue that mild cases across the psychiatry realm detract from focus on severe cases (2021). Many services and medical interventions flow toward mild to moderate problems that may be best resolved without any intervention. The authors suggest a transdisciplinary approach to addressing "psychiatrization." Psychiatric drug consumption in the United States is higher than ever and there is a push to export mental health care to the global regions that do not currently use the U.S. approach to diagnosis. (Beeker, et al., 2021). The expansion is sold as a positive, providing access to mental health care. In the United States, the industry of ADHD drugs markets to those who may see improvement on the drugs rather than those who are severely impaired. Quizzes suggest impairment and are designed to make people think they have the disorder (Schwarz, 2013), attracting mild cases, i.e., people with normal behavior, to the ADHD umbrella.

Beyond opportunity cost: Medicalization as a standalone ethical lapse

Pinpointing why medicalization is an ethical problem is challenging. Many people do not find it problematic and happily pathologize all moods and use medications for mild anxiety and depression as well as for poor focus. Beyond even the opportunity costs is a feeling, the ethical analysis of which is more difficult. An industry has built up around ADHD. The profit margins are huge. Utilitarian approaches are often invoked in bioethics. They look at the pros and cons, the overall utility, doing the most good for the most people, or reducing harm. They inform the opportunity costs described above.

One reason medicalization is bad is that it diverts attention, funding, and awareness from social conditions. But placing behavior in the medical sphere can be itself a moral bad, even it did not divert resources. Arguably there is not an easy universal moral rule to apply, no Kantian fix. But it is bad perhaps to expect that a medical fix, quite often a drug, will resolve something as multi-caused and multifactorial as behavior. Parents should not have their hopes set so high. Seeing medicine as so powerful is misplaced: it is not really curing a disease in the case of ADHD.

An obligation to exhaust all other options should be an imperative, avoiding unnecessary risk of the side effects of the drugs, but it is not. A doctor should use his or her position to do good, but good has been lost in the shuffle. A Kantian analysis might condemn medicalization as it universally undermines trust in the scientific community. The concept of looking to medicine first when a child acts out diverts social resources and places a huge burden on children. Shifting the emphasis from individual behavior to the experience of behavior in society alters the burden of childhood behavior and highlights the ecosystem.

The social determinants of health (and mental health) need resources and attention. A many-billion-dollar industry is a red flag. A growing number of cases is another red flag. Medicalization is not harmless. Society should be more accepting of a wider range of behaviors, willing to engage in kind and thoughtful discipline or alternative learning styles, and patient both in allowing kids to be kids and in viewing maturity as a solution to rambunctious behavior.

Proposed solutions

Attention to the social problems and the ecosystem. Add more recess and gym to everyone's school day. Decrease class sizes. Add tools to use to practice attention span. Teach and allow time for resilience building. Allow mistakes and undesirable grades to be learning experiences. Increase diets of whole, natural foods; exercise.

The qualities defining ADHD are also common responses to trauma. Resolving and eliminating childhood trauma and encouraging people to build resilience when they have traumatic experiences would help.

Allow certain services without a diagnosis!

Make a different cutoff for evaluations: Look to those who are two standard deviations from the middle-of-the-road attentive child or more (based on literature that evaluates large populations, not just comparisons to members of the child's class at school) and take the one end of graph, where people have much less ability to pay attention, and consider asking what qualities they exhibit that those just left of the mean, or in the one to two standard deviations from the mean do not.

Within that small group, the most extreme cases could be isolated. Perhaps evaluations for cognitive or medical problems would be wise or medically called for in less than one percent. By reducing the number of people evaluated and then developing criteria to establish the worst off socially or behaviorally within that subset, ADHD could be limited to only severe cases. That would at least draw a line at evaluating, at most, 2.3 percent of children, and diagnosing many fewer, a big jump from the almost ten percent of the childhood population diagnosed with ADHD now.

Diseases with biological evidence do not need cutoffs, nor should they have them. But in the case of ADHD, a limit could help. In states like Kentucky, Arkansas, and Louisiana, even if every pediatrician in the state were to agree each diagnosis is accurate and deserved according to the AAP and the DSM-5, I simply cannot go along. They are diagnosing poverty, stress, overcrowded classes, lack of fields, too little free time, too much free time without appropriate resources, and too few athletics. Let's not call it ADHD and let's destigmatize high energy children.

Conclusion

Medicalization, this idea that so many problems can be solved within the biomedical arena or with medication, harms society and reduces complex issues to groupthink, perpetuating an ideology that glorifies the simple medical approach and accepts its dangers.

The distraction from the underlying social, economic, or environmental problems is a huge opportunity cost. We also harm these children, experimenting on them without proof of safety, interfering with their resilience and social problem-solving skills. By diagnosing at the request of wealthy parents gaming tests, ADHD diagnosis furthers a socioeconomic divide. And by overprescribing to those in low-income brackets, doctors admit policymakers, teachers, and parents do not have the time or energy to improve their circumstances.

It is not easy to pinpoint and verbalize why medicalization is ethically problematic. After all, when applied to terrible illnesses and the pain and suffering accompanied by them, we see the benefits of a thriving pharmaceutical industry: the ability to treat disease and save lives. But medicalization refers to the overreach, the kneejerk reaction to address nonmedical or quasi-medical problems using a medical lens and almost inevitably, medication.

The financial conflicts of interest that rightly spark distrust of science and the pharmaceutical industry contribute to medicalization: profits go to the continued cycle of persuading society that medicine is the right approach to many problems. The ideology of medicalization is shared by much of the public. There is too much buy-in. Directing more attention to social policy and the many nonmedical prerequisites of health and wellness takes the ability to critique the current model responsibly. Attention has been diverted from creating social conditions conducive to children's behavior; developing such conditions takes patience, creativity, social and environmental change, and time. The best solution may be to let kids be kids.

References

American Psychiatric Association (2013). Diagnostic and Statistical Manual of Mental Disorders, 5th edition. Arlington, VA.: American Psychiatric Association.

Beeker, T., Mills, C., Bhugra, D., Te Meerman, S., Thoma, S., Heinze, M., & von Peter, S. (2021). Psychiatrization of Society: A Conceptual Framework and Call for Transdisciplinary Research. *Frontiers in Psychiatry*, 12, 645556. https://doi.org/10.3389/fpsyt.2021.645556

Cadwalladr, C. (2015). Students used to take drugs to get high. Now they take them to get higher grades. *Guardian* https://www.theguardian.com/society/2015/feb/15/students-smart-drugs-higher-grades-adderall-modafinil

Cecil, C. (2018). It Starts with a Step. New Degree Press.

Centers for Disease Control (2022). ADHD Treatment Recommendations. https://www.cdc.gov/ncbddd/adhd/guidelines.html, citing American Academy of Pediatrics, Subcommittee on Children and Adolescents with Attention-Deficit/Hyperactivity Disorder. ADHD: Clinical practice guideline for the diagnosis, evaluation, and treatment of children and adolescents with attention-deficit/hyperactivity disorder. Pediatrics, September 30th, 2019.

Centers for Disease Control (2020). State-Based Prevalence of ADHD Diagnosis and Treatment. https://www.cdc.gov/ncbddd/adhd/data/diagnosis-treatment-data.htm).

Cha, A. (March 14, 2016). Kids with August birthdays are more likely to get an ADHD diagnosis. Here's why. *Washington Post.*

Cha, A. (May 3, 2016). CDC warns that Americans may be overmedicating youngest children with ADHD. *Washington Post.*

Chen, M., Lan, W., Pan, T., Chen, T., Hsu, J. (2016). Influence of Relative Age on Diagnosis and Treatment of Attention-Deficit Hyperactivity Disorder in Taiwanese Children. *Journal of Pediatrics.* Vol. 172, 162-167.E1. https://doi.org/10.1016/j.jpeds.2016.02.012

Cooper J. (2004). Disorders are different from diseases. *World psychiatry: official journal of the World Psychiatric Association (WPA)*, 3(1), 24.

Cortese, S. (2019). The Association between ADHD and Obesity: Intriguing, Progressively More Investigated, but Still Puzzling. *Brain Sci.* 9(10):256. doi: 10.3390/brainsci9100256. PMID: 31569608; PMCID: PMC6826981.

Cosgrove, L., Krimsky, S. (2012) A Comparison of DSM-IV and DSM-5 Panel Members' Financial Associations with Industry: A Pernicious Problem Persists. PLoS Med 9(3): e1001190. https://doi.org/10.1371/journal.pmed.1001190

Domaradzki, J. (2013). Extra Medicinam Nulla Salus. Medicine as a Secular Religion. *Polish Sociological Review.* 181, 21–38. http://www.jstor.org/stable/41969476

Eagle, Ruth. (November 4, 2020). What are the Effects of Ritalin? MedicalNewsToday.https://www.medicalnewstoday.com/articles/ritalin-effects#Serious-side-effects

Fenton Communications for the Robert Wood Johnson Foundation (2007). Recess Rules: Why the undervalued playtime may be America's best investment for healthy kids and healthy schools. *Robert Wood Johnson Foundation*.https://www.rwjf.org/en/library/research/2007/09/recess-rules.html

Hart, K. C., Massetti, G. M., Fabiano, G. A., Pariseau, M. E., & Pelham, W. E., Jr. (2011). Impact of group size on classroom on-task behavior and work productivity in children with ADHD. *Journal of Emotional and Behavioral Disorders*, 19, 55-64.

Hyman, M. (2008). The UltraMind Solution. New York: Scribner.

Hyman, M. (2015). Seven Strategies to Address ADHD, website https://drhyman.com/blog/2015/10/21/7-strategies-adhd/.

Jarrett, O. (2019). A Research-Based Case for Recess: Position Paper (2019) *US Play Coalition in collaboration with American Association for the Child's Right to Play* (IPA/USA) and the Alliance for Childhood https://usplaycoalition.org/wp-content/uploads/2019/08/Need-for-Recess-2019-FINAL-for-web.pdf

Kazda, L., Bell, K., Thomas, R., McGeechan, K., Sims, R., Barratt, A. (2021) Overdiagnosis of Attention-Deficit/Hyperactivity Disorder in Children and Adolescents: A Systematic Scoping Review. *JAMA*. 4(4): e215335. doi:10.1001/jamanetworkopen.2021.5335 Kids with August birthdays are more likely to get an ADHD diagnosis. Here's why.

Kuo F.E., Taylor, A.F. (2004). A potential natural treatment for attention-deficit/hyperactivity disorder: evidence from a national study. *Am J Public Health*. 94(9):1580-6. doi: 10.2105/ajph.94.9.1580. PMID: 15333318; PMCID: PMC1448497.

Landrigan, P. (August 23, 2011). How environmental exposures can contribute to autism and ADHD. *MedPage Today KevinMD.com*.

Landrigan, P., Schechter, C., Lipton, J., Fahs, M., and Schwartz, J. (2002). Environmental Pollutants and Disease in American Children: Estimates of Morbidity, Mortality, and Costs for Lead Poisoning, Asthma, Cancer, and Developmental Disabilities. *Environmental Health Perspectives*. Vol. 110, No 7.

Lantz, P.M., Lichtenstein, R.L., Pollack, H.A. (2007). Health Policy Approaches to Population Health: The Limits of Medicalization. *Health Affairs*, 26, 1253-1257. doi: 10.1377/hlthaff.26.5.1253.

Macht, J. (2017). The Medicalization of America's Schools [electronic resource]: Challenging the Concept of Educational Disabilities New York: Palgrave Macmillan; Secaucus: Springer [Distributor] Chapter 4.

Market Data Forecast. (January 2022). https://www.marketdataforecast.com/market-reports/attention-deficit-hyperactivity-disorder-therapeutics-market)

Marvin, R. The Endless Scroll: How to Tell if You're a Tech Addict. *PC Mag. com.* https://www.pcmag.com/news/the-endless-scroll-how-to-tell-if-youre-a-tech-addict

Mosendz, P. and Melby, C. (2022). ADHD Drugs Are Convenient to Get Online. Maybe Too Convenient. *Bloomberg*. https://www.bloomberg.com/news/features/2022-03-11/cerebral-app-over-prescribed-adhd-meds-ex-employees-say.

O'Neil, C. (2016). Weapons of Math Destruction. New York: Broadway Books.

Pellegrini, A. D., & Bohn, C. M. (2005). The Role of Recess in Children's Cognitive Performance and School Adjustment. Educational Researcher, 34(1), 13–19. http://www.jstor.org/stable/3699908

Ra C.K., Cho, J., Stone, M., et al. (2018). Association of Digital Media Use with Subsequent Symptoms of Attention-Deficit/Hyperactivity Disorder Among Adolescents. *JAMA*. 320(3):255–263. doi:10.1001/jama.2018.8931

Ridgway, A., J., Northup, A., Pellegrin, A., LaRue, R., and Hightshoe, A. (2003). Effects of recess on the classroom behavior of children with and without attention-deficit hyperactivity disorder. *School Psychology Quarterly* 18(3): 253–268).

Rosen, L. and Gazzaley, A. (2016). The Distracted Mind: Ancient Brains in a High-Tech World. Cambridge, MA: The MIT Press.

Rose S. L. (2013). Patient advocacy organizations: institutional conflicts of interest, trust, and trustworthiness. *The Journal of Law, Medicine & Ethics, 41*(3), 680–687. https://doi.org/10.1111/jlme.12078

Schwarz, A. (December 14, 2013). The Selling of Attention Deficit Disorder. *New York Times.*

Schwarz, A. (May 16, 2014) Thousands of Toddlers Are Medicated for A.D.H.D., Report Finds, Raising Worries. *New York Times.*

Shapin, S. (1995). Trust Honesty, and the Authority of Science. In Bulger, R., Bobby, E., and Fineberg, H. (Eds.) Society's Choices: *Social and Ethical Decision Making in Biomedicine.* Washington D.C.: National Academy Press (388-408).

Talbot, M. (2009). Brain Gain: The Underground World of "Neuroenhancing" Drugs. *The New Yorker* https://www.newyorker.com/magazine/2009/04/27/brain-gain. Also published for the Guardian under separate title: Talbot, M. (2009). Can a daily pill really boost your brain power? *The Guardian.* https://www.theguardian.com/science/2009/sep/20/neuroenhancers-us-brain-power-drugs

Taylor, A. F., and Kuo, M. (2011). Could Exposure to Everyday Green Spaces Help Treat ADHD? Evidence from Children's Play Settings? *Applied Psychology: Health and Well-Being.* 3(3): 281-303. DOI: 10.1111/j.1758-0854.2011.01052.x

Timimi, Sami. (2002. ebook 2014). Pathological Child Psychiatry and the Medicalization of Childhood. London: Routledge.

Vallee, M. (2013). Perpetuating a Reductionist Medical Worldview: The Absence of Environmental Medicine in the American ADHD Clinical Practice Guidelines. *Advances in Medical Sociology,* Vol 15, 241-264.

Walker, T. (2019). Educators and Parents Reset the Class Size 'Debate'. *National Education Association, NEA News.* https://www.nea.org/advocating-for-change/new-from-nea/educators-and-parents-reset-class-size-debate

Wayt, T. (2022). Startups push ADHD meds through TikTok ads, concerning doctors. *New York Post.* March 13, 2022.

Whalen, C.K., & Hencker, B. (1980) The Social Ecology of Psychostimulant Treatment: A Model for Conceptual and Empirical Analysis. In C.K. Whalen & B. Hencker (Eds.) Hyperactive Children: The social ecology of identification and treatment. New York: Academic Press.

Wired (2015). How ADHD Became a Multi-Billion Dollar Industry (Video) https://www.wired.com/video/watch/how-adhd-became-a-multi-billion-dollar-industry

Woods, B. (August 18, 2009) Chasing the Red Queen in Academia. Student Voices blog. *Scitable by Nature.* https://www.nature.com/scitable/blog/student-voices/alice_through_the_ivory_tower/

Yuste, R., Genser, J., and Herrmann, S. (2021). It's Time for Neuro-Rights, *Horizons* No. 18.

Zola, I. (1972) Medicine as an Instrument of Social Control. *The Sociological Review*. 20(4): 487-504. (quoted).

ADHD Goes Global: An American Export

Patrick Hahn

A 2007 review[1] found that the United States, with less than five percent of the world's population, accounted for a staggering eighty percent of the world's consumption of ADHD meds. The figure was even higher in terms of dollars, with the US accounting for ninety-two percent of global spending.[2] Per capita, the US had more than twice as many prescriptions than its nearest rival, Canada.[3] More recently, the 2014 report of the International Narcotics Control Board found that the US accounted for eighty percent of the total world consumption of methylphenidate.[4]

There is no objective test for ADHD, and the criteria for diagnosing this condition are hopelessly subjective and context-dependent. Reported incidence rates are known to vary by a factor of fifty.[5] In a 1992 study, mental health professionals from four different countries

---

Patrick D. Hahn is an affiliate professor of Biology at Loyola University Maryland.

ADHD Goes Global is adapted from chapter eighteen in *Obedience Pills: ADHD and the Medicalization of Childhood.* Samizdat Health Writer's Cooperative, April 29. 2022.

[1] Richard M. Scheffler et al., "The Global Market for ADHD Medications," *Health Affairs* 26, no. 2 (March/April 2007): 450-457, https://doi.org/10.1377/hltaff.26.2.450

[2] Ibid., 451.

[3] Ibid., 453.

[4] International Narcotics Control Board, "Report 2014," Tuesday, March 3, 2015, https://www.incb.org/incb/en/publications/annual-reports/annual-report-2014.html

[5] Sami Timimi, "ADHD is Best Understood as a Cultural Construct," *British Journal of Psychiatry* 184, no. 1 (January 2004): 8, https://doi.org/10.1192/bjp.184.1.8

– the United States, Japan, China, and Indonesia – watched videos of four boys, playing both by themselves and with other children, and rated the boys' conduct on an eighteen-item checklist for disruptive behaviors. Clinicians from China and Indonesia found significantly more disruptive behaviors than did their colleagues in the United States or Japan, indicating that notions of what is considered "disruptive" vary a great deal between cultures.[6]

So, is ADHD just another American cultural export, like rock-and-roll or the Super Mario Brothers? A 2007 meta-analysis by Joseph Biederman and his colleagues[7] purported to debunk this notion. They looked at incidence rates in 102 studies comprising 171,756 subjects from North America, Europe, Asia, South America, Oceania, the Middle East, and Africa. A variety of criteria were employed to diagnose this condition, including from the *DSM-III, the DSM-IIIR, the DSM-IV, and the World Health Organization's International Classification of Diseases (ICD-10).*

The *ICD-10* category corresponding to ADHD is called Hyperkinetic Disorder (HKD), and is defined by much stricter criteria. A 2006 study found that one hundred percent of boys diagnosed with HKD also met the criteria for ADHD, while only twenty-six percent of boys diagnosed with ADHD met the criteria for HKD.[8]

---

[6] E.M. Mann et al., "Cross-Cultural Differences in Rating Hyperactive-Disruptive Behaviors in Children," *American Journal of Psychiatry* 149, no. 11 (November 1992): 1539-1542, https://doi.org/10.1176/ajp.149.11.1539

[7] Guilherme Polanczyk et al., "The Worldwide Prevalence of ADHD: A Systematic Review and Metaregression Analysis," *American Journal of Psychiatry* 164, no. 6 (June 2007): 942-948, https://doi.org/10.1176/ajp.2007.164.6.942

[8] Benjamin B. Lahey et al., "Predictive Validity of ICD-10 Hyperkinetic Disorder Relative to DSM-IV Attention Deficit Hyperactivity Disorder Among Younger Children," *Journal of Child Psychology and Psychiatry* 47, no. 5 (2006): 472-479, https://doi.org/10.1111/j.1469-7610.2005.015900.x

The researchers' estimate of the worldwide-pooled prevalence rate of ADD/ADHD/HKD was 5.29%. Moreover, they concluded that most of the variation was due to different diagnostic criteria, and after controlling for this, rates were essentially the same throughout much of the world. Significant differences remained between the United States and Africa, between the United States and the Middle East, between Europe and Africa, and between Europe and the Middle East.[9]

The authors then re-analyzed their data by means of an "additional model" said to "increase statistical power" and this time they found no remaining significant differences.[10] These results were replicated by associates of Dr. Biederman in two subsequent meta-analyses.[11]

It is beyond the scope of the present work to comment on the statistical wizardry needed to make a fifty-fold difference in incidence rates disappear. It was all a tempest in a teapot anyway. There is no evidence of any long-term benefit to drugging children for ADHD. Nor is there evidence for the existence of a subset of children so labeled who benefit. So, the question of whether the incidence of ADHD (as defined by *DSM-IV* criteria or any other) is the same throughout the world is a moot point. It is not clear what this would prove if it were true, given there is no non-psychiatric illness that follows this pattern.

---

[9] Polanczyk et al., "Prevalence," 945.

[10] Ibid., 945-946.

[11] Erik G. Wilcutt, "The Prevalence of DSM-IV Attention-Deficit Hyperactivity Disorder: A Meta-Analytic Review," *Neurotherapeutics* 9, no. 3 (July 2012): 490-499, https://doi.org/10.1007/s13311-012-0135-8; Guilherme V. Polanczyk, Erik G. Wilcutt, Giovanni A. Salum, Christian Kieling, and Luis A. Rohde, "ADHD Prevalence Estimates Across Three Decades: An Updated Systematic Review and Meta-Regression Analysis," *International Journal of Epidemiology* 43, no. 2 (April 2014): 434-442, https://doi.org/10.1093/ije/dyt262

The global migration of ADHD

While the United States continues to lead the world in prescribing stimulant drugs for kids, the rest of the world is catching up. In 1993, thirty-one countries had adopted the use of ADHD medications, but by 2003 that number had swollen to fifty-five. Low-use countries exhibited annual growth rates as high as forty-six percent, while moderate-use countries had growth rates of twenty percent.[12]

In a 2014 review,[13] sociologists Peter Conrad and Meredith R. Bergey attributed the global migration of ADHD to five factors: 1) The transnational pharmaceutical industry, 2) The increasing influence of American psychiatry, 3) The adoption of the DSM criteria for diagnosing ADHD, 4) The internet, and 5) ADHD advocacy groups. Each of these tends to reinforce the others.

While the United States may be nearing saturation point in terms of ADHD diagnosis and treatment, the rest of world still represents, in the eyes of the drugmakers, a largely untapped market. A review by Global Data gushed:

> *Between 2010 and 2018, the global ADHD market is expected to grow at a CAGR of 8%. During this forecast period, patents for various drugs such as Adderall XR, Daytrana, Concerta (methylphenidate), Strattera (atomoxetine) and Kapvay are set to expire. However, the losses due to the expiry of these patents would be compensated by new drugs entering the market such as Vyvanse and Intuniv.*[14]

---

[12] Scheffler et al., "Global Market," 451.

[13] Peter Conrad and Meredith R. Bergey, "The Impending Globalization of ADHD: Notes on the Expansion and Growth of a Medicalized Disorder," *Social Science and Medicine* 122, (December 2014): 31-43, https://doi.org/10.1016/j.socscimed.2014.10.019

[14] Ibid., 36.

Not to be outdone, Global Industry Analysts noted that "the global market for ADHD drugs is severely constrained by the lack of awareness of the disorder, even in developed countries such as the UK, Germany and Japan." To remedy this dire situation, they called for more marketing and education directed at physicians and, where possible, potential consumers.[15] This call has not gone unheeded.

The ADHD Institute, "an educational platform developed and funded by Takeda," offers "ADHD resources" for "patients, parents, educators, and professionals" with country-specific information for Canada, Germany, Spain, Sweden, and the UK.[16] All these "ADHD resources" were developed by Takeda, which in 2019 acquired Shire PLC, manufacturer of Vyvanse and Adderall XR.

Janssen Global, which markets the ADHD drug Concerta, provides country-specific information on its products for no fewer than fifty different nations. The website for Xian-Janssen, the company's branch in China, provides these helpful details about Attention Deficit Hyperactivity Disorder:

> *ADHD is common in school-age children, will continue to adolescence and adulthood, and has a wide negative influence on one's academic, career and social life. There are two main methods of ADHD management: (1) pharmacological treatment; (2) non-pharmacological treatment: including behavioral therapy, parent training, etc. For more information see your Doctor or Healthcare Professional.*[17]

---

[15] Ibid., 36.

[16] ADHD Institute, accessed September 10, 2021, https://adhd-institute.com

[17] Xian Janssen, "Attention Deficit Hyperactivity Disorder," accessed September 10, 2021, https://www.xian-janssen.com.cn/en/therapy/adhd

What is being sold here is not so much a specific drug, nor even a specific diagnosis, as a specific worldview: one in which human distress is the manifestation of drug-treatable brain disease, and one in which the drugmakers are benevolent, objective sources of information.

ADHD advocacy groups are active online, too. ADHD Europe offers a position statement "ADHD Myths and Facts,"[18] conveniently translated into French, Spanish, Greek, Italian, and Hungarian. A "Fact Sheet"[19] produced by ADHD Australia warns readers that "ADHD is currently under-diagnosed, particularly in girls and the adult population." The Center for ADHD Awareness Canada informs us that "Overwhelming scientific evidence has led all major medical associations and government health agencies to recognize ADHD as a major medical disorder."[20] The website for ADHD New Zealand instructs teachers on how to identify this condition and communicate their concerns to the parents.[21]

The website for ADHD UK offers its "Adult ADHD Self-Screening Tool."[22] Sample questions include "How often do you have trouble wrapping up the final details of a project, once the challenging parts have been done?" "How often do you make careless mistakes when you have to work on a boring or difficult project?" and "How often do you have difficulty keeping your attention when doing boring or

---

[18] ADHD Europe, "ADHD Myths and Facts," accessed September 10, 2021, https://adhdeurope.eu/awareness/myths-and-facts

[19] ADHD Australia, "What is ADHD," accessed September 10, 2021, https://www.adhdaustralis.org/about-adhd/what-is-attention-deficit-hyperactivity-disorder-adhd/

[20] Center for ADHD Awareness Canada, "ADHD Facts – Dispelling the Myths," accessed September 10, 2021, https://caddac.ca/understanding-adhd/in-general/facts-stats-myths/

[21] ADHD New Zealand, "Managing ADHD in Schools," accessed September 10, 2021, https://www.adhd.org/nz/adhd-in-schools.html

[22] ADHD UK, "Adult ADHD Self-Screening Tool," accessed September 10, 2021, https://adhduk.co.uk/adult-adhd-screening-survey/

repetitive work?" all rated on a five-point Likert scale. Users who score high on this quiz are advised, not to find work that doesn't bore them, but to discuss the results with a clinician.

And that highlights the problem with checklists such as this: they decontextualize human experience, draining it of any larger meaning and reducing every variety of human distress to a drug-treatable medical disorder.

Global acceptance of this medical model of ADHD likely is facilitated by the numerous international medical graduates who currently fill one-third of residency positions in psychiatry in the United States.[23] While many of these residents choose to remain in this country, those who return to their homelands will have been schooled in the diagnostic categories in the DSM – and every iteration of that volume has broadened the number of children eligible for that diagnosis.

The latest version of the ICD, ICD-11, which came into effect 1 January 2022,[24] has replaced the old category of "Hyperkinetic Disorder" with Attention Deficit Hyperactivity Disorder, bringing the rest of the world into line with American psychiatry. Just as in the DSM, this condition is divided into three subtypes: Predominantly Inattentive, Predominantly Hyperactive, and Combined. Whereas hyperactivity was the defining feature of HKD, the new category of ADHD gives equal emphasis to hyperactivity or inattention. The maximum age of onset, previously defined as "early onset (usually

---

[23] R. Rao Gogineni, April E. Fallon, and Nyapati R. Rao, "International Medical Graduates in Child and Adolescent Psychiatry: Adaptation, Training, and Contributions," *Child and Adolescent Psychiatric Clinics of North America* 19, no. 4 (October 2010): 833-853, https://doi.org/10.1016/j.chc.2010.07.009

[24] World Health Organization, "WHO Releases New International Classification of Diseases," June 18, 2018, https://who.int/news/item/18-06/2018/who-releases-new-international-classification-of-diseases-(icd-11)

in the first five years of life)" has been changed to twelve years, again bringing the rest of the world into line with American psychiatry.

No doubt this will increase the number of children worldwide considered eligible for stimulant drugs.

The market continues to expand. The following insights come from an April 2020 report from Persistence Market Research, a company which entices customers with its promised "Expertise in Life Sciences and Transformational Health":

> *Rising prevalence of ADHD across the globe, owing to the low threshold of diagnostic criteria, is expected to fuel growth of the global attention-deficit hyperactivity disorder (ADHD) therapeutics market over the forecast period.*
>
> *The COVID-19 pandemic is certainly a difficult time for individuals with attention-deficit hyperactivity disorder, owing to their vulnerability to the distress caused by the pandemic and physical distancing measures. As a result of these measures, individuals with ADHD might exhibit increased behavioral problems. On the back of this, ADHD therapeutics will witness significant growth in sales.*
>
> *Increasing introduction of innovative ADHD therapeutic products such as fruit-flavored chewable pills for children will favor the growth of the global attention-deficit hyperactivity disorder therapeutics market.*
>
> *The attention deficit hyperactivity disorder therapeutics market is expected to grow twofold between 2021 and 2031.*[25]

[25] Persistence Market Research, "ADHD Therapeutics Market to Expand Twofold by 2030, Deprioritized Status of ADHD in Hospitals Due to Covid-19 Pandemic Surging Market Growth," April 2020, https://www.persistencemarketresearch.com/market-research/attention-deficit-hyperactivity-disorder-therapeutics-market.asp

Three nations

It is beyond the scope of this chapter to provide an exhaustive account of the history of the ADHD diagnosis in every country in the world where it is used. Instead, we will look at three nations with very different approaches to this label: one which has embraced the medical model of ADHD almost as enthusiastically as the United States; one in which the medical model has barely begun to penetrate; and one in which that model has encountered stiff resistance but still has penetrated to a certain extent.

ADHD in Canada

The diagnostic category known as ADHD, and the practice of prescribing stimulant drugs for this condition, is almost exclusively an American invention. However, the switch in emphasis from hyperactivity to inattention (which guaranteed that many more children, including girls, would receive this label) came not from American doctors but their professional counterparts in Canada, led by clinical psychologist Virginia Douglas and her colleagues at McGill University and Montreal Children's Hospital. Dr. Douglas summarized this work in her 1972 Presidential Address to the Canadian Psychological Association.[26]

Dr. Douglas and her colleagues assessed the performance of children labeled "hyperactive" at a variety of tasks, and compared the results with those of their peers not so labeled. In one "automated concept learning" task, the performance of children labeled "hyperactive" equaled that of controls under a continuous reward scheme, but plummeted under an intermittent reward scheme.[27]

---

[26] Virginia I. Douglas, "Stop, Look, and Listen: The Problem of Sustained Attention and Impulse Control in Hyperactive and Normal Children," *Canadian Journal of Behavioural Science* 4, no. 4 (1972): 259-282.

In plain English, these boys (almost all of her subjects were boys) were perfectly capable of paying attention to the assigned task *when there was something in it for them*. So, what is being measured here is not attention but rather obeisance to adult authority. It is not clear what is to be gained by regarding the lack of such obeisance as a manifestation of brain pathology.

Of course, while Canadian researchers have played a key role in shaping the modern concept of ADHD, the flow of ideas between Canada and its much larger neighbor to the south has by no means been in one direction. In a book chapter aptly titled "In the Elephant's Shadow,"[28] Canadian sociologists Claudia Malacrida and Tiffani Semach discuss the many ways which American influences have shaped the debate on ADHD in Canada, both in the popular media and professional forums.

Most parenting magazines sold in Canada are of American origin, as are the majority of books about parenting, psychology, and self-help. The lion's share of Canadian television programming is produced in America. Most of the experts quoted in stories about ADHD are American as well.[29]

ADHD skeptics get a hearing as well, but here too the debate is dominated by American voices, notably Dr. Breggin, whose books have sold well in Canada.[30]

---

[27] Ibid., 263-264.

[28] Claudia Malacrida and Tiffani Semach, "In the Elephant's Shadow: The Canadian ADHD Context," in *Global Perspectives on ADHD: Social Dimensions of Diagnosis and Treatment in Sixteen Countries*, ed. Meredith R. Bergey et al., (Baltimore: Johns Hopkins University Press, 2018), 34-53.

[29] Ibid., 35.

[30] Ibid., 36.

In regard to patient advocacy, the picture is mixed. In the 1990's, the American-founded advocacy group CHADD boasted of forty chapters in Canada,[31] but since then the national organization has dissolved. CHADD Vancouver, the last remaining chapter of that organization in Canada, has re-named itself the ADD Vancouver Support Group. As of 19 September 2021, the organization's home page informs readers "Out of concern for our participants and speakers, we have decided to postpone the ADD Vancouver Support Group meetings until further notice." The website's content is sparse, and many links are broken.[32]

By contrast, the Center for ADHD Awareness Canada (CADDAC) is thriving. Incorporated in 2006 as a national not-for-profit organization, CADDAC lobbies in support of ADHD-related legislation; provides networking between ADHD groups across Canada; sponsors workshops, conferences, and webinars as well as live shows for kids, teens, and adults with ADHD and their families and friends; produces educational materials for individuals and families affected by ADHD as well as for medical professionals and educators; promotes the "Canadian ADHD Awareness Week"; and operates an extensive, content-rich website in addition to the organization's Facebook and Twitter pages.

Under "Funding Policy," they offer this meaningless disclaimer: "CADDAC only accepts funding for projects that we propose, or that we deem to be of benefit to our patient population,"[33] and then goes to list some of their sponsors, including Takeda Canada and Janssen, not to mention Purdue Pharma, whose subsidiary Adlon Therapeutics is the manufacturer of Adhansia XR.

---

[31] Ibid., 46.

[32] ADD Vancouver Support Group, accessed September 19, 2021, addvancouversupport.ca

[33] CADDAC, accessed September 19, 2021.

On 1 September 2021, Purdue Pharma was dissolved by a federal bankruptcy court judge in the wake of mounting overdose deaths associated with its blockbuster drug Oxycontin.[34]

CADDAC's annual report, "2019 Accomplishments," repeats a familiar bait-and-switch argument: "Left untreated, ADHD can have devastating effects over the course of one's lifetime," going on to mention mood and anxiety disorders, substance use disorders, transportation accidents, suicides, injuries, teenage pregnancies, unemployment, underemployment, and incarceration – neatly sidestepping the question as to whether any of these outcomes is averted by drug treatment.

In regard to the educational and health services industries, here too the influence of the United States is obvious. US professional organizations for doctors, psychiatrists, psychologists, and teachers are much larger than their Canadian counterparts and actively recruit Canadian members, and US drugmakers actively target Canadian doctors for their marketing campaigns.[35]

However, again Canadians have attempted to put their own unique stamp on things. The Canadian ADHD Resource Alliance (CADDRA) was incorporated as a not-for-profit national organization in 2006. The organization publishes the Canadian ADHD Practice Guidelines; hosts the annual CADDRA ADHD Conference; facilitates an annual ADHD Research Day; lobbies for increased resources for health care professionals and patients; and operates an "eLearning Portal" with webcasts, audio podcasts, ePosters, and article reviews. Membership is available only to practicing physicians, psychologists, and other

---

[34] Jan Hoffmann, "Purdue Pharma is Dissolved and Sacklers Pay $4.5 Billion to Settle Opioid Claims," *New York Times*, September 2, 2021.

[35] Malacrida and Semach, "Context," 36.

health care professionals. The board of directors consists of eight medical doctors and one psychologist.

CADDRA's webpage[36] lists among its sponsors Janssen, Shire Canada, and Purdue Pharma, and offers this curiously defensive statement of self-exoneration:

> *As many medical organizations do, we also receive some funding from pharmaceutical companies through sponsorship of our annual conference and educational grants for specific projects proposed to the funder by CADDRA.*
>
> *Funding is not conditional on incorporating messaging that benefits the company or promotes their products – in fact this is strictly prohibited according to the Rx& D Stakeholder Relations Collaborative Partnership Guiding Principles available on the Rx& D website. Conference sponsors have no input into the accredited conference program or schedule. CADDRA stipulates in all agreements with corporate, or any other type of funders, that the organization has full control of content and messaging in proposed projects.*
>
> *No outside funding is sought or accepted for development, review and publication of the Canadian ADHD Practice Guidelines. CADDRA continues to work towards diversification of its funding base to obtain financial support for education, training and advocacy projects from a variety of private and public funded sources.*

The first iteration of the Canadian ADHD Practice Guidelines was issued in 2011. The guidelines reviewed similar documents issued by both the United States and United Kingdom and noted that the

---

[36] Canadian ADHD Resource Alliance, accessed September 19, 2021, https://www.caddra.ca

two countries have radically different approaches to this condition. In the UK, medication is used only for extreme cases, as a last resort, while in the US medication typically is the first resort. The CADDRA guidelines called for a "holistic-based care, individualized to the patients," including education for patients and families, behavioral strategies, psychological treatment, and educational accommodations, with medication used as a way to facilitate the other interventions. The clear implication was that the Canadians intended to steer a middle course between those charted by the US and the UK.[37] How has that worked out?

Canadians are proud of their generous federally-funded health care system.[38] ADHD patients with complex needs can be referred to "centers of excellence." Telehealth and air transport of patients facilitate delivery of care across that nation's wide-open spaces.[39]

However, public health funding does not cover the services of psychologists, educators, or social workers, which means that low-income patients do not have the same access to non-medical treatment that patients from high-income families enjoy. ADHD diagnosis and treatment in Canada are managed almost exclusively by medical personal, leading Malacrida and Semach to conclude "In practice it is unlikely that such [nondrug] interventions will be implemented as part of a sustained, collaborative treatment approach."[40] Despite promises of holistic, patient-based care, the rate of diagnosis and drugging for ADHD in Canada is second only to that of the United States.[41]

---

[37] Malacrida and Semach, "Context," 42.

[38] Canadian Press, "Poll: Canadians are Most Proud of Universal Medicare," Sunday, November 25, 2012, https://www.ctvnews.ca/canada/poll-canadians-are-most-proud-of-universal-medicare-1.1052929

[39] Stephen P. Hinshaw et al., "International Variation in Treatment Procedures for ADHD: Social Context and Recent Trends," *Psychiatric Services* 62, no. 5 (May 2011): 459-464, https://doi.org/10.1176/ps.62.5.pss6205_0459

[40] Malacrida and Semach, "Context," 45.

[41] Scheffler et al., "Market."

ADHD in Ghana

A team of three Dutch researchers – sociologist Christian Bröer, anthropologist Rachel Spronk, and psychotherapist Viktor Kraak – conducted the first study on the use of the ADHD diagnosis in Ghana, or indeed in any sub-Saharan African country besides South Africa.[42] They contacted all the major mental health clinics, private clinics, and university departments and asked them to identify all clinicians who use that diagnosis. The search yielded ten clinicians (four psychiatrists, four clinical psychologists, and two pediatricians), and the researchers were able to speak to eight. Only one (a psychiatrist) operated outside the capital city of Accra. All but one had been educated in Western countries.

The number of children treated for ADHD each year by each of these clinicians ranged from two to several hundred. All but one of them rendered the diagnosis by means of unstructured observations and verbal reports.[43]

In Ghana, all citizens are covered by National Health Insurance. ADHD is recognized in the Standard Treatment Guidelines, and the only medication recommended is methylphenidate. Nevertheless, that drug is rarely prescribed. Instead, children with that label commonly are prescribed tranquilizing drugs, notably haloperidol and chlorpromazine, as well as the anticonvulsant carbamazepine, the tricyclic antidepressant imipramine, and the "non-stimulant" ADHD drug atomoxetine.[44]

---

[42] Christian Bröer et al., "Exploring the ADHD Diagnosis in Ghana," in *Global Perspectives on ADHD: Social Dimensions of Diagnosis and Treatment in Sixteen Countries,* ed. Meredith R. Bergey et al., (Baltimore: Johns Hopkins University Press, 2018), 354-375.

[43] Ibid., 362-363.

[44] Ibid., 363.

Prescriptions for haloperidol, chlorpromazine, carbamazepine, and imipramine all are subsidized under the National Health Insurance Scheme, whereas those for atomoxetine and methylphenidate are not. The cost of a month's supply of methylphenidate in Ghana is approximately eighty dollars, whereas a month's supply of atomoxetine retails for two hundred dollars. In a nation with an annual per capita GDP of $1,770, obviously these prices are out of reach for all but the wealthiest citizens.[45]

Dr. Bröer and his colleagues surveyed the popular media in Ghana and could find no references to that diagnostic category prior to 2008. Since then there have been a few tentative efforts by NGO's to raise awareness of ADHD in that country. The UK-based CarePlus Ghana has used Janssen's promotional video materials, and in 2010 the Ghanaian African Social Development Foundation, in collaboration with the Dutch National Committee for International Cooperation and Sustainable Development, produced a seminar on ADHD in Ghana.[46]

From the foregoing, it should be obvious that the concept of ADHD has barely begun to penetrate the national consciousness in Ghana, and there only in a tiny minority of affluent, western-leaning citizens in the nation's two largest cities. In the rest of the country, childish misbehavior is dealt with as it always has been, through corporal punishment, spiritual interventions, and prayer.

In theory, public education in Ghana is free, but in practice many children end up staying home due to their parents' inability to afford school fees or supplies.[47] Child labor is still a huge problem, [48] and

---

[45] Ibid., 363.

[46] Ibid., 364.

[47] Personal observations.

[48] United States Department of Labor, "Child Labor and Forced Labor Reports," 2019, https://dol.gov/agencies/ilab/resources/reports/child-labor/ghana

the reader could be forgiven for wondering whether efforts to raise "ADHD awareness" should be considered a priority.

ADHD in France

In a book chapter, French sociologists Madeline Akrich and Vololona Rabeharisoa reviewed the history of ADHD in that country – or TDAH, for *Le Trouble Déficit de l'Attention avec ou sans Hyperactivité*, the name by which that diagnostic category is known there.[49]

The first book on this subject published in France, *L'Hyperactivité chez l'Enfant*, by Michel Dugas, was released in 1987.[50] The new American import was slow to catch on, but all that began to change in the early 2000's, perhaps because of the efforts of HyperSupers, the French advocacy group for ADHD founded in 2000. Since that time the number of books, news articles, and scientific papers about ADHD has soared.[51]

The tone of the articles has changed as well. Between 1998 and 2004, two-thirds of the papers expressed doubts about the validity of this diagnostic category, with one researcher sarcastically referring to ADD as "American Democratic Disability." But three-fourths of papers published between 2005 and 2012 treated the condition as a bona fide neurological disorder.[52]

In 2011, psychologist Stephen Faraone, in collaboration with two French researchers, published the first (and still the only) estimate of

---

[49] Madeline Akrich and Vololona Rabeharisoa, "The French ADHD Landscape," in *Global Perspectives on ADHD: Social Dimensions of Diagnosis and Treatment in Sixteen Countries*, ed. Meredith R. Bergey et al., (Baltimore: Johns Hopkins University Press, 2018), 233-260.

[50] Ibid., 235.

[51] Ibid., 235-237.

[52] Ibid., 239.

the incidence of ADHD in that country. [53] The researchers concluded that 3.5% of children had a diagnosis of ADHD, with a preponderance of boys bearing that diagnosis, concluding "Our work suggests that the epidemiology of ADHD in France is similar to the epidemiology of ADHD as reported by other countries."[54]

As acceptance of the diagnostic category of ADHD has risen in France, so have prescriptions for Ritalin. Sales of that drug have risen from 50,000 boxes in 2000 to 280,000 in 2008 to 500,000 in 2013.[55]

Prescriptions for Ritalin are comparatively difficult to obtain.[56] The drug is classified as a "narcotic" with a high potential for abuse and dependency. The initial prescription must be written by a specialist (i.e., a psychiatrist, neurologist, or pediatrician) and the drug must be re-prescribed every twenty-eight days by the attending physician and every year by the specialist. Until very recently, the initial prescription had to be obtained in a hospital, but that rule was waived in September of 2021.[57]

The slow but growing acceptance of the medical model of ADHD by no means has eclipsed alternative approaches to that condition. Indeed, French psychiatry has a long-standing tradition of treating the complaints that fall under the diagnostic rubric of "mental illness" with empathy and compassion. This approach dates at least as far back as the Eighteenth Century, with Phillipe Pinel's efforts to humanize care at the Sâlpetieré.[58] Many French psychiatrists have

---

[53] Michel Lecendreux, Eric Konofal, and Stephen V. Faraone, "Prevalence of Attention Deficit Hyperactivity Disorder and Associated Features among Children in France," *Journal of Attention Deficit Disorders* 15, no. 6 (August 2011): 516-524, https://doi.org/10.1177/1087054710372491

[54] Akrich and Rabeharisoa, "Landscape," 248-249.

[55] Ibid., 239.

[55] Ibid., 238.

[57] HyperSupers TDAH France, "Fin de la Prescription Initiale Hospitaliére (PIH) pour le Méthylphenidate," September 13, 2021, https://tdah-france.fr

[58] Phillipe Pinel, *A Treatise on Mental Alienation,* trans. Gordon Hickish, David Healy, and Louis C. Charland (Chichester: J. Wiley and Sons, 2008).

viewed medication warily, as a distraction from the real business of finding out what is going on in a child's world. In 2005, *Le Monde* ran a piece on ADHD which quoted Bernard Golse, head of the psychiatry unit at a children's hospital in Paris:

> *With Ritalin, the mystery remains unsolved since the meaning of the disorder still has to be worked out in regard to each child's history* .[59]

This multiplicity of approaches is reflected in the actions of the advocacy group HyperSupers, which takes an agnostic view regarding the nature of that condition and an eclectic approach to treatment.[60] In 2011, that group conducted the first and only survey of how French children and their families deal with ADHD and found that thirty-nine percent of patients were engaged in psychotherapy, twenty-seven percent in speech and language therapy, and nineteen percent in psychomotor therapy. Forty-four percent of these children had received an individualized education plan at their schools, while twenty percent had been excluded from school at least once, thirty percent had repeated at least one grade, and half of the parents reported having a difficult or very difficult relationship with teachers.[61]

Given the diversity of views in France regarding the nature of the complaints which fall under the diagnostic rubric of ADHD, it is little wonder that while prescriptions for Ritalin have skyrocketed in recent years, per capita consumption of the drug remains less than five percent of what it is in the United States.[62]

---

[59] Akrich and Rabeharisoa, "Landscape," 238.

[60] Claire Edwards et al., "Attention Deficit Hyperactivity Disorder in France and Ireland: Parents' Groups' Scientific and Political Framing of an Unsettled Condition," *Biosocieties* 9, no. 2 (2014): 153-172.

[61] Akrich and Rabeharisoa, "Landscape," 253.

[62] Ibid., 239.

In October of 2021, the French government held a two-day conference on mental health and psychiatry which an article by the news network France24 described as "an attempt to rejuvenate a failing branch of the French medical establishment."[63]

The article quoted child psychiatrist Marie-José Durieux, who lamented the decline of French psychiatry:

> *Just 30 years ago, psychiatry was practiced with a lot of interest and excitement. We associated psychiatry with imaginative sciences like philosophy, psychoanalysis, sociology and literature.*

Dr. Durieux blamed the decline on drugs and that American import, the *DSM*. "Medication alone is not enough to solve existential problems," she averred. Whether these concerns will lead to lasting changes remains to be seen.

Finding the right niche for ourselves

When I asked Dr. Healy why Europe and the rest of the world has yet to embrace the disease model of ADHD to the extent that North America has, he related that reluctance to the Jungian concepts of introversion and extraversion – concepts which, he says, never really caught on here.

In an essay, Dr. Jung characterized the introvert as reflective, with a tendency toward caution, while the extravert is prone to impulsivity and novelty seeking.[64] The psychiatrist Hans Eysenck conceptualized

---

[63] Aude Mazoue, "French Psychiatry Has Gone Downhill in Part Because of American Influence," France24, October 3, 2021, https://www.france24.com/en/france/20211003-french-psychiatry-has-gone-downhill-in-part-because-of-american-influence

[64] Carl Jung, *Two Essays on Analytical Psychology*, trans. R.F.C. Hull (Princeton: Princeton University Press), 41-63.

the two types as lying at opposite ends of a continuum, and suggested that the avoidant behavior of the introvert, and the novelty-seeking of the extravert, reflect largely inborn differences in arousability, with the nervous system of extravert being less arousable, while that of the introvert more so.[65]

Modern research has since confirmed that the introversion-extraversion dichotomy is biologically-based. Scores on introversion-extraversion scales predict individual responses to anaethesia.[66]

Dr. Healy explained:

> *The ones who come along talking about being anxious or depressed, they're the introverts, and the ones coming along figuring they've got ADHD and that they need meds for their ADHD are the extraverts. Half of the people come along to me and complain about having too much focus. And the other half are people who come along and say It seems I don't have focus enough.*

Dr. Healy explained that these different personality styles used to be seen as part of the normal range of human variation, rather than as pathologies in need of medical treatment:

> *There's some of us who focus more than we should, and need to loosen up, and there's others who maybe aren't as quite focused and there are times when the answer may be they need to focus more. And, you know, the world needs people who can focus well, and also those who maybe don't focus quite as much.*

---

[65] Gordon Claridge and David Healy, "The Psychopharmacology of Individual Differences," *Human Psychopharmacology: Clinical and Experimental* 9, no. 4 (July/August 1994): 285-298, https://doi.org/10.1002/hup.470090408

[66] David Healy, *Shipwreck of the Singular: Healthcare's Castaways*, Samizdat Health Writer's Co-operative (2021).

He went on to tell the story of a patient of his, a young man studying at university who was bright, personable, had big ideas, and knew how to get other people excited about his ideas. This young man dreamed of being an entrepreneur, and he got the idea that the way to do that was to study business and get a job at a giant corporation and work his way up the career ladder. But he found his coursework required him to spend long hours working on spreadsheets – a task which bored him and failed to inspire him. So, he began taking ADHD meds to improve his concentration, and he managed to finish his degree and get a job at a giant corporation, only to find himself doing – more spreadsheets!

> *You will never become an entrepreneur while working at a corporation like this. The idea of getting on with life is to find the right niche for ourselves. And if you're more extraverted and you've got a loose kind of focus, you're going to be more creative and entrepreneurial, and you don't want to go into corporations. On the other hand, if you're more introverted, more of a detail person, spreadsheets may be just the thing for you.*
>
> *But whether you're introvert or extravert, really both types are up against the same kind of problem, which is: These days the world doesn't want people to be varied. It's wants us to be homogenous, it's got to be pro forma tick boxes, we all have to be meeting the same quality standards. The idea of a team has gone out the window, you know, the idea that we need people who can score goals and people who can make sure the other team don't score goals. That's all gone out the window. We just want everybody to fit into the same mold which isn't a good situation for either introverts or extraverts, okay?*
>
> *In Europe, there's probably a little more understanding of this way of speaking. There's no one over here that talks this way. Over here people are a lot more categorical. You know, this is why DSM-III to*

> *some extent worked so well, with a bunch of labels. The people over here want their labels, they don't want to take these things away.*
>
> *It's a curious kind of situation. People like me who want to tell people that they're not mentally ill but they're actually pretty capable, they've had a bad deal from life but they've done all too well coping with it – I mean they're not mentally ill in the sense of brokenness, and they probably know the drugs are going to disable rather than enable them – that kind of message doesn't go down all that well. And this is not drug company crooks or ADHD experts bringing it, it's the way the world is going, and as with a bunch of these things, the world seems to go that way a lot quicker in the United States than anywhere else.*

Indeed. But given the confluence of factors we have discussed here, we may expect the number of children diagnosed and drugged for "ADHD" will continue to skyrocket, around the globe for years to come.

Reconstructing Truth, Deconstructing ADHD: Badiou, Onto-Epistemological Violence and the Diagnosis of ADHD

Mattias Nilsson Sjoberg

Psychiatric/neurodevelopmental diagnoses have expanded in number and scale with increased influence over matters of education and upbringing. One of the most common psychiatric diagnoses among children and adolescents is attention deficit hyperactivity disorder (ADHD). The dominant perspective of ADHD is biomedical, where ADHD is defined as a neurogenetic dysfunction and disorder of the brain.

Due to the absence of biological markers, the diagnosis is legitimized on the basis of a humanitarian principle: as an ideology. Through the diagnosis, which is construed in this chapter as a form of onto-epistemological violence, the unique subject is forced into an object and a second-class citizen who undergoes instrumental techniques of behavior modification.

The overall leitmotif of this chapter is to shift the focus from 'chemical imbalances' to 'power imbalances' (see UN, 2017) to counteract reductionism, disempowerment and medical behaviorism. Theoretically, it draws upon the *French* philosopher Alain Badiou's ontological examination of being *qua* being, wherein the aim is to critically examine the onto-epistemological violence following the diagnosis of ADHD and to seek out a less violent pedagogy.

Mattias Nilsson Sjöberg works in the Childhood-Education-Society Department at Malmö University, Sweden.

The violent diagnosis of ADHD

This chapter argues that the diagnosis of ADHD is violent. The term violent does not refer to the pharmaceutical violence well documented and problematized by others (e.g. Mills, 2014). What is referred to here as *onto-epistemological violence* emerges from a reading of the diagnosis of ADHD through Badiou's ontological examination of being qua being and his (mathematically deductive) method for deconstructing every one-effect of being (as explained below).

Epistemological violence refers to a scientific position rendering a fragmentary and reductionist knowledge production. It is derived from the belief that by using technology, and thus from a neutral and objective position, it is possible to find answers and represent nature consistent with the human idea about it (Shiva, 1988). Thus, onto-epistemology is a theoretical construct of Karen Barad (2007), who argues that different kinds of epistemological mattering cannot be separated from the ontological 'articulation' of the world. Therefore, Barad asserts that onto-epistemological practices always include ethical concerns (see further Nilsson Sjöberg, 2017).

Onto-epistemological violence, in turn, is something that has emerged through my reading of Badiou and his ontological examination of being. Badiou suggests that mathematical set theory is the only presently available language whereby it is possible to speak about being without 'violently' (in a constructible manner) reducing the universal principle of all ontological categories. Epistemological violence is not considered separate from the ontological violence, as it is somewhat presented in the analysis below. This distinction is made for analytical clarification.

The critique of ADHD is extensive, and the presentation below is far from exhaustive. Much educational inquiry has focused on a technological rationality and various forms of powerful dividing practices, where the diagnosed individual emerges as a technological object and a fragmentary subject through specific knowledge apparatuses. What Badiou is able to bring to this critique is his metaphysical 'turn' toward the ontological. Dahlbeck (2018) argues that educational researchers should not stop asking metaphysical – eternal – questions 'because our different ways of answering them will continue to shape how we live' (p. 1462). Slee (2006) pinpoints that much work still needs to be done because dominant ideas of inclusion have been cemented in segregating and excluding practices. Because a diagnosis like ADHD follows specific ontological assumptions about the world, Slee adds that the time is here to 'let's get metaphysical' (p. 117).

In this chapter, I argue that thinking about being in new ways is crucial, as is the need to seek out a less violent educational model other than the one facing an (ever-increasing) group of diagnosed individuals. Badiou's ontological examination of being and its effects are presented in more detail below. Before that, we examine how the diagnosis of ADHD constitutes an ethical dilemma in educational processes starting with notions concerning knowledge and truth.

The one, the other and the truth

Since ancient times, the relation between the individual and the state has been of utmost philosophical and educational concern. In particular, those members of society who challenged and reluctantly conformed to the (desirable) order of the state have caused educational concerns and effort. Moral assumptions and educational models always reflect the cultural contexts within which they come to exist; indeed, they reflect the ontological presuppositions they are derived from. It has been widely suggested that a technological rationality has come to play a crucial role in rendering production in society more efficient, thereby leading to an enormous apparatus of classification and an increased belief in the instrumentalization of educational processes (e.g. Biesta, 2010). Inseparable from this is the 'eternal' philosophical and educational question of how to live and work toward a true and good life.

Badiou repeatedly answers the above by stating that we have to take responsibility for the actual which is constantly generated by (four) various truth procedures – science, politics, art, love – making up the world we live in. Badiou, who sides with Plato against sophistry, seeks to reinstate a universal concept of truth in the sense that a truth is the result of a local and generic procedure. As such, a truth is always particular and comes into existence depending on the local structures within a situation. This 'immanence of truths' thus implies a universal value (Badiou, 2016: 71). However, the dominant view today is a universal morality directed at the general and not the particular. According to Badiou (2002), this implies an ethics based on the humanitarian principle of human rights where certain interests take it upon themselves to pity and intervene against what, from the perspective of a dominant 'One,' is presented as an a *priori* existing 'Other.'

What Badiou highlights is not only a matter of tolerating 'the Other' but also biopolitical control: an intervention in minority bodies/ brains to re/produce a social order in accordance with the privileged position of a dominant 'One' (see Badiou, 2009, preface). This bioethics, he claims, is based on a logic of identity in order to make society more efficient. Here, Badiou finds the basis for a hierarchical social system. Crucial then is to identify and disrupt those dominant truths, and truth procedures, which generate the world we live in. The reason for this is that a truth generated by certain dominant interests has a tendency to maintain an unequal social order if it passes by unnoticed.

Below is a brief overview of the critique of the dominant 'truth' about ADHD. Thereafter, follows an analysis of the so-called onto-epistemological violence, which refers to how certain truths about ADHD are forced into the world by specific (techno-positivistic) truth procedures. At the same time, when attempts to totalize being are made, the world by a dominant 'One' is forced into a kind of 'unequal distortion.' Badiou (2018) emphasizes that such a distortion or scandal in the world (in what we tend to think of as a given 'real'), reveals that there is another 'Real' possible to strive for; an event that gives the opportunity to collectively create new truths and to let the world appear in other less 'distorted' ways. Thus, it is in the impossibility to totalize being that the possibility of change is to be found. This is why we should never cease questioning those who try to totalize being from the perspective of 'One' and, at the same time, never give up on the idea of change. The reverse would be to act as a reactive subject and to continue to live at the level of a human animal and not as an active 'truth-making' subject in the world.

Parenthetically, Badiou's philosophy is a theory of change and in the end a philosophy that seeks a new humanity. Because Badiou states that mathematics is ontology, it is also, according to Pluth (2010), a formalized in-humanism. In Badiou's philosophy, the human animal does not differ from any other living animals. Ontologically, all is infinite multiplicity and in the end, nothing, a no-thing. Animal life consists of bodies and language, but to become a human *subject* it requires fidelity to (the universal idea of) truth. According to Badiou, this is what 'negates' the human subject from the human animal and other living animals (Pluth, 2010, pp. 8-12, 182-185).

The 'critical' case of ADHD

Psychiatric diagnoses such as ADHD have increased globally and expanded since the 1980s to reach an almost explosive rate during the first decades of the 21st century (e.g. Bergey et al., 2018). In the dominant biomedical paradigm, ADHD is defined as a genetic and/or neurochemical dysfunction manifested as a mental/cognitive disorder (e.g. Gillberg, 2014, 2018). However, neurobiological markers for validating ADHD have yet to be discovered and distinguished (e.g. Timimi, 2018).

Psychiatric/neurodevelopmental diagnoses and interventions are anything but neutral (e.g. Rose, 2019). Regarding ADHD, this is obvious when the (normative) diagnostic criteria grounded in diagnostic manuals such as DSM-5 (APA, 2013) are scrutinized (Freedman & Honkasilta, 2017). Various researchers have raised concerns that a psychiatric (or so-called neurodevelopmental) diagnosis serves a number of different interests at the same time as the diagnosed individual is transformed into a technological object, which in turn enables social control over, and instrumental modification of, behaviors not following a conformist order.

Hjörne (2016) argues that diagnostic categories entail segregating educational systems and excluding educational practices, even in Sweden: a country otherwise used as a leading example of democracy and social welfare. While Graham (2008) refers to the performativity of psychomedically influenced pedagogical discourses in the production of students as 'disorderly objects,' Harwood and Allan (2014) use the term 'psychopathologisation' to demonstrate a 'complex web of power relations' where a number of discursive and material practices partake in an epistemologically violent production of the 'ADHD-child.

The construction of 'truths' regarding ADHD extends far beyond the situations where the so-called symptoms appear (particularly at school). Laurence and McGallum (1998) argue that when electroencephalography (EEG) was introduced as a diagnostic technique it became a powerful tool 'which carved out new space – the space "inside the child's head" – for the operation of power' (p. 198). Baker (2002) states that the entire diagnostic project is nothing but repressive eugenics, where some children and youths are separated into different groups through the diagnostic process. Children (students) only become dysfunctional when they are not sufficiently productive (at school), after which they are to be seen and treated as a risk and a burden to society. The 'dysfunctional' group of children and youths is then subjected to various instrumental 'perfecting technologies' so as to conform to the dominant order.

Others emphasize that the dominant role of the biomedical model of ADHD leads to causal explanations being one-sided and that the uniqueness of the one diagnosed is downplayed (Erlandsson & Punzi, 2017). This entails educational concerns as the diagnosis is heterogeneous in nature and thus mystifies pedagogical relations rather than explains the unique situation of every living person/ student (Graham, 2010). As a result, Erlandsson, Lundin and Punzi (2016) suggest that the acronym ADHD should be placed inside quotation marks (='ADHD'). (This principle is applied from this point on and until otherwise indicated.) An additional remark is that the diagnosis of 'ADHD' is based on a variety of logical errors – a significant example being the circular logic where the observed behavior is explained by means of the neuropsychiatric diagnosis as a theoretical construct, and vice versa (Lindstrøm, 2012; Pérez-Álvarez, 2017; Tait, 2009).

This 'repressive illogic' described above brings us to an example I would argue is largely representative of the pro-diagnostic paradigm in relation to 'ADHD.' In other words, due to a lack of empirical evidence, the diagnosis is instead based on ideology. In the section below, it is shown that the diagnosis is legitimized on the basis of a utility-based humanitarian principle. Also presented below are the educational and ethical problems arising when inadequate representations of being are presented as absolute and adequate truths (see Nilsson Sjöberg & Dahlbeck, 2018).

The quasi-humanitarian and utility-based diagnosis of ADHD

A strong advocate of the neurogenetic perspective on 'ADHD' is Christopher Gillberg, who, in a Nordic context, has played an important role in the expansion of the diagnosis (Smith, 2017). Based on the US diagnostic manual for mental disorders (DSM-5), Gillberg (2014, 2018) claims that 'ADHD' is an innate neurological dysfunction manifesting itself in a mental and behavioral disorder. Gillberg includes 'ADHD' under the diagnosis of ESSENCE.

This term "diagnosis" is used for describing and explaining a set of behaviors that must be exhibited by children and youths in order for certain measures to be taken. These measures mainly apply to children and youths not performing sufficiently well in school, and who are thus assumed to be at risk of developing future social problems. This implied future threat to public order, seen by Gillberg (2014) as 'one of the major public health issues of our time' (p. 75), legitimizes the diagnosis as an instrument for selection through which targeted measures, not infrequently pharmaceutical, are enabled and may be applied at an early age.

In the absence of biological markers for making a diagnosis, diagnostics are not only based on medical/physiological and psychological/ cognitive examinations, but also on interviews and various types of diagnostic questionnaires based on how parents and teachers assess the child's behaviour. Additionally, specific technological examinations in clinical laboratory settings may also be used for measuring attention and impulsivity (Gillberg, 2014, pp. 174-186).

Notwithstanding the lack of specific biological markers, Gillberg states that people with 'ADHD' must be approached on the basis of systematic psycho-medical knowledge providing an adequate understanding of 'ADHD' as a neurological dysfunction. However, there is no consensus on the causes behind the diagnosis (aetiology), which may explain why 'ADHD' manifests itself heterogeneously. While pointing out that everyone with 'ADHD' is unique, Gillberg adds that people said to have 'ADHD' frequently see themselves as normal, while the so-called disorder is to be found in the opinions of others (2014, p. vi).

To legitimize the diagnosis, Gillberg invokes a humanist ideal. The neuropsychiatric diagnosis is used in the belief that it will prevent stigmatization and that the individual may experience a sense of belonging to the community. Gillberg believes that the diagnosis serves to integrate rather than to segregate.
Although the knowledge concerning 'ADHD' is inadequate, it is said that the diagnosis plays an adequate role in the sense that it assigns a name to something otherwise uncertain. A crucial argument presented is that if we cannot know for certain what causes 'ADHD,' then a diagnosis cannot be all that bad after all:

> *[M]ost people forget that a diagnosis is a form of treatment in itself. Having a name for the difficulties one is experiencing can never be worse than fumbling in the dark. The name also comes with information about causes, risks, and reasonable approaches. Even if – at worst – nothing else can be offered, that is still not a bad treatment effort! (Gillberg, 2014, p. 185)*

Lacking scientific and empirical evidence, Gillberg takes support from the philosopher Ludwig Wittgenstein by stating, 'What we cannot speak about we must pass over in silence' (Gillberg, 2018, p. 158)4 He uses this quote to support why a diagnosis should be deemed necessary and important: without diagnosis, we/he cannot talk about the 'thing' (or 'essence') that ADHD is considered to correspond with, and certain 'interventions' cannot be legitimized.

It is clear that the diagnosis of 'ADHD' does not primarily exist as a result of medical-psychiatric and techno-scientific progression. Instead, a reverse type of logic applies: the diagnosis as a theoretical construct seeks medical-psychiatric and techno-scientific validation at the same time as the diagnosis serves certain functions in relation to individual and society as formulated by dominant interests. The diagnosis is pure ideology, and as such it supports an educational model emphasizing identity over diversity. The current principle, as well as a crucial argument, is that the diagnosis represents a humanitarian utility aspect. Utility outweighs risk, according to the prognosis determined via the diagnosis.

The following is an analysis of the onto-epistemological violence (re)produced by Gillberg – here used as an example of something obviously much larger than Gillberg himself – when he argues in favor of the existence of the neuropsychiatric diagnosis on the basis of a utility-based humanitarian principle. The following examples are taken from the neurobiological laboratory, as this is where a large part of the knowledge concerning 'ADHD' is produced as truths.

Following Badiou and his ontological examination of being, I will now scrutinize how certain truth procedures force the fragmented 'ADHD-subject' into the world, thereby simultaneously reducing 'ADHD' (the unique subject) to the level of a manipulated laboratory rat.

Treated as a rat: onto-epistemological violence and the fragmentary ADHD-subject

In a philosophical sense, being is that which is, whereas an ontological examination of being *qua* being entails searching for what is universal for everything that exists. There is a long tradition in philosophy arguing that the way in which we understand being is fundamental for the actions that follow. For the purposes of this chapter, he highlights an increasing contemporary belief in an ideologically driven techno-scientific positivism seeking to make us uncritically seduced in its attempt to totalize being (Badiou, 2011). However, Badiou is not anti-technological (see Badiou with Tarby, 2013, pp. 92-104); neither is he anti-scientific, as his ontological position in itself is mathematical, thus scientific (Brassier, 2010). Badiou himself states that 'mathematics = ontology' (2005, p. 6); 'It [mathematics] makes it possible to take on an ontology of the pure multiple without renouncing the truth ...' (Badiou, 1999, p. 104).

Based on the language of mathematics, and more specifically set theory, Badiou argues that being is an infinite multiple. Infinite multiplicity is pure alterity, and as such it is 'the regime of being' (Badiou with Tarby, 2013, p. 57). In other words, the substance of being is void: void is an indiscernible no-thing, an unnameable that is completely neutral beyond technological and literary definitions, but which through various forms of situational operations, generic truth procedures, are forced into the world as hierarchical differences.

As explained in more detail below, the void is also named the empty set. Void, or the empty set, relates to the infinite multiplicity that Badiou (2005) thinks of as universal for all ontological categories. Infinite multiplicity as pure alterity is not difference; it is nothingness, the unnameable, and this is what I relate to the uniqueness (the 'Real Being') of each and every one. Thus, being is neither one nor multiple. It is a multiple of multiplicities and as such, in the end, it is nothing, a no-thing.

What Badiou argues is that each attempt to capture an elusive being generates new truths. Generic truth procedures work as organizing practices with a 'one-effect'. This means that being qua being as infinite multiplicity, a 'no-thing,' is forced into the world as 'one,' presented as a different and distinct 'some-thing.' And this, according to Badiou, is an absolute and universal statement that is derived from his 'absolute ontology' (Badiou, 2016, pp. 74–77).

With the Platonic cave allegory in mind, from the Real a distorted real is forced into the world by certain dominant interests, where these dominant interests also do what it takes to re/produce a specific (capitalist) state of order presented as the best possible of all alternatives (Badiou, 2018).

Above I have highlighted a contemporary biomaterialism where the process of becoming is reduced to a biological level. The labelled person is transformed – commodified – into a dysfunctional object through the use of biotechnological apparatuses. Badiou speaks of different degrees of identification making a specific object appear in the world in a certain way. Thus, some objects become existent while others remain non-existent; in any given situation, some things can be said to exist more than others. Using the movie theatre as a modern example of the Platonic cave allegory, Badiou (2012) describes how what we might think of as the real truth is projected on the movie screen towards which everybody turns their heads.

But what is projected on the screen and presented is only a kind of sensible (visible and audible) reduction of the True, of the 'Real', but which is most often presented and taken for an undisputable fact: "This … audience has no way of deducing that the substance of True is anything other than the shadow of a simulacrum' (p. 213). This 'shadow of simulacrum' are by some 'dominant' groups with specific interests made to appear on the movie screen and is presented as an absolute truth to the one labelled as 'ADHD' and to a wider audience. Neurobiological research, different types of MRI-scans, and psychiatric/neurodevelopmental diagnoses easily fits into this model.

To examine how certain truths about 'ADHD' are generated in neurobiological research, I use the example of a study by Hoogman et al. (2017), where the truth about 'ADHD' through biotechnological innovations is presented as absolute. Hence, the study tries to capture and totalize being. On the basis of their so-called 'mega-analysis', the research team consisting of a total of 84(!) professionals claim that they have found evidence that 'ADHD' is a 'disorder of the brain'. On the basis of a limited number of people having undergone certain brain scans in many different sites, Hoogman et al. interpret and present their results in a way that (almost) leads us to believe that the truth regarding 'ADHD' has now been established. Notwithstanding the dubious representation, or misinterpretation (e.g. Batstra et al., 2017), a result of this presentation is that a new distorted/fragmented truth is forced into the world – one that makes a specific state of being come into existence. However, this truth is not a final answer as to what causes 'ADHD.' Rather, it sets being in motion and thus makes the one labelled as 'ADHD' and the world appear in a certain way.

According to Badiou, the sets that constitute being are infinite and always constructible. Hence, the truth presented by Hoogman et al. (2017) is just one of many truths that are generated – today at a rapid pace. And it turns out to be a truth that divides humanity in two: a generic truth procedure that forces the otherwise indifferent multiplicities at the level of being into differences possible to organize into a hierarchically stratified order of society. It is a truth, according to Hoogman et al., well worth presenting to the world: 'This message [that ADHD is a disorder of the brain] is clear for clinicians to convey to parents and patients, which can help to reduce the stigma of ADHD and improve understanding of the disorder'

(2017, p. 2).

The study of Hoogman et al. is just one of a large number of empirical studies using modern technology in clinical laboratory environments to generate certain kinds of truths. The truth procedure used by Hoogman et al. is also a prime example of the (onto-) epistemological violence discussed in this article. This is the case as laboratory experiments take place far away from the situations in which the so-called symptoms of 'ADHD' appear and turn into a problem. This (onto-)epistemological violence is equivalent with a decontextualization and fragmentation that reduces 'ADHD' into a neurogenetic dysfunction (re)presented on a computer screen as a 'hard fact' and unquestionable truth.

Hoogman et al. uses biotechnology not only to represent 'ADHD', but also to present and thus force a certain kind of truth into the world. While it is presented as absolute, such a techno-positivistic presentation is only representing a 'shadow of simulacrum' (Badiou, 2012, p. 213), thus it is a fragmentation of 'ADHD' made by the research team. Only certain truths, or beings/existences, are forced into and made appearing in the world, however, whereas other still remain non-existent. In relation to educational processes of becoming, this is of utmost importance as this form of inadequate knowledge is used and presented as an adequate truth (e.g. in the 'pedagogic' act of so-called psychoeducation). Simultaneously, the empirical facts are generated by certain interests to legitimize and support 'ADHD' as a theoretical construct.

Despite the limited space provided in a chapter, it seems relevant to include yet another example, once again from the neurobiological laboratory. Here, researchers are looking to distinguish and differentiate genetic and neuromolecular entities from each other in order to find a causal answer as to what causes 'ADHD' (Gallo & Posner, 2016).

Gallo and Posner argue that human life – particularly 'unwanted life,' such as 'ADHD,' they note – should be reduced to the minimum possible genetic-molecular functions to better enable the identification of a linear causality. Thus, various animal models are used, not infrequently rats (Sagvolden & Johansen, 2011). The rats are first manipulated so that they exhibit symptoms comparable to human 'ADHD.' They are then injected with so-called designer drugs, once again altering the behavior of the rats in accordance with what those working in the laboratory consider a normal/functional behavior for a rat. If the rats' response to the chemical substance corresponds with the response of people diagnosed with 'ADHD' when 'medicated,' not only are the different animal models seen as valid for using in experiments of this kind, but the diagnosis is also confirmed (Gallo & Posner, 2016; Sagvolden & Johansen, 2011).

The life of those who are labelled as 'ADHD' is here equated with the life of manipulated laboratory rats. As such it constitutes a (onto-) epistemological violent act with not least significant socio-political consequences. Apparently, the laboratory is also where a pedagogy for managing these 'ADHD rats' is created by means of clinical experimentation, since we know that a large portion of children and youths (and adults) diagnosed with 'ADHD' face the same 'treatment/intervention' as the rats: a medical behaviorism. On the basis of the above examples, it is no longer possible to stop thinking about neophrenology and repressive eugenics.

But what about those that appear on the other side of the (onto-) epistemological violence? Honkasilta (2016) emphasizes that children/youths diagnosed with 'ADHD' seek out and find explanations *beyond* a psychomedical discourse, while parents and other adults stand *behind* the assumption that an individual diagnosis defined as a neurological dysfunction is to be seen as adequate support that offers the best way forward for educational success and a reduction in stigma. Singh (2013) highlights that children/youths with a diagnosis do not see themselves as neurologically dysfunctional; instead they see themselves as agents (not) responsible for their actions. The examples could be multiplied.

On an overarching level the UN (2017) not only notices the dominance of the biomedical paradigm but also sees it as important to shift the focus from 'chemical imbalances' to 'power imbalances'. This assertion is partly derived from how the biomedical model has been highly disputed by psychiatrized subjects, sometimes referred to as 'survivors' or 'users.' The counter-response created by this (onto-)epistemological ('psychiatrized') violence is highlighted thus:

If epistemic violence is to deny being, then the response to the violence is to construct ways that bring psychiatrized people back into existence. If epistemic violence is understood as the non-recognition of being, then the resistance to epistemic violence would mean bringing into being that which is denied existence. (Liegghio, 2013, p. 127)

First, Liegghio separates the epistemological from the ontological; at the same time, it is stated that the two are not separable. Second, if the (onto-)epistemological violence *denies being* and leads to an act of violence against all of those whose full existence is not recognized as a result of psychiatrization, then the counter-response would be to *restore being*. I now discuss what Badiou's ontological examination of being, on the basis of my reading, has to say about the onto(-epistemological) violence exercised by the diagnostic culture in which we live. I also draw up the outlines of a less violent pedagogy beyond the diagnosis.

Counting for inclusion: onto-epistemological violence and the diagnosis of 'ADHD'

Badiou claims that being qua being is pure and infinite multiplicity, a conclusion reached by means of mathematical deduction and, more precisely, of mathematical set theory. Mathematics then is the kind of formalization we may use to reach an absolute understanding of being as such: 'mathematics is ontology, i.e., the independent study of the possible forms of the multiple as such, of any multiple, and therefore of everything that is – because everything, that is, is in any case a multiplicity' (2016, p. 68).

Moreover, mathematical set theory is used by Badiou to deconstruct every possibility to organize life on the basis of being as One: 'It thereby deconstructs any one-effect; it is faithful to the non-being of the one…' (2005, p. 33). A premise for Badiou (2005) is if something may appear in a multiple form, then it must imply that 'the One' is not a characteristic of being. What Badiou's absolute ontology helps to understand is that if 'the One' does not exist, neither can 'the Other' (Badiou, 2002).

As a materialistic philosopher arguing on the basis of mathematical set theory, Badiou presents the thesis that being consists of infinite and indifferent multiplicities that are forced into the world as difference(s), or distinct sets, through certain types of generic truth procedures. The basic principle in mathematical set theory is that a set is a collection, *nota bene*, of arbitrary elements that may be counted as one. If a set may be constructed by any types of elements that may be counted as one, then all sets are always constructible. Furthermore, two sets may be equal and identical if, for instance, set A is composed of exactly the same elements as set β.

In all cases of sets that are not identical to one another, they constitute subsets of each other, whereby one set becomes superior to other sets. In set theory, different subsets always include other subsets, which follow in infinity. This is possible since the construction of a set is always followed by a new subset, which in turn is made up of another constructible subset, and so on. This is where Badiou finds what he refers to as the *empty set,* or the null set (denoted by the symbol Ø). One might never capture this empty set; it is indiscernible. The empty set is what Badiou denotes as void, and void is nothingness – the unnameable.

But if being is pure multiplicity, how is it possible for something to appear as 'one,' as an existing object? Badiou finds the answer in the structure of the present order. It is through specific truth procedures that the pure multiple – multiplicities that on the level of being are indifferent to each other – are forced into the world and emerge as difference. As clarified above, 'ADHD' is a diagnosis constructed to bring structure to life in accordance with a dominant order (the diagnosed child is to be included in a greater whole, not the other way around), and there are some who take it upon themselves to do so by means of a diagnostic process.

Here, the empty set (Ø) becomes very important. Badiou sees Ø as the utmost nothingness of being. When the diagnosis becomes the answer for managing the nothingness of being, the uncertainty of life, then the empty set is not taken into account. And why the empty set is not taken into account is because it is indiscernible. Instead, the neuropsychiatric diagnosis of 'ADHD' constitutes a totalization of being; or it is at least presented that way when the knowledge concerning 'ADHD' is in fact inadequate.

But when the diagnosis from 'the One' to 'the Other' is presented as an adequate truth, it becomes a totalitarian principle as a result of the perspective of the world (of 'ADHD') made by a 'dominant One.' In this process, the otherwise unique subject is reduced to a neurological disordered object and forced into the world as 'the Other'. And it is the position of a 'dysfunctional Other.'

This process turns the empty set (Ø: the unique and unnameable subject) into a closed set. So, with regard to whether or not the diagnosis is stigmatizing, it is sufficient to go to the origin of the word to see how the classified subject – which at the level of being is a pure multiple and therefore indifferent to other multiplicities – through the diagnosis emerges as a 'negative difference,' identified and labelled as a disordered/dysfunctional object. Through the diagnostic classification, the unnameable subject (Ø) is made into a closed set and nameable object. What we see is onto(-epistemological) violence and this is the case as the closed set, according to Badiou (2002), is the enemy of true subjectivities.

Let us now investigate the onto(-epistemological) violence following the classifying principle of the diagnosis, as well as the problem of unique individuals, through psychiatric classification, are forced together into the same category. Hjörne (2016), for instance, highlights how diagnostic categories affect educational practices. Stereotypical prejudices, segregation and exclusionary practices most often follow the process of categorization.

In mathematical set theory, as used by Badiou (1999, 2005), elements with a certain arbitrarily selected characteristic are brought together. Let us here focus on the element U as in a U(nique being), but whose characteristics are the behaviors inattention and hyperactivity-impulsivity; and when brought together, they constitute the subset B as in B(ehavior). The subset B(ehavior) thus consists of x number of U(nique beings), which we may here denote as {U}. In relation to the subset B(ehavior), an additional set has been constructed, which is A as in A(DHD). The element {U} then becomes subordinate to the subset B(ehavior), which is subordinate to the subset A(DHD). The subset A(DHD), in turn, is subordinate to the subset NPD[6], which is subordinate to H(umanity) – the principle should be very clear by now. What happens as a result of this classification and categorization is that all individuals exhibiting certain behaviors

– so-called symptoms – resembling each other, when brought together in a new set, are moved toward a general character and an abstraction *away* from the individual element *toward* what the new set has in common.

On the basis of the examples provided above, we now understand that classifying a heterogeneous group of unique individuals, and placing them into a category so that schools can offer an individual and inclusive pedagogy, is based on highly questionable reasoning. When made into the subset A(DHD), the unique individual is included in a greater quantity, but at the same time s/he no longer belongs to her- or himself. It becomes clear that simply placing 'ADHD' inside quotation marks is not sufficient (see Erlandsson, Lundin & Punzi, 2016). If we follow Badiou's ontological examination of being and its subsequent effects, 'ADHD' must be addressed on the basis of the principle ADHD. In this way, it is possible to move beyond the onto(-epistemo)logical violence of the neuropsychiatric diagnosis so a less violent educational model can come into existence.

Parenthetically, the diagnosis of ADHD belongs to the Swedish acronym NPF. NPF, in this article translated to NPD, refers to the Swedish term 'neuropsykiatrisk funktionsnedsättning,' which is best translated as 'neuropsychiatric disorder' or 'neuropsychiatric dysfunction', in turn closely related to the definition 'neurodevelopmental disorder' as used in DSM-5 (APA, 2013), or 'a disorder of the brain.'

Conclusion, or what we cannot speak about we must pass over in silence

Almost half a century ago, Conrad and Schneider (1980) wrote that '[...] "counterpower" to medical social control needs to be created' (p. 260), with regards to the diagnosis of hyperkinesis/MBD, a predecessor to 'ADHD'. In hindsight, we see that the impact of this counterpower has been rather limited as the biomedical paradigm and neuropsychiatric discourse and diagnoses have steadily grown and become normalized. For precisely this reason, further critique is made relevant.

Turning to Badiou's metaphysics and ontological examination of being *qua* being, this article has engaged in the counterpower to the biomedical paradigm with a particular interest in the diagnosis of 'ADHD.' On a related note, Badiou (2002) argues that we live in a social order sustained by differentiated objects of various kinds: an identity politics of sorts. It is in the constant invention of new objects – identities – where such a system finds support and creates investments in the market.

Besides this identity politics, a normalization politics aiming to achieve uniformity among citizens seems to be dominant (Richardson, 2005). Normalizing identity politics are completely dominant when it comes to neuropsychiatric diagnoses such as 'ADHD.' Within formal education, there has been a worldwide push for performance and efficiency: a technological rationality enforced by the use of standardized curriculums and measurements squeezing students into conformity rather than focusing on unique subjectification (e.g. Biesta, 2010). In combination with the neuropsychiatric dogma and its expansive influence in education and upbringing, we have to deal with an (enormous) classification apparatus striving for uniformity among students.

Paradoxically, in the pursuit of uniformity, a constant flow of new psychiatric identities are created, resulting in a hierarchical and stigmatized situation of us-and-them (see Runswick-Cole, 2014). What also needs to be emphasized is that the diagnosis is many other things but individual, as it is closely intertwined with professional, political, economic, and ideological interests. Hence, from what has been demonstrated above, 'ADHD' should be understood as an anthropomorphic and biosociotechnological construct rather than a 'disorder of the brain'.

In this chapter, it is argued that a dominant 'One' has excluded the empty set in the quest to capture and totalize being (or 'ADHD'). However, according to Badiou, being is elusive and cannot be totalized. This indeterminate aspect of being is determined by the absoluteness of mathematical set theory, as suggested by Badiou. Following this, the equation 'diagnosis = inclusion' is based on a questionable reasoning. The diagnosis of 'ADHD' also appears as a violent humanitarian act because the diagnosis equates the one labelled as 'ADHD' with a manipulated laboratory rat. The diagnosed individual is made into a kind of animal-like state of being and is thereby not considered sufficiently human and thus in need of instrumental perfecting technologies to become a functional member of society.

Indeed, it is a violent pedagogy, which, it turns out, is also evil. This is so because evil, for Badiou, is the 'desire to name [the unnameable] *at any price*', and when one truth attempts to totalize the others, it is nothing but a disaster (Badiou, 2008, p. 127, italics in original). The diagnosis turns the unique subject, the empty set, into a closed set, thereby totalizing void. And as pinpointed by Badiou, the enemy of true subjectivities is none other than the closed set. Hence, in the quest for a less violent and evil pedagogy, the diagnosis of 'ADHD' should no longer be used, nor should it be placed inside quotation marks. If we want a less violent and evil world, the diagnosis should no longer be used (~~ADHD~~).

When suggested that educators (and others) should drop the language of disorder and the diagnosis as such, it seems much easier to say than to do. It is so because the diagnosis is a significant 'cog' – the diagnosis is of a high value use for many involved parties – in a complex professional, political, economic, and ideological apparatus more than it is a diagnosis that corresponds with a transcendental essence ever possible to find 'out there'.

Even if the diagnosis (of ADHD) is irreducible to the emergence of compulsory school, the educational domain certainly works as a catalyst for the growth of disability categories. For example, the 'hunt for disability' described by Baker (2002), Graham (2008, 2010), and Harwood and Allan (2014) is inexorably linked to school finance. This seems to be the case also in the Nordic countries, though not a legal requirement (Hjörne, 2016; Honkasilta, 2016).

The diagnosis is considered an 'inclusive' necessity to continue production towards a world which by a dominant 'One' is deemed the best possible and all other alternatives impossible. At the same time, the process of psychopathologisation is supposed to destigmatize underperformance in school and society by forcing some individuals into the world as 'dysfunctional/disordered Others' suitable for different kinds of instrumental perfecting technologies such as psychotropic neuroenhancement.

However, it is here that Badiou's ethics and political subject becomes highly significant, when he pushes to never give up the Idea: the idea of change towards equality. When certain behaviors – in school, for example – present themselves in a way that is defined and perceived by a dominant order as a 'dysfunction/disorder,' it is precisely this rupture within the given order that reveals a non-equal reality or structure.

Such a scandalous rupture (Badiou, 2018), or disastrous trace within a situation (Badiou, 2005), is the very place to start if we want to remake the world. Such a 'disaster,' or 'dysfunction,' of the world reveals a given 'real' in it, but at the same time such a rupture reveals that there is another 'Real" that is possible to, in a constructible manner, be (ever) searched for. Such a truth-making procedure should, however, be a collective work, Badiou argues, and indeed follow the Idea of an egalitarian experimentation towards equality within the world.

Let me summarize by returning to Gillberg, who uses a quote from Wittgenstein – 'What we cannot speak about we must pass over in silence' – to legitimize the diagnosis when the empirical evidence runs short. It leads to the conclusion that what we have inadequate knowledge about, we must be careful of how we pass over (see Nilsson Sjöberg & Dahlbeck, 2018). What then requires, if we follow Badiou, is courage and hard work, because it requires courage and hard work to learn how to 'fumble in the dark' together and thus change the world from the perspective of 'Two' rather from 'the One' (see Nilsson Sjöberg, 2018).

References

APA (2013). *Diagnostic and Statistical Manual of Mental Disorders* (DSM-5). 5th ed. Washington, DC: American Psychiatric Association.

Badiou, A. (1999). *Manifesto for Philosophy*. Albany, N.Y.: State University of New York Press.

Badiou, A. (2002). *Ethics – An Essay on the Understanding of Evil*. London: Verso.
Badiou, A. (2005). Being and Event. London: Continuum.

Badiou, A. (2008). *Conditions*. London: Continuum.

Badiou, A. (2009). *Logics of Worlds. Being and Event II*. London: Continuum.
Badiou, A. (2011). *Second Manifesto for Philosophy*. Cambridge, UK: Polity.
Badiou, A. (2012). *Plato's Republic*. Cambridge, UK: Polity.

Badiou, A. with Tarby, F. (2013). Philosophy and the Event. Cambridge, UK: Polity. Badiou, A. (2016). *In Praise of Mathematics*. Cambridge, UK: Polity.

Badiou, A. (2018). In Search of the Lost Real. In A. J. Bartlett & J. Clemens (Eds.), *Badiou and His Interlocutors. Lectures, Interviews and Responses*, (pp. 7-16). London: Bloomsbury.

Baker, B. (2002). The Hunt for Disability: The New Eugenics and the Normalization of School Children. *Teachers College Record*, 104(4): 663-703.

Barad, K. (2007). *Meeting the Universe Halfway: Quantum Physics and the Entanglement of Matter and Meaning*. Durham, NC: Duke University Press.

Batstra, L., Meerman, S., Conners, K. & Frances, A. (2017). Subcortical brain volume differences in participants with attention deficit hyperactivity disorder in children and adults. *Lancet Psychiatry*, 4(6): 439.

Bergey, M. R., Filipe, A. M., Conrad, P. & Singh, I. (Eds.) (2018). *Global Perspectives on ADHD. Social Dimensions of Diagnosis and Treatment in 16 Countries*. Baltimore: Johns Hopkins University Press.

Biesta, G. (2010). *Good Education in an Age of Measurement: Ethics, Politics, Democracy*. Boulder: Paradigm Publishers.

Brassier, R. (2010). Science. In A. J. Bartlett & J. Clemens (Eds.), *Alain Badiou: Key Concepts*, (pp. 61-72). Durham: Acumen.

Conrad, P. & Schneider, J. W. (1980). *Deviance and Medicalization. From Badness to Sickness*. St. Louis: Mosby.

Dahlbeck, J. (2018). At the wake, or the return of metaphysics. *Educational Philosophy and Theory*, 50(14): 1462-1463.

Erlandsson S. & Punzi, E. (2017). A biased ADHD discourse ignores human Uniqueness. *International Journal of Qualitative Studies on Health and Well-being*, 12:sup1, 1319584. DOI: 10.1080/17482631.2017.1319584

Erlandsson S., Lundin, L. & Punzi, E. (2016). A discursive analysis concerning information on 'ADHD' presented to parents by the National Institute of Mental Health (USA). *International Journal of Qualitative Studies on Health and Well-being*, 11. DOI: dx.doi.org/10.3402/qhw.v11.30938

Freedman J. E. & Honkasilta, J. M. (2017). Dictating the boundaries of ab/normality: a critical discourse analysis of the diagnostic criteria for attention deficit hyperactivity disorder and hyperkinetic disorder. *Disability & Society*, 32(4): 565-588.

Gallo, E. F. & Posner, J. (2016). Moving towards causality in attention-deficit hyperactivity disorder: overview of neural and genetic mechanisms. *Lancet Psychiatry*, 3(6): 555-567.

Gillberg, C. (2014). *ADHD and Its Many Associated Problems*. Oxford: Oxford University Press.

Gillberg, C. (2018). *ESSENCE. Om ADHD, autism och andra utvecklingsavvikelser*. [ESSENCE. ADHD, Autism and other Developmental Disorders.] Stockholm: Natur & Kultur.

Graham, L. J. (2008). From ABCs to ADHD: The Role of Schooling in the Construction of Behavior Disorder and Production of Disorderly Objects. *International Journal of Inclusive Education*, 12(1): 2–33.

Graham, L. J. (2010). Teaching ADHD? In L. J. Graham (Ed.), (De)Constructing ADHD: *Critical Guidance for Teachers and Teacher Educators* (pp. 1-20). New York, NY: Peter Lang.

Harwood, V. & Allan, J. (2014). *Psychopathology at School. Theorizing Mental Disorders in Education*. New York: Routledge.

Hjörne, E. (2016). The narrative of special education in Sweden: History and trends in policy and practice. *Discourse: Studies in the Cultural Politics of Education*, 37(4): 540-552.

Honkasilta, J. (2016). *Voices Behind and Beyond the Label: The Master Narrative of ADHD (De)constructed by Diagnosed Children and Their Parents* (Doctoral dissertation). University of Jyväskyla: Jyväskyla Studies in Education, Psychology and Social Research.

Hoogman, M. & 81 co-endorsers (2017). Subcortical Brain Volume Differences in Participants with Attention Deficit Hyperactivity Disorder in Children and Adults: A Cross-Sectional Mega- Analysis. *Lancet Psychiatry*, 4(4): 310-319.

Laurence, J. & McCallum, D. (1998) The Myth-or-Reality of Attention-Deficit Disorder: a genealogical approach. *Discourse: Studies in the Cultural Politics of Education*, 19(2): 183- 200.

Liegghio, M. (2013). A Denial of Being: Psychiatrization as Epistemic Violence. In B. LeFrançois, R. Menzies & G. Reaume (Eds.), *Mad Matters. A Critical Reader in Canadian Mad Studies*, (pp. 122-129). Toronto: Canadian Scholars Press.

Lindstrøm, J. A. (2012). Why Attention-Deficit/Hyperactivity Disorder Is Not a True Medical Syndrome. *Ethical Human Psychology and Psychiatry*, 14(1): 61-73.

Mills, C. (2014). *Psychotropic Childhoods: Global Mental Health and Pharmaceutical Children*. Children & Society, 28(3): 194–204.

Nilsson Sjöberg, M. (2017). (Un)becoming dysfunctional: ADHD and how matter comes to matter. *International Journal of Inclusive Education*, 21(6): 602–615.

Nilsson Sjöberg, M. (2018). Toward a Militant Pedagogy in the Name of Love: On Psychiatrization of Indifference, Neurobehaviorism and the Diagnosis of ADHD – A Philosophical Intervention. *Studies in Philosophy and Education*, 37(4): 329–346.

Nilsson Sjöberg, M & Dahlbeck, J. (2018). The inadequacy of ADHD: a philosophical contribution. *Emotional and Behavioural Difficulties*, (23)1: 97–108.

Pérez-Álvarez, M. (2017). The Four Causes of ADHD: Aristotle in the Classroom. *Frontiers in Psychology*, 8(928). DOI: 10.3389/fpsyg.2017.00928

Pluth, E. (2010). *Badiou: A Philosophy of the New*. Cambridge, UK: Polity.

Richardson, D. (2005). Desiring Sameness? The Rise of Neoliberal Politics of Normalisation. *Antipode, 37(3): 515-535.*

Rose, N. (2019). *Our Psychiatric Future. The Politics of Mental Health*. Cambridge: Polity.

Rose, N. & Abi-Rached, J. M. (2013). *Neuro: The New Brain Sciences and the Management of the Mind*. Princeton: Princeton University Press.

Runswick-Cole, K. (2014). 'Us' and 'them': the limits and possibilities of a 'politics of neurodiversity' in neoliberal times. *Disability & Society, 29*(7): 1117-1129.

Sagvolden, T. & Johansen, E. B. (2011). Rat Models of ADHD. In C. Stanford & R. Tannock (Eds.), *Behavioral Neuroscience of Attention Deficit Hyperactivity Disorder and Its Treatment. Current Topics in Behavioral Neurosciences*, (pp. 301-315). Berlin, Heidelberg: Springer.

Shiva, V. (1988). Reductionist Science as Epistemological Violence. In A. Nandy (Ed.) *Hegemony and Violence. A Requiem for Modernity*, (pp. 232-256). Tokyo: United Nations University.

Singh, I. (2013). Brain talk: power and negotiation in children's discourse about self, brain and behaviour. *Sociology of Health & Illness*, 35(6): 813-827.

Slee, R. (2006). Limits to and possibilities for educational reform. *International Journal of Inclusive Education*, 10(2/3): 109-120.

Smith, M. (2017). Hyperactive Around the World? The History of ADHD in Global Perspective. *Social History of Medicine*, 30(4): 767-787.

Tait, G. (2009). The logic of ADHD: a brief review of fallacious reasoning. *Studies in Philosophy and Education*, 28(3): 239-254.

Timimi, S. (2018). Attention-deficit hyperactivity disorder: a critique of the concept. *Irish Journal of Psychological Medicine*, 35(3): 257-259.

United Nations, UN (2017). *Report of the Special Rapporteur on the right of everyone to the enjoyment of the highest attainable standard of physical and mental health.* Retrieved December 11, 2017, from http://ap.ohchr.org/documents/dpage_e.aspx?m=100

Wittgenstein, L. (1922). *Tractatus Logico-Philosophicus*. Oxon: Routledge & Kegan Paul.

The Ontology of ADHD: Discovery or Invention?

Christoffer Hornborg and Soly Erlandsson

Modern societies have undergone considerable changes in recent decades. For example, the perception of what constitutes "normal behavior" has changed, with implications on our view of how children (and adults) should and should not behave. This is not unique for the era we are living in, however, since behaviors that are considered deviant tend to vary over time. The Swedish medical historian, Karin Johannisson (1944-2016) drew our attention to the fact that diagnoses and disease images are created and recreated in parity with society's norms and values. What is considered "sick, healthy, normal and deviant" changes continuously and "diagnoses are born, make careers and die" (Johannisson, 2006).

Historian Paula Fass (2016) is of the opinion that parents in the American society are disappointed with their "perfectly normal" children, because the children do not live up to their expectations. She declares that children, for that reason among other things, are no longer allowed to have a childhood. The rapidly growing tendency to perceive children as dysfunctional may thus reflect a striving or a search for the "desired life-world" (Erlandsson & Punzi, 2017). Nilsson Sjöberg (2016) makes a similar observation

---

Christoffer Hornborg is a licensed clinical psychologist, and a licentiate candidate in Sociology at the University of Gothenburg, Sweden.

Soly Erlandsson is senior professor of Psychology at University West, Sweden.

about school settings, where children who for various reasons can't adjust to expectations and demands risk being seen as inherently dysfunctional. For some children, hardships as a result of parents' separation and, not infrequently, a break from a familiar environment with school, peers and other circumstances can imply delusion and less security. A failure to live up to norms, demands and expectations of adults can hence lead to children being at risk of turning into *patients*, with a lifelong neuropsychiatric diagnosis.

Over the last two decades, the phenomenon of ADHD has gained increasing attention in the academic sphere as well as in public debate. In many countries, including Sweden, there has been an escalation in the frequency of diagnosis (Polyzoi, Ahnemark, Medin & Ginsberg, 2018). This is particularly obvious among children and young adults, who seek help for various perceived difficulties in fitting into the norms set by society. In a report from 2015, the Swedish Medical Ethics Council explained the importance of continuing to discuss and reflect on the ethical aspects of the number of ADHD diagnoses, where there has been a sharp increase since the 1990s (Smer report, 2015).

The report highlights the increased prescription of drugs in connection with the diagnosis of ADHD, and whether this is reasonable or not. The authors also emphasized the importance of understanding cognitive and emotional development from a societal perspective: "ADHD actualizes several value conflicts, where the individual's needs must be set against society's expectations, demands and priorities." Council members were hesitant to the term "neuropsychiatry" being used as a definition of the diagnosis, since it can be perceived that the biological mechanisms have a greater explanatory value in ADHD than in other psychiatric diagnoses. Undoubtedly, the concept neuropsychiatry is used almost exclusively - both by professionals, by the media, as well as by the general public.

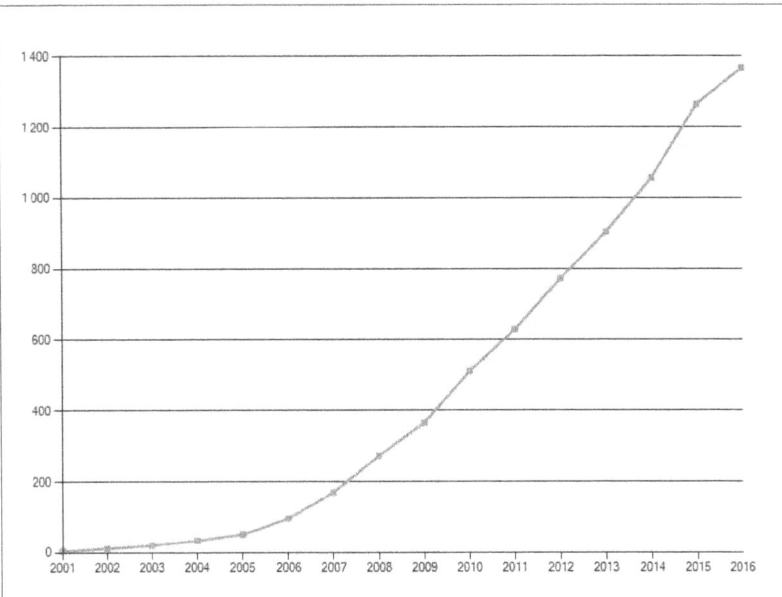

TABLE 1:
Outpatient diagnosis of F90 hyperactivity disorders in Sweden, ages 20-29, both sexes, number of patients/100 000 inhabitants (National Board of Health and Welfare, 2018).

ADHD was initially a medical category designed for hyperactive children but through time it has expanded to include "ADHD Adults" (Conrad & Potter, 2000). The massive epidemiological change among young adults, illustrated in Table 1, has generated an extensive academic and medical debate on how this change should be understood. One side of the debate has argued that ADHD is a universally occurring medical condition that exists regardless of linguistic concepts and societal conditions. This position dominates within biomedical science (Barkley et al., 2002; Faraone, 2021). The other side has problematized ADHD as a medical term and instead emphasized the societal and cultural processes that have led to an expanded use of this classification and diagnosis. Such a position is often represented by researchers in social sciences, among them, Conrad & Potter (2000); Péres-Álvarez (2017); Honksilta & Koutsoklenis (2022) and critics in psychiatry (Timimi & Leo, 2009; Timimi, 2015).

The two different perspectives outlined above have tangible implications for the interpretation of scientific data, as they are often based on contrasting ontological and epistemological assumptions: realism versus nominalism and naturalism versus constructionism (Rhodes, 1990). Has society *discovered* more cases of disorder among a large number of children and young adults, who have previously been undiagnosed? Or has it *changed* the view of what should be considered a disorder? These contradictory perspectives have resulted in a battle of knowledge about whether ADHD exists or not, which has unfortunately limited the possibilities of conducting a profound intellectual discourse on the topic.

Rather than acknowledging what both perspectives can contribute to an understanding of the phenomenon, the debate has been dominated by a conflict about which perspective is correct (Carlberg, 2014). However, the dominant view is found within a materialistic paradigm in which symptoms of inattentiveness and hyperactivity are associated with an 'underlying' biological dysfunction. Péres-Álvarez (2017) contributes with a critical position towards the current, well-established but controversial ADHD diagnosis requesting a new, meta-scientific position in which both the science of ADHD and its social applications are scrutinized.

Skeptics and enthusiasts around an elephant that thrives

The controversy surrounding ADHD can be likened to the story of the blind men who approach the elephant from different directions, each believing that he has acquired a complete picture of the elephant (Saxe, 1963). The man who encounters a tusk describes the elephant as a spear, while the man who explores the trunk describes it as a snake, and so on. Depending on the way in which the men approach the elephant, different images of its constitution emerge. No matter how many blind men explore the trunk and no matter how many detailed descriptions they generate, they will not reach a full understanding of the elephant, nor will they agree with the blind men who are exploring the elephant's tusks. And vice versa. The Danish psychologist Svend Brinkmann (2014) has described this as a dilemma where both the skeptics and the enthusiasts' ontological approaches to ADHD tend to be too simplified. Brinkmann instead refers to Ian Hacking's philosophy of science, for which the most fruitful approach is to see ADHD as a real phenomenon, but that it is dependent on certain socio-cultural conditions.

Hacking (1998) studied the diagnosis of *fugue* as it appeared during the late 1800s, when people suddenly and unexpectedly walked miles away from their home or workplace and were unable to remember their past. Instead of seeing the diagnosis as either valid or merely socially constructed, Hacking sought to understand the contextual factors that allowed the diagnosis to arise and thrive over time and space. To do this he used the concept of *ecological niche*, a metaphor derived from biology. Just as biological organisms only will survive in a niche with the right conditions, the same applies to certain types of disease categories. For example, the diagnosis of dyslexia could not flourish in a society without a written language. It is possible to argue that the symptoms of ADHD always have existed, but Hacking's idea of the ecological niche helps to illuminate under which conditions something becomes a medical condition.

The ecological niche of a diagnosis can rarely be understood in terms of a single cause. Rather, there are several simultaneously acting factors that make the niche and the condition possible, factors that Hacking calls *vectors*. It is the combination of vectors that creates the conditions for the diagnosis. When they disappear, the niche is destroyed, and the condition no longer thrives (in the sense of an ailment). From this perspective, epidemiological change in ADHD can better be understood by a combination of external vectors than by an increased frequency of symptoms within the population. In relation to ADHD, this argument can be supported by epidemiological studies, suggesting that the variation in diagnosis over time and space depends on different methodological and clinical approaches, rather than differences in prevalence (Polanczyk et al., 2014). Accordingly, in a Swedish longitudinal study, there was no evidence that ADHD traits increased in the population between 2004 and 2014 (Rydell, Lundström, Gillberg, Lichtenstein & Larsson, 2018).

Instead of arguing that society has become more effective in detecting the etiology behind a relatively heterogeneous cluster of symptoms, it is reasonable not to reduce psychiatric epidemiology into an overly simplified explanation. ADHD, like many other disorders, is not something that one simply either has or does not have. Most of the problems designated by the ADHD diagnosis are continuously distributed throughout the population. To quote Asherson with colleagues (2010): "most people have symptoms of ADHD at some time. The disorder is diagnosed by the severity and persistence of symptoms." The degree and persistence are thus crucial for a diagnosis, while at the same time people with an ADHD diagnosis can experience periods of life in which they do not have symptoms (Brinkmann, 2016). What constitutes ADHD is thus dependent on social norms about where the boundaries between normality and deviation should be drawn. Freedman and Koutsoklenis (2017) have pointed out how the eighteen diagnostic criteria for ADHD are described in DSM 5 (“often” or “is often”). Since there is no clear threshold in the diagnostic manual it becomes problematic to determine what is normal and what is not.

In clinical assessments of ADHD, a most unfortunate aspect is that etiology tends to be confounded with the patient's level of functioning (criteria D). The question of determining whether someone with certain symptoms "has ADHD" or not, thus becomes contingent on mere severity, i.e., clinical significance: *As long as the individual is impaired enough, a diagnosis is justified*. This is where the mainstream psychiatric paradigm is lacking a profound intellectual discourse on the nature of disease versus diversity. As a comparison, it is important to remember that homosexuality wasn't removed from DSM until 1973. Arguably, belonging to a sexual minority can reduce the quality of social, academic, or occupational functioning, more so in some nations, communities, or families than others, but this association with suffering does not imply a discourse on how being different than the norm should be considered a disorder located in the brain.

The ontology of a psychiatric category, such as ADHD, is therefore about establishing a shared understanding of *what we want* to be considered as a disease. In doing so, it is important to be aware of how diagnostic classification and medicalization may lead to stigmatization when suffering is decontextualized and those who suffer are viewed as chronically disabled (Timimi & Leo, 2009).

According to Karin Johannisson, psychiatric diagnoses began to grow rapidly from the beginning of the 21st century (Johannisson, 2006). In her view, medical science positions the body and the understanding of the disease on a biological stage. It exists only when we agree on its existence, and through affirmation and naming, a process applicable to the birth and naming of ADHD (without a name, the disease has no place to survive).

With the diagnosis, the disease becomes real for the sufferer and for the various surrounding institutions that are involved. In some instances, the diagnosis can mean a tangible reward for the ones who carry it and for the presumptive receiver of the diagnosis, not least because of various patient associations that are formed, and that contribute to keeping the diagnosis alive. The diagnosis also has the power to attract people who are perceived to carry the typical symptom picture (ibid). What also matters is where in the body the diagnosis is located. The higher up and the clearer the location, the higher its status (Album, 1990).

We can observe that ADHD linked to a brain dysfunction has become an important research topic for the neuro-biological field of research. Diagnoses are first and foremost a way to understand and relate to illness at a given time and a given state of knowledge as well as a specific meaning-bearing context (Johannisson, 2006). To derive the meaning-bearing context - many children and young people who receive an ADHD diagnosis also often have psychological problems. So, what comes first? Has the child's emotional development been inhibited due to a particular event (perhaps not even having to be a serious trauma, but an event that the child interpreted and experienced as a trauma)?

The multiple realities of ADHD

Clinical assessors of ADHD observe a patient heterogeneity that is hard to reconcile with the academic idea of a universal core symptom (such as reduced working memory, inhibitory dysfunction, memory problems, emotional dysregulation, or difficulties within a specific area of attention). Simply put, it is not easy to find a common variable for the diagnosis ADHD that matches all patient profiles, except that for all individuals it represents a form of disability when it comes to handling different demands in everyday life.

A central aspect of how the prevalence table above should be interpreted is thus that there has been a marked increase in the extent to which humans are described as clinically impaired in terms of certain cognitive and behavioral attributes. This increased 'need' to categorize people as clinically impaired of course calls for a consideration of socioeconomic disadvantage and psychiatric functioning. In a recent descriptive study on Global Mental Health and ADHD, Ortega and Rodrigues Müller (2020) illustrated a huge variation of the prevalence of ADHD in different regions in Brazil and clarified that the prevalence is higher in socioeconomically disadvantaged populations. On a group level, it *could* perhaps be possible to find biological components that characterize people diagnosed with ADHD. This has been sought by investigating differences in dopaminergic function between individuals diagnosed with ADHD and a control group (Volkow et al., 2009; Wang et al., 2013). However, there are at least two objections regarding the clinical relevance of such results.

Firstly, it is difficult to generalize this kind of research to specific contexts where the phenomenon of ADHD primarily exists. Since brain imaging is not used as a diagnostic tool in psychiatry, schools, or assessment units, it would be a mere guess to comment on the brain of a particular person in a clinical setting, even in cases where symptoms of ADHD would be identified in the diagnostic process. Although neuropsychological tests can be used, they do not have the sensitivity to discriminate ADHD from the traits of a normal population. Hence, diagnosis is always an assessment based largely on the acquisition of patient history and the presence of disability over time.

Clinicians simply have no idea whether the patient they diagnose has a brain that deviates in a specific way, even though the narrative of the brain is a central component for how ADHD is conceptualized. The same category that explains concentration difficulties in the classroom can indicate impulsive behavior in the schoolyard, a strong drive to perform at the workplace, a low working memory as measured by the test results in the psychologist's office, and so on. It is only in a limited context, for a small category of people such as neuroscientists, that ADHD emerges as a color image of the brain. Yet, as Brinkmann (2016) points out, it is unthinkable that the brain would not be implicated in ADHD, since it is active in all psychological processes. Regarding this highly contextual appearance of ADHD, it is first and foremost the person and her behavior in a given setting that constitutes the phenomenon ADHD, even though the individual's brain is indispensable for its occurrence.

Secondly, an important reservation regarding brain imagery is that it risks being misunderstood as evidence of causality. Thus, in Sweden's largest morning newspaper Dagens Nyheter, the research of Volkow and her colleagues was described under the heading: "New finding solves the mystery of ADHD" (Bratt, 2009; own translation). However, just as the tusk only constitutes one observation point for describing the elephant, brain imagery (as well as self-assessment and behavioral observations) constitutes an isolated measurement rather than an etiological explanation. It is unlikely that observations of how individuals with an ADHD diagnosis perform in self-assessment forms (Ustun et al., 2017) would be interpreted as a "solution" to what ADHD is.

This way of talking about ADHD unravels a cultural logic, in which the elephant's tusks are considered to represent a deeper reality than the trunk. As a counterpoint, Pérez-Álvarez (2017) has formulated a hypothesis that cerebral variation in many cases can be seen as a dependent variable reflecting the behavior of the individual in his environment rather than an independent variable. For example, a study conducted among taxi drivers in London showed deviations in specific areas of the brain compared with the normal population (Maguire, Woollett & Spiers, 2006). In the same way, it is unlikely that brain deviation would be a reason why some individuals drive a taxi. The color brain images identifying ADHD can be understood as a *reflection* of the behavioral repertoire of the subject, rather than an indicator of genetically determined hardware.

Even if minor differences in brain size do exist between diagnosed and non-diagnosed children, Batstra and colleagues (2014) have questioned that this implies abnormal development, and that it should not be referred to as "fixed states but to slower anatomical development that mostly catches up later in life" (ibid, p. 2). Timimi (2015) has a similar argument and address that it is clinically impossible to confirm in medical tests where the line between a normal and an anormal brain should be drawn. Despite this, there is undoubtedly a solid discourse aimed at reifying the medical category of ADHD as a neurological condition, where the behaviors are caused by an 'underlying' disorder.

Te Meerman (2019) has described this view as an example of circular reasoning. He points out that children "can be classified with ADHD because these are the very behaviors that are used to define the disorder. It is circular to suggest that the name for these behaviors is the cause of these behaviors" (ibid, p. 94). A similar notation i.e., that the symptoms are a guarantee of the diagnostic category, and at the same time used as an explanation to the symptoms "in an endless loop" was brought up by Perez-Álvarez (2017, p 2). Such a conflation of ADHD, as both cause and effect, has also been noted in an analysis of how the National Institute of Mental Health (USA) on an online document informs parents about ADHD (Erlandsson, Lundin & Punzi, 2016).

We argue that it is important to avoid an epistemological hierarchy that assigns unequal ontological value to the different parts of the elephant, so to speak. The category of "ADHD" can emerge in a color image of the brain, in the scores of standardized forms, or in an individual's everyday behavior, but one of these phenomena should not be seen as a consequence of another. Such an ontological approach is inspired by the Dutch philosopher Anne-Marie Mol, who concludes that "there is no deeper reality behind the one we live with" (Mol, 2000: 82).

Pragmatism as an ontological approach to ADHD

In pragmatic philosophy, truth is not something we can lean back on, but rather programs for action aiming to achieve certain results (Whyte, 1999). Pragmatism is thus forward-looking and on its way somewhere. From this perspective, it becomes less relevant to establish a static truth about what ADHD is, and more relevant to ask what the function of the category is and what it results in. What results are achieved with an ADHD diagnosis? Which actors want to use it, which do not, and why?

Based on a pragmatic approach, we cannot dwell in the truth that ADHD is always associated with a specific parameter, e.g., that the "ADHD patient" sitting in front of the clinician has a brain that functions in a particular way, but we can see that this assumption is functional only in a context where it is favorable to treat the claim as credible or "true". Similar arguments have previously been proposed for other diagnoses, such as schizophrenia. British psychology professor Mary Boyle (1990) has thus questioned the homogeneity and the scientific status of the syndrome, but at the same time argued that both psychiatrists and patients and their families in some cases need the diagnosis of schizophrenia.

Brinkmann (2017) has pointed out that we need to find a way of reconciling essentialism and constructionism in order to better understand psychiatric conditions. As mentioned, there is a tension between those who claim that ADHD is a valid medical diagnosis and those who emphasize how ADHD is socially constructed (Barkley et al, 2002; Timimi et al., 2004). In understanding this tension, it is important to note that studies of classification as a social and cultural process do not suggest that the categorized phenomena are not meaningful or "real". A thousand-dollar bill is palpably real and can even have the potential to make the difference between life and death in some contexts, even though its form and value are constructed in a social context.

Few would doubt that thousand-dollar bills exist and have a real impact on the world. Similarly, both the category and the diagnostic criteria for ADHD have been constructed by people in a spatial and temporal setting, but this does not make the diagnosis less real in the context in which it occurs. Psychiatric diagnoses may be overlapping, vague, and contested throughout history, but they can nonetheless be seen as socially accepted idioms of distress that are functional in the sense that they provide access to treatment and resources in society (Nichter, 2010). As Hacking (1998) reminds us, we need to ask not whether a disorder is "real" but whether it is *motivated.*

Looking at the increasing rate of ADHD diagnoses, the diagnosis seems to have taken on a life of its own. It has become a colossus on clay feet and cannot be moved in any direction, even if its survival is dependent on an industry with various actors. Whether ADHD is a motivated phenomenon then becomes subordinated to the brain discourse with its sole mission of showing us what is "real", and a more profound intellectual and ethical debate on what we as health professionals and as society want to accomplish, is renounced. In 2015, the media reported that the UN Committee on the Rights of the Child was concerned about the increasing prescription of central stimulants (Ritalin and Concerta) to children in Sweden and the harmful effects of these drugs. Despite warnings, also addressed to the Swedish government who were advised to follow the Convention on the Rights of the Child and prioritize other measures, the prescription of central stimulants increased for both children and adults diagnosed with ADHD.

In times when we more than ever need to recognize and understand that human experiences may differ as a result of social conditions, increased focus on diagnostics and a brain that is dysfunctional contributes to marginalize people. For a child with obvious behavioral problems, the ADHD diagnosis can be perceived as a kind of recognition. However, the diagnose is not a confirmation of one specific child—all children receiving the ADHD diagnosis are seen through the same lens (Erlandsson & Punzi, 2017). It is understandable that assessments and diagnoses of children with disabilities reflect different professional areas of knowledge, but generally these diagnoses are mainly based on subjective assessments and products of a system with interests and influence from many different arenas (political, economic, professional, etc., see Frances & Widiger, 2012; Leo & Lacasse, 2015). It is a huge problem that the biomedical discourse has an interpretative priority over the humanistic/psychosocial discourse in the understanding of mental health (Erlandsson and Punzi, 2016).

In understanding how the prevalence of psychiatric diagnoses expands locally as well as globally, there is a risk of viewing patients as passive recipients of an imperialist psychiatric ideology (Watters, 2010). But clinical experience and qualitative studies remind us that people are agents who actively seek out a psychiatric diagnosis (cf. Brinkmann, 2014; Nielsen, 2017). A pragmatic approach therefor needs to consider the fact that many individuals actively and meaningfully relate to their diagnosis. In the case of ADHD though, many of those being subject to a diagnosis are children and young people who are usually not involved in the decision-making process, and it might be parents or teachers rather than the 'patient' who is primarily seeking a label (cf. Clarke & Lang, 2012; Doré & Cohen, 1997).

Furthermore, it is not unusual for parents of children with behavioral dysfunctions to obtain information about ADHD from the Internet (Bussing et al., 2012). Parents are, however, vulnerable to misguidance without adequate evaluation skills (Lundin & Erlandsson, 2017). Lundin and Erlandsson analyzed parents' life experiences shared as posts online using a narrative psychological method. The structure of the parents' narratives reflected a daily life dominated by their children's behavior. In their role as parents, they experienced a lack of self-confidence and sometimes seemed to have lost confidence in the health care system. Therefore, the only light in the tunnel for most of them was to rely on a diagnose and medical treatment as a solution to the experienced difficulties with the child (ibid).

Downplaying suffering and symptoms as "normal" might not be desirable for a large proportion of those seeking help. For example, the diagnosis can be a strategic resource for maneuvering the reality of their suffering, or as doctor and medical sociologist Cecil Helman (2007) puts it: "a way of giving meaning to experiences of ill health, of placing it in... the wider themes of the culture and society in which they live... [i.e.] a basic way of organizing an experience... [and establishing] a sense of coherent order on the chaos of the patient's symptoms and feelings "(ibid, p. 140). Or to quote Brinkmann (2014: 128): "It is bad enough to suffer, but if one's suffering appears as lacking in meaning, it is even worse, so people look for explanations that change the meaningless into something meaningful."

Here, Brinkmann acknowledges how a narrative of patient's difficulties are not just a labeling but also a treatment intervention per se. And for some patients, it is undoubtedly a great relief to get an ADHD diagnosis. The question is whether patients (and parents) report relief because the clinician *found the actual cause*, or because the patient was provided with an explanation that is culturally approved, which has implications such as reduced self-blame, social acceptance, and so on. Based on the reasoning above, about circular arguments and logical fallacies on *cause* (te Meerman, 2019), we naturally adhere to the second hypothesis. As an example, relief of self-blame and guilt in parents was found in a qualitative study performed by Dauman, Haza and Erlandsson (2019). In focus were French parents, affected by their children's problematic conduct, interacting with parents in similar situations over two Internet communities. The online posted narratives provided detailed descriptions of the everyday life experiences as parents. *Liberating parents of guilt* appeared as the core category of the Grounded Theory analysis. Objectives of the Internet communities were foremost to remove feelings of guilt in the parents by emphasizing a genetic origin of ADHD.

There is a risk that the dominant, medical paradigm in mental health depletes valuable knowledge about children's and adults' most basic needs. Our mission as health professionals (psychologists as well as physicians) lies in bringing order to chaos - not just by offering a label, but by helping the clients to gain a deeper insight into what their suffering means and why it might occur. This is in line with a more health-oriented definition of disease in which comprehension, manageability, and, not least, meaningfulness constitutes key elements for reducing suffering (Antonovsky, 1979). This recognition of these elements leads to the next question: whether the static and individualized gene-brain discourse is the most suitable and ethically adequate narrative for people suffering from the cognitive and emotional symptoms labeled as "ADHD". Or are there any better ways to make sense of the symptoms, feelings and suffering associated with inattentiveness and hyperactivity?

Conclusion

In theory, an individual can experience the entire list of ADHD symptoms without meeting the criteria for diagnosis, as long as the symptoms do not interfere with reduced functioning according to criteria D (American Psychiatric Association, 2013). A diagnosis is therefore not a measure of "how much ADHD" a person has, but how well her life is working out. The lack of sensitive measurement methods or biomarkers means that record taking about how the person has functioned over time usually constitutes the primary variable behind diagnosis. ADHD can thus be seen as a consequence of the patient's level of functioning during his or her life story, rather than vice versa. Furthermore, the diagnosis can operate as a semantic tool for helping people with chronic life problems.

From a biomedical perspective, the picture painted above might be interpreted as a denial of the realness of suffering that people with ADHD struggle with, or the importance of treatment. From a pragmatic perspective, instead, we must acknowledge that the patient group exists, but that it is heterogeneous. Honkasilta and Koutsoklenis (2022) emphasize that the group of children diagnosed with ADHD is highly diverse, best exemplified in high rates of comorbidity.

Ontologically, ADHD can be understood as a *human* or *interactive* kind rather than a *natural* kind (Hacking, 1992). It should not be conceptualized as a *cause* of symptoms, but rather an umbrella term for symptoms, and its increased prevalence fills a pragmatic purpose only as long as it helps to improve health through different forms of treatment, increased opportunities for community support, and an increased sense of coherence. To take Hacking's theory into consideration, studying the social and cultural context is advisory in order to examine what variables are creating a perceived need for an epidemiological explosion of incongruous proportions.

If we find that context is decisive (even complex and heterogeneous), can we then write off the idea that ADHD should be classified as a neuropsychiatric condition? Johannisson asks what society earns or loses from providing diagnoses and her answer is that the diagnose can obscure the view of non-medical explanations to a given problem. The more variations of the self that we medicalize, the more the limits of normality are pushed (Johannisson, 2006).

Declaration of conflicting interests

The authors declared no potential conflicts of interest with respect to the research, authorship, and/or publication of this article.

References

Album, D. (1991). Sykdommers og medisinske spesialiteters prestisje (The prestige of diseases and medical specialists). Nordisk Medicin 106: 232-236.

Antonovsky, A. (1979). *Health, stress and coping*. San Francisco: Josey-Bass.

American Psychiatric Association. (2013). *Diagnostic and statistical manual of mental disorders (5th ed.)*. Washington DC: American Psychiatric Association.

Asherson, P., Adamou, M., Bolea, B., Muller, U., Morua, S. D., Pitts, M., ... & Young, S. (2010). Is ADHD a valid diagnosis in adults? Yes. *BMJ: British Medical Journal* (Online), 340.

Barkley, R., Cook, E. H., Diamond, A., Zametkin, A., Thapar, A., Anastopoulos, A. D., & Pelham, W. (2002). International consensus statement on ADHD. *Clinical Child and Family Psychology Review*, 5, 89–111.

Batstra, L., Nieweg, E. H., & Hadders-Algra, M. (2014). Exploring five common assumptions on attention deficit hyperactivity disorder. **Acta Paediatrica**, 103(7), 696–700. doi:10.1111/apa.12642.

Boyle, M. (1990). *Schizophrenia: A scientific delusion*. London: Routledge.

Bratt, A. (2009, September 8). Fynd löser gåtan ADHD (Findings solve the mystery of ADHD). *Dagens nyheter*. Retrieved from http://www.dn.se/nyheter/vetenskap/fynd-loser-gatan-adhd.

Brinkmann, S. (2014). Psychiatric diagnoses as semiotic mediators: The case of ADHD. *Nordic Psychology*, 66(2), 121-134.

Brinkmann, S. (2016). Toward a cultural psychology of mental disorder: The case of attention deficit hyperactivity disorder. *Culture & Psychology, 22*(1), 80-93.

Bussing R, Zima BT, Mason DM, Meyer JM, White K, et al. (2012). ADHD knowledge, perceptions, and information sources: Perspectives from a community sample of adolescents and their parents. *J Adolesc Health*, 51, 593-600.

Carlberg, I. (2014). En diagnos det stormat kring: Adhd i ett historiskt perspektiv. Stockholm: Socialstyrelsen. From https://www.socialstyrelsen.se/publikationer2014/2014-10-40.

Clarke, J.N. and Lang, L. (2012). Mothers Whose Children Have ADD/ADHD Discuss Their Children's Medication Use: An Investigation of Blogs. *Social Work in Health Care*, 51: 5. https://doi.org/10.1080/00981389.2012.660567.

Conrad, P., & Potter, D. (2000). From hyperactive children to ADHD adults: Observations on the expansion of medical categories. *Social Problems*, 47(4), 559-582.

Dauman, N. Haza, M. & Erlandsson, SI. (2019). Liberating parents from guilt: A grounded theory study of parents' internet communities for the recognition of ADHD. *International Journal of Qualitative Studies on Health and Wellbeing*. https://doi.org/10.1080/17482631.2018.1564520.

Doré, C. & Cohen, D. (1996). La prescription de stimulants aux enfants « hyperactifs »: une étude pilote des incitatifs et des contraintes pour les parents, les médecins et les enseignants [The prescription of stimulants to "hyperactive" children: a pilot study of incentives and constraints on parents, teachers, and physicians]. *Santé mentale au Québec*, 22(1), 216-238.

Erlandsson, SI., Lundin, L., & Punzi, E. (2016). A discursive analysis concerning information on "ADHD" presented to parents by the National Institute of Mental Health (USA). *International Journal of Qualitative Studies on Health and Well-Being*, 11(1), 30938. [Google Scholar]

Erlandsson, SI. & Punzi, E. (2016). Challenging the ADHD consensus. Guest Editorial in: *International Journal of Qualitative Studies on Health and Well-being 2016, 11*: 31124 - http://dx.doi.org/10.3402/qhw.v11.31124

Erlandsson, SI. & Punzi, E. (2017). A biased ADHD discourse ignores human uniqueness. *International Journal of Qualitative Studies on Health and Well-being, 2017 VOL. 12*, 1319584 https://doi.org/10.1080/17482631.2017.1319584

Faraone, SV. & Larsson, H. (2019). Genetics of attention deficit hyperactivity disorder. *Molecular Psychiatry*, 24:562–575 https://doi.org/10.1038/s41380-018-0070-0

Fass, P.S. (2016). The end of American childhood: A history of parenting from life on the frontier to the managed child. Princeton, NJ: Princeton University Press. [Google Scholar]

Frances, A. & Widiger, T. (2012). Psychiatric diagnosis: Lessons from the DSM-IV Past and Cautions for the DSM-5 Future. **Annual Review of Clinical Psychology**, 8: 109-130.

Freedman, J. E., and Honkasilta, J. (2017). Dictating the boundaries of Ab/normality: a critical discourse analysis of the diagnostic criteria for attention deficit hyperactivity disorder and hyperkinetic disorder. *Disabil.* Soc. 32, 565–588. doi: 10.1080/09687599.2017.1296819 §

Hacking, I. (1992). World making by kind-making: Child abuse for example. In M. Douglas & D. Hull (Eds.), *How Classification Works: Nelson Goodman among the Social Sciences* (pp. 180-238). Edinburgh: Edinburgh University Press.

Hacking, I. (1998). *Mad Travellers: Reflections on the Reality of Transient Mental Illnesses*. London: Free Association Books.

Helman, C. (2007). *Culture, Health and Illness (5th ed.)*. Oxford: Butterworth-Heinemann.

Honkasilta, J. and Koutsoklenis, A. (2022). The (un)real existence of ADHD – criteria, functions, and forms of the diagnostic entity. *Frontiers in Sociology*, doi: 10.3389/fsoc.2022.814763.

Johannisson, K. (2006). Hur skapas en diagnos. Ett historiskt perspektiv (How is a diagnosis created? A historical perspective). In: G. Hallerstedt (Ed.), *Diagnosens makt. Om kunskap, pengar och lidande (The power of diagnosis. About knowledge, money and suffering)*. (pp.29-41). Daidalos AB, Gothenburg, Sweden.

Leo, J. & Lacasse, JR. (2015). The New York Times and the ADHD epidemic. *Society*, 52: 3-8.

Lundin, L. & Erlandsson, SI. (2017). Parental discussions online through the medical discourse-lens. Journal of Childhood & Developmental Disorders. Vol. 3 (4):15, http://childhood-developmental-disorders.imedpub.com. DOI:10.4172/2472-1786.100053.

Maguire, E. A., Woollett, K., & Spiers, H. J. (2006). London taxi drivers and bus drivers: a structural MRI and neuropsychological analysis. *Hippocampus*, 16(12), 1091–1101. https://doi.org/10.1002/hipo.20233

te Meerman, S. (2019). ADHD and the power of generalization. Exploring the faces of reification. PhD Thesis, Rijksuniversiteit, Groningen, Netherlands.

Mol, A. (2000). Pathology and the clinic: An ethnographic presentation of two atheroscleroses. In M. Lock, A. Young & A. Cambrosio (Eds.), *Living and Working with the New Medical Technologies: Intersections of Inquiry* (pp. 82-102). Cambridge: Cambridge University Press.

National Board of Health and Welfare. (2018). *Diagnoser i öppen vård, Antal patienter/100 000 inv, F90 Hyperaktivitetsstörningar, Riket, Ålder*: 20-29, Båda könen. Retrieved May 29, 2018, from Socialstyrelsen, http://www.socialstyrelsen.se/Statistik/statistikdatabas/

Nichter, M. (2010). Idioms of distress revisited. *Culture, Medicine, and Psychiatry*, 34(2): 401-416.

Nielsen, M. (2017). My ADHD and me: Identifying with and distancing from ADHD. *Nordic Psychology*, 69(1), 33-46.

Nilsson Sjöberg, M. (2016). (Un)becoming dysfunctional – ADHD and how matter comes to matter. International Journal of Inclusive Education. Published online ahead of print. doi:10.1080/13603116.2016.1251977 [Taylor & Francis Online], [Google Scholar]

Ortega, F. and Rodrigues Müller, M. (2020). Global Mental Health and Pharmacology: The Case of Attention Deficit and Hyperactivity Disorders in Brazil. *Front. Sociol. 5:535125. doi: 10.3389/fsoc.2020.535125.*

Pérez-Álvarez, M. (2017). The four causes of ADHD: Aristotle in the classroom. *Frontiers in Psychology*, 8:928.

Polanczyk, G. V., Willcutt, E. G., Salum, G. A., Kieling, C., & Rohde, L. A. (2014). ADHD prevalence estimates across three decades: An updated systematic review and meta-regression analysis. *International Journal of Epidemiology, 43*(2), 434-442.

Polyzoi, M., Ahnemark, E., Medin, E., & Ginsberg, Y. (2018). Estimated prevalence and incidence of diagnosed ADHD and health care utilization in adults in Sweden – a longitudinal population-based register study. *Neuropsychiatric Disease and Treatment*, 14, 1149-1161.

Rhodes, L. (1990). Studying biomedicine as a cultural system. In T. M. Johnson & C. Sargent (Eds.), *Medical Anthropology: Contemporary Theory and Method* (pp. 159-173). New York: Praeger.

Rydell, M., Lundström, S., Gillberg, C., Lichtenstein, P., & Larsson, H. (2018). Has the attention deficit hyperactivity disorder phenotype become more common in children between 2004 and 2014? Trends over 10 years from a Swedish general population sample. *Journal of Child Psychology and Psychiatry*, 59(8), 863-871).

Saxe, J. G. (1963). *The blind men and the elephant*. New York: McGraw-Hill.

Statens medicinsk-etiska råd. ADHD – etiska utmaningar. Stockholm 2015. Smer rapport 2015:2.

Timimi, S. (2015). Children's mental health: time to stop using psychiatric diagnosis. *Eur J Psychother Cound*, 17: 342-358.

Timimi, S., & Leo, J. (Eds.). (2009). *Rethinking ADHD: From brain to culture*. New York: Palgrave Macmillan.

Timimi, S., Moncrieff, J., Jureidini, J., Leo, J., Cohen, D., Whitfield, C., & White, R. (2004). A critique of the international consensus statement on ADHD. *Clinical Child and Family Psychology Review*, *7*(1), 59-63.

Ustun, B., Adler, L. A., Rudin, C., Faraone, S. V., Spencer, T. J., Berglund, P., ... & Kessler, R. C. (2017). The World Health Organization adult attention-deficit/hyperactivity disorder self-report screening scale for DSM-5. *Jama psychiatry*, 74(5), 520-526.

Volkow, N. D., Wang, G.-J., Kollins, S. H., Wigal, T. L., Newcorn, J. H., Telang, F., & Swanson, J. M. (2009). Evaluating dopamine reward pathway in ADHD. *JAMA*, 302(10), 1084-1091.

Wang, G.-J., Volkow, N. D., Wigal, T., Kollins, S. H., Newcorn, J. H., Telang, F., ... & Fowler, J. S. (2013). Long-term stimulant treatment affects brain dopamine transporter level in patients with attention deficit hyperactive disorder. *PloS one*, 8(5), e63023.

Watters, E. (2010). *Crazy like us: The globalization of the american psyche*. New York: Simon & Schuster.

Whitaker, R. (2010). *Anatomy of an epidemic: Magic Bullets, Psychiatric Drugs, and the astonishing rise of mental illness in America.* New York: Crown.

Whyte, S. R. (1999). Pragmatisme: Akademisk og anvendt. *Tidsskriftet Antropologi,* 40, 129-138.

What *is* the Evidence for ADHD and its Treatment?

Robert Foltz

Every morning, millions of children and teenagers across the U.S. take a medication for ADHD. Day in, and day out, parents and youth rely on the "science" of psychiatry to improve their outcomes. Whether the hoped-for outcomes are improved academic achievement, improved impulse control, better focus, more sociability, or fewer disruptive symptoms, families rely on experts to make decisions based on the best evidence to inform treatment strategies.

As a parent or policy maker, you are probably thinking, "but the psychiatrist is the expert ... so they must be prescribing the medication that is needed ... at the right dose ... for the time it is needed." The evidence, however, is less reliable than you may think. Because the primary intervention strategy for ADHD is medication (most often a psychostimulant), the focus of this chapter will be on the evaluation of this class of medication. In examining the depth and breadth of the evidence, it will be important to discern the short-term benefits from our standard practice. That is, while medication research will be examined here, long-term study of the effectiveness of these medications is rare, though the typical child receiving stimulants for ADHD is on them for many months, if not years. And with regard to these medications, short-term advantages do not generalize to long-term improvements.

Robert Foltz, Psych.D., is associate professor of clinical psychology at the Chicago School of Professional Psychology, USA.

Originally conceptualized as a disorder of childhood, the Diagnostic and Statistical Manual, Fifth Edition, Text Revision (DSM-5-TR, APA, 2022) describes the prevalence of ADHD into adulthood. While the DSM continues to maintain that ADHD symptoms must begin in childhood (before the age of 12), their persistence into adulthood – while a likely outcome for many people diagnosed – is also a reflection of our failed treatments. The APA reports that ADHD occurs in 2.5% of the adult population (nearly 6.5 million adults in the U.S.).

In the DSM-IV, ADHD symptoms were required to result in "clear evidence of clinically significant impairment in social, academic, or occupational functioning" (APA, 1994, p. 84). In our recent conceptualizations of ADHD (with the DSM-5 and DSM-5-TR), it is now sufficient that symptoms "reduce the *quality* of social, academic, or occupational functioning" (italics added) (2022, p. 69). The subjective measure of "quality" increases the likelihood of a broader application of the diagnosis versus an objective measure of "unable to maintain employment," for example.

How reliable is the ADHD diagnosis? In this context, being "reliable" means being able to consistently identify the disorder. That is, are the diagnostic criteria developed in a way to consistently identify the disorder of ADHD. One of the inherent vulnerabilities here, is that the ADHD diagnostic criteria *all* begin with the word "often." As used here, "often" is used as a measure of frequency that then ties to impairment in social, academic, or home settings. But "often" for a teacher is different than "often" for a soccer coach which is different than "often" for a parent.

Because of this, all of those stakeholders could report the behavior is "often" even though it may be occurring at dramatically different rates in those settings. For example, if a child's math teacher, seeing the child one hour a day, reflects on the child's blurting out answers, he may conclude that the child often blurts out the answer if it occurs several times a week. This observation is also in the context of other children blurting out answers, of course. But if you ask the child's parent how often he or she blurts out answers, the parent may observe multiple times in an hour, each morning and evening, every day of the week, etc. But both adults would endorse "often." The subjectivity in measuring these symptoms increases the likelihood of being able to identify this "disorder" but also reduces the validity of identifying this cluster of symptoms as a discernable condition, because so many of these behaviors would also be observed in other disorders and children without a diagnosis.

Another way to evaluate the diagnosis is through considering inter-rater reliability. In the case of diagnosing, inter-rater reliability reflects the agreement between multiple clinicians in identifying the same diagnosis. Achieving high inter-rater reliability indicates that most people observing the behaviors or symptoms would agree that it is, indeed, XXX disorder. The current diagnostic criteria for ADHD achieve an inter-rater reliability kappa score of 0.61 (Frances, 2017) which is generally considered "acceptable." Let's unpack that. A kappa score of 0.61 "can immediately be seen as problematic. Almost 40% of the data in the dataset represent faulty data…" and if the value of kappa is .60 - .79, it indicates that 35 – 63% of the data is reliable (McHugh, 2012, p. 278). Conversely, approximately a third to two-thirds of the data is unreliable. This brings us back to the issue of reliability. And as there is no specific diagnostic test (blood test, brain scan, psychological evaluation) for the disorder, it's fair to conclude that there are substantial concerns with the reliability, and thus the validity, of the ADHD diagnosis, despite it being applied to millions of children every year.

Another complication in the ADHD diagnosis is its ability to disappear under certain circumstances. Keep in mind, the condition is considered a neurodevelopmental disorder; a brain condition influenced across a developmental continuum. The American Psychiatric Association (2022) concedes that despite the purported neurological and developmental underpinnings, "signs of the disorder may be minimal or absent when the individual is receiving frequent rewards for appropriate behavior, is under close supervision, is in a novel setting, is engaged in especially interesting activities, has consistent external stimulation (e.g., via electronic screens), or is interacting in one-on-one situations (e.g., the clinician's office)" (p. 70). This information should be particularly relevant when we are weighing our treatment options. Rather than years of exposure to a psychostimulant, it may indeed be worth reconsidering our funding of educational environments, for example, in the availability of technologies and one-on-one learning opportunities for children.

Finally, a word of caution to parents: The DSM also provides the opportunity to diagnose children with ADHD even if they fail to meet the criteria. A condition labeled "Unspecified Attention-Deficit/Hyperactivity Disorder" is permitted in situations where behaviors characteristic of ADHD are present, causing impairment, but "do not meet the full criteria for ADHD" (p. 76).

Convincing headlines?

We're all susceptible to good headlines and marketing. If they feed our confirmation bias, we're even more accepting of the claims. Good marketing strategies embrace this, and while pharmaceutical companies save lives every day, they are also exceptionally well-skilled in selling their products and generating substantial profits. To that end, Tom Insel, M.D., former Director of the National Institute of Mental Health, noted recently, "It's difficult to show that outcomes, measured by morbidity and mortality, are better today than in 1975. In terms of mental health care, the last four decades have been much better for the pharmaceutical industry than for the public" (Insel, 2021, p. 45).

Here are some examples of these marketing strategies:

Concerta

"Concerta is proven to help manage the symptoms of inattention, hyperactivity, and impulsivity. With these symptoms under control, your child can focus better and pay closer attention to the things he or she is doing throughout the day."

Vyvanse

"Vyvanse helped treat ADHD throughout the day in children (aged 6 – 12). In one study of kids (aged 6 – 12) with ADHD, Vyvanse demonstrated ADHD symptom control for up to 13 hours, starting 1.5 hours after taking it ... Vyvanse demonstrated ADHD symptom control throughout the day and into the evening – even at 8pm."

Evekeo

"How does Evekeo work to treat children with ADHD? Evekeo is a type of ADHD medicine called a stimulant. Stimulants help networks in the brain communicate with each other better. Taking a stimulant for ADHD symptoms might make it easier to pay attention and focus, and control hyperactive and impulsive behavior."

Quillivant

"Rapid ADHD symptom control. Quillivant XR has been proven to start working in 45 minutes. In a clinical study, children 6 to 12 years old with ADHD who took Quillivant XR had improved attention and behavior through the day compared with those who took a sugar syrup ... Did you know ...? Quillivant is banana flavored."

CHADD: (Children and adults with attention-deficit / hyperactivity disorder)

"ADHD is a disorder in certain areas of the brain and is inherited in the majority of cases. It is not caused by poor parenting or a chaotic home environment, although the home environment can make the symptoms of ADHD better or worse ... there is no single cause that explains all cases of ADHD and that many factors may play a part ... ADHD is clearly a brain-based disorder. Currently research is underway to better define the areas and pathways that are involved."

Is this making sense yet?

Whether you are a staunch proponent of the ADHD diagnosis or an enthusiastic skeptic, there is no doubt that many children and teens struggle in our educational environments. These difficulties can also affect them socially, at home, and can be long-lasting. But to claim that this cluster of difficulties is "neurodevelopmental" remains to be proven. The claims within advertising deserve further scrutiny. "Helping networks in the brain communicate with each other ... clearly a brain-based disorder ... symptom control ... helping treat throughout the day" and similar claims must be scrutinized. Based on these claims, even if we aren't sure what to call this condition, maybe the medications do effectively address behaviors that challenge youth around the world? How should we think about that possibility?

In examining the use of methylphenidate (Ritalin) globally, it raises more questions than answers. The global use of methylphenidate and other drugs is monitored by the International Narcotics Control

Board (INCB). All of the stimulants used in the treatment of ADHD are controlled substances (Schedule II as designated by the DEA). The INCB provides an overview of manufacture and consumption of these drugs and in doing so, can provide a glimpse into how the U.S. compares to other countries in our utilization of these medications. In 2020, the global manufacturing of methylphenidate was 62.9 tons. The U.S. accounted for 78% of this overall total (49 tons) (INCB, 2021). Now, your first thought may be: 'well, we have manufacturing and technology capabilities that enable us to create more than others, so we probably export most of our supply to support the treatment of ADHD globally,' right? Remarkably, the U.S. only exported 12.8 tons in 2020, using the remaining supply for domestic consumption. In other words, the U.S. consumed 36.2 tons of methylphenidate, which means *we use almost 60% of the world's Ritalin supply.*

Methylphenidate and its different forms (e.g., Concerta and Quillivant) are very popular. However, another class of stimulants (the amphetamines and their derivatives) are also very popular and heavily advertised. Summarized by the INCB (2021), the U.S. remains the largest consumer of amphetamine and dexamphetamine for medical purposes (primarily in the treatment of ADHD). The INCB reports this consumption as S-DDD (defined daily doses for statistical purposes). For amphetamines, the global consumption was 13.3 S-DDD per 1000 inhabitants per day. The U.S. represents 8.15 S-DDD of that total. In other words, the U.S. uses over 60% of the world's amphetamine supply for medical purposes. Related to dexamfetamine, the U.S. is the leading consumer and of the top 10 countries, the U.S. represents 70% of the utilization (INCB, 2021).

The implications may be concerning. If ADHD is a neurodevelopmental disorder and the experts indicate that medication offers the best chance at treating it, one may conclude that the neurodevelopment of our youth is heavily compromised compared to populations around the world. It is not as if other countries don't have access to our diagnostic paradigms. Nor is it the case that they don't have access to medication treatments. Indeed, if the demand was there, manufacturing would increase. This leaves us in a position to wonder why the U.S. is so afflicted with neurodevelopmental disorders in our youth, or else question what else may be going on.

FDA trials for ADHD meds

Obtaining approval from the Food and Drug Administration (FDA) is a complicated, time-consuming process. There are different phases to drug development beginning with the chemical composition of the drug to animal trials, ultimately leading to the testing of the medication in the targeted clinical population to determine appropriate dosing, effectiveness, and side-effects. As noted above, pharmaceutical companies play an essential role in healthcare and save lives every day. Yet in the realm of psychiatry, the outcomes may not reflect those achieved in other areas of medicine.

As we imagine how drug trials are conducted, we may assume that by the time a drug is approved, thousands of children have been tried on the drug and careful scrutiny has occurred over many months, if not years, to determine if the drugs work and to what extent young people experience side-effects. Children and teens remain on these medications for extended periods of time, so of course it would be important to observe effectiveness over time and any impact on development over the dynamically changing central nervous system, hormones, etc.

The following is a summary of drug trials conducted to obtain FDA approval for drugs used to treat ADHD. This table summarizes information that is available within the Package Inserts (available online) for any of the approved medications. While this is only a partial list, it represents the most popular medications being used currently.

Medication	Generic name	Studies Conducted Sample size Duration
Vyvanse	Lisdexamfetamine Dimesylate	N = 52 3-week optimization, 2-week crossover N = 290 4 weeks N = 129 4-week optimization, 2-week crossover
Concerta	Methylphenidate HCL	N = 416 3 weeks N = 177 4 weeks
Quillivant	Methylphendiate HCL	N = 45 4-week optimization, 2-week crossover
Evekeo	Amphetamine Sulfate	N = 105 8 weeks N = 97 2-week crossover
Adderall X	Dextroamphetamine Sulf-Saccharate	N = 327 4 weeks N = 584 3 weeks

As you can see, these trials are not conducted for months (or years) and do not involve thousands of children and teens. While most of the samples are large enough to achieve statistical significance, the short duration across a range of developmental periods in youth raise questions about how informative they are regarding safety and effectiveness.

Measures of "effectiveness"

In medication trials, a variety of tools are used to measure "success" or "effectiveness." One of the most popular tools is called the SKAMP (Swanson, Kotkin, Agler, M-Flynn, and Pelham Scale). The SKAMP is designed for clinicians to document their observations of ADHD symptoms. The reliability and validity for the SKAMP tool were established in 1992. There are additional forms available, such as the T-SKAMP, designed for teachers (Murray et al., 2009). And the SKAMP-D represent items 5 through 8 on SKAMP.

"The SKAMP is a 10-item scale designed to assess impairment associated with specific context-bound ADHD classroom behaviors. Teachers rate the severity of 10 items (6 for attention, such as "difficulty getting started on classroom assignments"; and 4 for deportment, such as "difficulty remaining quiet according to classroom rules") on a 4-point scale: *0 = not at all, 1 = just a little, 2 = pretty much, to 3 = very much*. It should be noted that subsequent versions of the SKAMP have been developed, including one with a 7-point scale and the addition of an individualized write-in item" (Murray et al., 2009, p. 196). There are ways to then analyze the scores. Some research summarizes the entire score across items, while as noted, the SKAMP-D looks at items 5 though 8.

The 10-item SKAMP is published in Murray et al. (2009, p. 206). As noted above, concerns around the use of "often" in the ADHD diagnostic criteria persists. And the SKAMP, in its measure of medication effectiveness also utilizes a continuum of frequency descriptors that may be of concern. For example, if you imagine the range of behaviors in classrooms across the country, quantifying them with these anchors may be problematic.

Sample SKAMP item	Not at All	Just a Little	Pretty Much	Very Much
Difficulty staying on task for a classroom period	0	1	2	3
Problems in completion or work on classroom assignments	0	1	2	3
Difficulty attending to an activity or discussion of the class	0	1	2	3

For a medication to be determined "effective," scores on the SKAMP would demonstrate improvement over time, compared to placebo. As noted in the DSM, there are also other strategies that can minimize, if not make disappear, the symptoms of ADHD. The SKAMP has been in use for approximately 30 years and remains one of the primary measures of medication effectiveness. While this remains the "gold standard" for medication trials, it is worth considering why the field has not been able to improve the precision in measuring treatment effectiveness.

The longest ADHD study – What's the evidence from the MTA study?

The Multimodal Treatment of ADHD study has generated many publications and remains the foundation for providing evidence for the use of stimulants in the treatment of ADHD. The MTA study examined treatment across 579 children. One group received methylphenidate alone, one group received Behavioral Treatment, one group received a Combination of methylphenidate and behavioral treatment, and there was a group receiving routine community care.

It is true that in the short-term, Combined Treatment achieved the most symptom reduction (in measures of ADHD symptoms and overall Impairment). But while this difference may have achieved statistical significance, the clinical significance may be less noteworthy. Moreover, after the initial phase of data collection, the benefits of methylphenidate alone and combined treatments began to dissipate. Indeed, at 36 months, all treatment conditions were equally effective in their control of symptoms (Jensen et al., 2007).

Thankfully, the MTA researchers continued to monitor these young people. However, they continued to find little value of the medication first achieved in the earliest phase of the study. Indeed by 8 years of follow-up, "in nearly every analysis, the originally randomized treatment groups did not differ significantly on repeated measures … The MTA participants fared worse than the local normative comparison group on 91% of the variables tested" (Molina et al., 2009, p. 484).

In 2017, MTA researchers released another analysis of the data (Swanson et al.). Again, they concluded medication benefits dissipate but "growth-related costs may remain statistically significant into adulthood" (p. 668), specifically noting "extended use of medication was associated with suppression of adult height but not with reduction of symptom severity" (p. 663).

More recently, a meta-analysis of medication treatments was completed. The authors noted that their findings "represent the most comprehensive available evidence base to inform patients, families, clinicians, guideline developers, and policy makers on the choice of ADHD medications across age groups" (Cortese et al., 2018, p. 727). However, this comprehensive review could only support the short-term use of stimulants (with preference toward methylphenidate) as the availability of reliable long-term data was scarce.

But medication must improve academic performance, right?

Children are often prescribed stimulant medications after behavioral, or performance problems are identified in their academic settings. Indeed, a child's full-time job is being a student. As such, the value of stimulant medications on academic performance is of interest though research on this topic is curiously lacking. For example, if a pharmaceutical company could demonstrate that academic performance could demonstrably improve based on the use of a medication, we would all likely take it. In 2006, the American Psychological Association released a report on psychotropic medications. Related to stimulant use, they pointedly noted, "stimulants have no effect on academic achievement in the short-term. No long-term effects have been reliably reported on any outcome measure" (p. 43). Most recently, Pelham et al. (2022) released their finding about the impact of stimulants on learning. In their sample of 173 children between 7 and 12 years old, these researchers found that while medication improved productivity, it did not translate to learning. In other words, medications were associated with behavioral control, but this did not enable improved accuracy on work products or the overall learning outcomes.

Conclusions

Clinicians, parents, policymakers, and educators must be critical consumers of information. A quick, effective remedy is attractive for any of us when facing the discomfort, distress, and disruptions that can result from emotional and behavioral disorders. But our system is profoundly imperfect. While we have interventions that may help, "cures" remain very elusive. The benefits of our strategies differ dramatically across those that engage in treatment. Some may have short-term, long-term, or no advantages from our "best" treatments. This should be seen as a reflection of our imprecise and imperfect treatments, rather than labeling it as an "untreatable" or "difficult-to-treat" condition.

As this discussion has focused on a condition most common in young people, our sensitivity to its successes and failures should be amplified. The use of psychotropic medications in young people is not without consequence in their developing central nervous systems, consequences that we largely do not understand. Of course, anyone offering treatments to children and families in distress are doing their best to reduce the impact of these conditions, but we are too often making assumptions over-estimating the safety and effectiveness of our treatments. It is recommended that we proceed with caution and humility. Consider the downstream effects of our interventions and their potential impact beyond the short-term gains that may be achieved.

References

American Psychiatric Association. (2022). Diagnostic and Statistical Manual of Mental Disorders, Fifth Edition, Text Revision. Washington, DC: American Psychiatric Association Publishing.

American Psychiatric Association. (1994). Diagnostic and Statistical Manual of Mental Disorders, Fourth Edition. Washington, DC: American Psychiatric Association.

APA Working Group on Psychoactive Medications for Children and Adolescents. (2006). Report of the Working Group on Psychoactive Medications for Children and Adolescents. Psychopharmacological, psychosocial, and combined interventions for childhood disorders: Evidence base, contextual factors, and future directions. Washington, DC: American Psychological Association.

CHADD. Website content retrieved from https://chadd.org/for-parents/overview/

Concerta. Website content retrieved from https://www.concerta.net/concerta-for-children.html#children-2

Cortese, S. et al. (2018). Comparative Efficacy and Tolerability of Medications for Attention-Deficit Hyperactivity Disorder in Children, Adolescents, and Adults: A systematic review and network meta-analysis. *The Lancet Psychiatry*, 5(9). 727-738.

Evekeo. Website content retrieved from https://www.evekeo.com/

Frances, A. (2017). Newsflash from APA Meeting: DSM-5 has flunked its reliability tests. Retrieved from https://www.huffpost.com/entry/dsm-5-reliability-tests_b_1490857

International Narcotics Control Board. (2021). Psychotropic Substances 2021. Retrieved from: https://www.incb.org/documents/Psychotropics/technical-publications/2021/21-08898_Psychotropics_2021_ebook.pdf

Insel, T. (2022). Healing: Our Path from Mental Illness to Mental Health. New York: Penguin Press.

Jensen PS, Arnold LE, Swanson JM, Vitiello B, Abikoff HB, Greenhill LL, Hechtman L, Hinshaw SP, Pelham WE, Wells KC, Conners CK, Elliott GR, Epstein JN, Hoza B, March JS, Molina BSG, Newcorn JH, Severe JB, Wigal T, Gibbons RD, Hur K. (2007). 3-year follow-up of the NIMH MTA study. *J Am Acad Child Adolesc Psychiatry*. 46(8):989-1002. doi: 10.1097/CHI.0b013e3180686d48. PMID: 17667478.

McHugh, M. (2012). Interrater reliability: the kappa statistic. Biochem Med (Zagreb). 22(3):276-82. PMID: 23092060; PMCID: PMC3900052.

Molina BSG, Hinshaw SP, Swanson JM, Arnold LE, Vitiello B, Jensen PS, Epstein JN, Hoza B, Hechtman L, Abikoff HB, Elliott GR, Greenhill LL, Newcorn JH, Wells KC, Wigal T, Gibbons RD, Hur K, Houck PR; MTA Cooperative Group. (2009). The MTA at 8 years: prospective follow-up of children treated for combined-type ADHD in a multisite study. *J Am Acad Child Adolesc Psychiatry*. 48(5):484-500. doi: 10.1097/CHI.0b013e31819c23d0. PMID: 19318991; PMCID: PMC3063150.

Murray, D., Bussing, R., Fernandez, M., Hou, W., Garvan, C., Swanson, J., Eyberg, S. (2009). Psychometric Properties of Teacher SKAMP Ratings from a Community Sample. *Assessment*, 16(2). 193-208.

Pelham WE, Altszuler AR, Merrill BM, Raiker JS, Macphee FL, Ramos M, Gnagy EM, Greiner AR, Coles EK, Connor CM, Lonigan CJ, Burger L, Morrow AS, Zhao X, Swanson JM, Waxmonsky JG, Pelham WE. (2022). The effect of stimulant medication on the learning of academic curricula in children with ADHD: A randomized crossover study. *J Consult Clin Psychol*. 90(5):367-380. doi: 10.1037/ccp0000725. PMID: 35604744; PMCID: PMC9443328.

Quillivant. Website content retrieved from https://www.trisadhd.com/quillivant-xr/

Swanson, J.M., Arnold, L.E., Molina, B.S., Sibley, M.H., Hechtman, L.T., Hinshaw, S.P., Abikoff, H.B., Stehli, A., Owens, E.B., Mitchell, J.T., Nichols, Q., Howard, A., Greenhill, L.L., Hoza, B., Newcorn, J.H., Jensen, P.S., Vitiello, B., Wigal, T., Epstein, J.N., Tamm, L., Lakes, K.D., Waxmonsky, J., Lerner, M., Etcovitch, J., Murray, D.W., Muenke, M., Acosta, M.T., Arcos-Burgos, M., Pelham, W.E., Kraemer, H.C. (2017). Young adult outcomes in the follow-up of the multimodal treatment study of attention-deficit/hyperactivity disorder: symptom persistence, source discrepancy, and height suppression. *J Child Psychol Psychiatr*, 58: 663-678. https://doi.org/10.1111/jcpp.12684

Vyvanse. Website content retrieved from https://www.vyvanse.com/usage-for-kids

ADHD In the Making: From 'Identifying' Symptoms to 'Symptomatic' Identities

Juho Honkasilta and Athanasios Koutsoklenis

There is a time to admire the grace and persuasive power of an influential idea, and there is a time to fear its hold over us. The time to worry is when the idea is so widely shared that we no longer even notice it, when it is so deeply rooted that it feels to us like plain common sense. At the point when objections are not answered anymore because they are no longer even raised, we are not in control: we do not have the idea; it has us (Kohn 1999, 3).

The above citation from Alfie Kohn's book *Punished by Rewards* reminds us how discourse functions after having gained hegemonic status. It normalizes our understanding of the phenomenon in question and legitimizes related practices. The contemporary "common sense" notion of attention deficit hyperactivity disorder (ADHD) as a complex, multifactorial neurodevelopmental disorder is naturalized and normalized by cultivating the psycho-medical discourse of deficit and disorder. In and through this discourse, ADHD exists as a neurobiological or neurodevelopmental condition

---

Juho Honkasilta, PhD, is a Lecturer at the Department of Education, University of Helsinki, Finland.

Athanasios Koutsoklenis is assistant professor of Inclusive Education at the Democritus University of Thrace, Greece.

This chapter is adapted from the article "The (Un)real Existence of ADHD—Criteria, Functions, and Forms of the Diagnostic Entity" that appeared in Frontiers in Sociology: https://doi.org/10.3389/fsoc.2022.814763

within an individual caused by development processes of nature over which etiology, individuals, society, or culture has no power.

In this chapter, guided by Kohn's notion and based on our previous research, we have striven to break down (1) how the hegemonic idea that ADHD is a condition and a disorder within an individual becomes formed and (2) how the idea becomes sustained and materialized in discourse practice in everyday lives (see Honkasilta & Koutsoklenis, 2022). We illustrate how institutional, social and (intra)personal lives are governed through the psycho-medical discourse of ADHD; and through the idea that a neurodevelopmental interpretation frame for behaviors, performance and functioning joined with psychiatric diagnoses are useful or even necessary in structuring and making sense of everyday struggles.

We applied a discursive approach to make sense of an *ADHD diagnostic entity* and its hegemonic status. The premise of this chapter is that ADHD *exists* in an abstract space of *text* and becomes real in the concrete space of practice through *recognition of a certain kind* (see Honkasilta, 2016). Our particular focus is on discourse practice, which refers to the processes of text production, distribution, and consumption in which sociocultural ideologies, beliefs, norms, and power relations are naturalized (Fairclough, 2004).

We have used the term diagnostic entity as a reference to the plurality of meanings that the ADHD concept is given in discourse practice, such as a condition, a disorder, a diagnosis, a trait, or a label. By using the term, we emphasize that although the Diagnostic and Statistical Manual of Mental Disorders (DSM) and similar classification manuals initially provide the language to communicate about human beings and lives, the language dynamically shapes human lives beyond the conceptual boundaries set in the manuals (see, Honkasilta & Koutsoklenis, 2022).

We first discuss how the idea of ADHD being a natural neurodevelopmental state within an individual is formed via text in the DSM created by the American Psychiatric Association (APA). Here the focus of governance is on how behaviors become symptoms of a disorder. The second part focuses on how this idea is performed in institutional and social practice through given meanings to and functions of the diagnostic entity. The focus of governance will be on top-down and bottom-up processes that constitute the boundaries of being a person of a certain kind.

ADHD exists in text – The making of ADHD as a neurodevelopmental disorder

ADHD has been included in the DSM (in one form or another) since its second edition, published in 1968[1]. From the publication of the third edition in 1980, DSM has been committed to a 'neo-Kraepelinian', cause-effect biomedical framework of psychiatry (Jacobs & Cohen, 2012). This framework embraces the assumptions that 'psychiatry is a branch of medicine and treats people who are sick, there is a boundary between the normal and the sick, there are discrete mental illnesses, psychiatrists should concentrate on biological aspects of mental illnesses, and diagnostic criteria should be codified' (Jacobs & Cohen, 2012, p. 88). The recently published revised edition of DSM-5 (its eighth facelift) keeps the faith in the neo-Kraepelinian paradigm by adhering to a cause-effect biomedical explanatory framework. Neo-Kraepeliniaism assumes biological discoveries in order to establish this cause-effect relationship (Jacobs and Cohen, 2012).

ADHD is defined in the DSM-5-TR (APA, 2022, p. 37) as 'a neurodevelopmental disorder defined by impairing levels of

[1] For a detailed history of ADHD as a diagnostic entity see Smith (2014).

inattention, disorganization, and/or hyperactivity-impulsivity. Inattention and disorganization entail inability to stay on task, seeming not to listen, and losing materials necessary for tasks, at levels that are inconsistent with age or developmental level. Hyperactivity-impulsivity entails overactivity, fidgeting, inability to stay seated, intruding into other people's activities, and inability to wait— symptoms that are excessive for age or developmental level'.

The conceptualization of DSM suggests that ADHD is a complex, multifactorial, neurodevelopmental disorder that represents the convergence of biological risk factors and social/environmental adversities. This individual-medical model of disability regards ADHD as a condition within an individual – something individuals have – that exposes them to being vulnerable to developing adverse life trajectories. However, as the authors of the DSM-5-TR themselves explicitly admit for ADHD, the discoveries that establish ADHD as a neurodevelopmental disorder are yet to materialize. Specifically, the DSM-5-TR authors state that 'no biological marker is diagnostic for ADHD' (APA, 2022, p. 73) and that 'meta-analysis of *all* neuroimaging studies do not show differences between individuals with ADHD and control subjects' (APA, 2022, p. 73), thus 'no form of neuroimaging can be used for diagnosis of ADHD' (APA, 2022, p. 73). In the absence of scientific evidence on psychopathology that would support the contemporary idea and conceptualization, ADHD cannot be understood as a complex neurodevelopmental disorder without a complex assemblage of political, economic, and cultural processes that deem such a conceptualization to be valuable and useful.

The DSM is an example of a powerful, influential, and authoritative text (Crowe, 2000). It is one of the most successful technologies in modern western mental health industry having an extraordinary success in states, professionals, media, and lay-people (Gambrill, 2014; Horwitz, 2021). The DSM plays a multifaceted role in 'the global spread of psychiatric ways of being a person and how we all come to understand ourselves within this register' (Mills, 2014, p. 51): a) it provides both the theory on and the language with which to communicate about human differences, b) it provides guidelines for technologies of identification and naming of these differences, and c) it provides directions for institutional and social practices to make use of the ideology of labelling (Honkasilta & Koutsoklenis, 2022). We next discuss how the hegemonic idea that ADHD is a disorder within an individual becomes formed and naturalized in discourse produced in the DSM by examining the accuracy of the diagnostic criteria for ADHD provided in the manual.

How do behaviors become symptoms?

The lack of the establishment of a biomedical cause-effect explanatory framework inevitably impacts the *accuracy* of the diagnostic criteria. By accuracy we mean the "bundle of questions about the clarity of definitions that distinguish one category from another, the conceptual coherence of these definitions, and the ability of users of the classification system to implement these distinctions consistently in practice" (Kirk, 2004, p. 255–256). In a recently published article (i.e., Honkasilta & Koutsoklenis, 2022) we have provided a thorough critique of the accuracy of DSM-5 diagnostic criteria for ADHD using as a blueprint the criticism for descriptive diagnoses articulated by Kirk et al. (2013). We will attempt to provide here an analogous critique for the DSM-5-TR.

Behaviors become symptoms through circular reasoning

Unable to establish a biomedical cause-effect explanatory framework, DSM-5-TR authors are confined to a descriptive framework. In such a descriptive approach to diagnosis, behavioral indicators called symptoms are used alone for the diagnosis without the requirement to understand nor identify any presumed underlying causes or dynamics of the behavior in question (Kirk et al., 2013). The behavioral Indicators are then rebranded as 'diagnostic criteria', and they form the basis for the definitions of the diagnosis (Kirk et al., 2015). This process entails circular reasoning in which symptoms guarantee the diagnosis while the diagnosis is called upon to explain the symptoms in a perpetual loop (Pérez-Álvarez, 2017; Tait, 2009). But as Jacobs and Cohen (2012, p. 89) note: 'Until diagnostic criteria are formulated in words that do not simply refer to other words, vagueness cannot disappear from a disorder's definition'.

Behaviors become symptoms via ambiguity

The diagnostic criteria for ADHD in the DSM-5-TR continue to be ambiguous. The most representative example of their ambiguity is the descriptors 'often' that is employed in all eighteen diagnostic criteria. Since no description or threshold for the frequency of the behaviors is provided anywhere in the manual, who meets each criterion is completely dependent on shared understandings of how much of a particular behavior is indeed too much (Freedman & Honkasilta, 2017). In an analogous manner, one may wonder at what point talking becomes 'excessive' or under which circumstances it is appropriate or inappropriate for children to run or climb.

Behaviors become symptoms via redundancy

Redundancy is evident in the formulation of the diagnostic criteria, that is, supposedly different criteria are similar but with alternative wording. Therefore, individuals subjected to assessment are likely to meet several criteria and as a consequence reach the diagnostic cut-off.

Behaviors become symptoms via arbitrariness

On the one hand, as in the DSM-5, the number of criteria required for an ADHD diagnosis has been set arbitrarily in the DSM-5-TR;

no scientific justification has been presented nor method used for deducing how many criteria should be required for the diagnosis. On the other hand, as in its predecessors, the age of onset of symptoms (i.e., 12 years) has been also arbitrarily decided in the DSM-5-TR. The authors of the DSM-5-TR state that 'the requirement that several symptoms be present before age 12 years conveys the importance of a substantial clinical presentation during childhood' (APA, 2022, p. 71) but at the same time they acknowledge that 'an earlier age at onset is not specified because of difficulties in establishing precise childhood onset retrospectively' (APA, 2022, p. 71). Commenting on the issue, Sanders et al. (2019) highlight the fact that setting the age of onset at 12 years of age was based on research that was judged to be at high risk of bias.

Behaviors become symptoms via the fortification of normality

The diagnostic criteria are lists of symptoms which exemplify the contraries of socially valued norms (Freedman & Honkasilta, 2017). The 'normal child' behaves in a 'normal' way when playing quietly, remaining seated, waiting patiently in line, not talking too much, not daydreaming often, and by completing homework most of the time. Children who aberrate from these 'normal' behaviors are at risk of a 'dangerous development' (Bailey, 2010, p. 584). Their actions consist of a threat not only for their social and educational future but also for the associated cultural values (Freedman & Honkasilta, 2017). As was mentioned above, certain behaviors are more likely to be interpreted as normal. The interpretation is the privilege of other 'normal' individuals who judge behaviors as rude, intruding, deviant, inadequate or inappropriate. But 'the actual criterion being used here is the annoyance threshold of the observer' (Honkasilta & Koutsoklenis, 2022, p. 5) since value judgements are dependent on the emotional and sociocultural threshold of the observers.

Behaviors become symptoms via decontextualization

The DSM-5-TR retains the sanitized and asocial view of the human condition of its predecessor. No attention has been paid to the social context of the behaviors themselves nor to the meanings that behaviors may have for each individual. Therefore, fidgeting, tapping hands or squirming in the seat is not interpreted as a possible sign of stress but as the immediate result of an internal dysfunction, that is of the neurodevelopmental disorder named ADHD.

Does the above critique cancel the embodied experiences of those diagnosed?

An abundance of research shows that ADHD is diagnosed with several other psychiatric disorders or impairments. The frequency of this so-called co-morbidity has been estimated to be as high as 63.8% for the USA (Danielson et al., 2018). Moreover, data from neuropsychological evaluations documents the heterogeneity of those diagnosed with ADHD (e.g., DeRonda et al., 2021; Kofler et al., 2019; Solovieva and Rojas, 2014, 2015). The abovementioned evidence suggests that the population of children diagnosed with ADHD is highly diverse. Therefore, ADHD is a heterogeneous diagnostic category which does not encompass nor represent as such the lived experiences of so-called 'ADHD-people' or people 'with ADHD-symptoms', that is, the grouping of certain kinds of people the DSM and similar manuals create via their 'identification' criteria.

This does not deprecate or ignore the embodied experiences by diagnosed individuals and their significant others, nor difficulties in everyday lives associated with ADHD diagnostic entity in general. For them, experienced difficulties are very much real in their consequences. Neurobiological and psychological traits gain their pathological meaning in a mismatch between what kind of behavior, performance, or functioning is expected by self, others, or institutions and one's capabilities to meet them accordingly. The question is not whether these traits and associated experiences are real but instead why do they become regarded and named as symptoms manifesting a disorder within an individual?

ADHD becomes real in practice – Identity governance via ADHD diagnostic entity

Ian Hacking (2006) describes how science creates kinds of people that in one sense did not exist before they were 'identified'. This is what he calls 'making up people'. The engines used in these sciences, such as statistical analysis of classes of people and the striving to recognize hidden medical, biological, or genetic causes for problems that beset a class of people, are not only engines of discovery but also, and fundamentally, engines for making up people of certain kinds – "ADHD-people" or people "with" ADHD.

The idea cultivated via DSM, that ADHD represents a natural neurodevelopmental state within an individual, structures institutional and social practices. The DSM is an example of a top-down process providing an interpretation frame and language through which human behaviors can be translated to neuro-governed value-neutral symptoms irrespective of history and culture. Each time the DSM is revised, the interpretation frame is redone, adjusted, or maintained, thereby governing how human behaviors and being should be perceived.

The hegemonic position of contemporary conceptualization of ADHD as presented in the DSM also results from a bottom-up process deriving from people's intentional, dynamic, and situationally sensitive uses of psychiatric diagnoses as a gateway for navigating institutions and everyday interactions. Thus, no matter how influential the idea of ADHD as a natural state within an individual is (i.e., text produced in the DSM), it only materializes if *recognized* as such in *practices* of institutions (e.g., law, healthcare, welfare, education, and parenting), pertinent professionals (clinicians, physicians, educators, social workers, etc.), or laypeople (e.g., family members, peers, or the ones diagnosed). The idea of ADHD as a complex, multifactorial neurodevelopmental disorder becomes real via performance or enaction in material interactions with ideological conventions and power relations, with agents empowered to push these ideologies to action (e.g., clinicians, teachers, parents, interest groups) and with the ones being diagnosed.

Next, we approach ADHD as an identity category so as to illustrate the dynamic ways the ADHD diagnostic entity functions as an instrument of governance. We conceptualized identity as dynamic ways of becoming recognized as certain kinds in certain ways in social interaction. Approaching ADHD as an identity category is thus not about being a certain kind but becoming certain kinds.

ADHD identity governance via institutional practices

We applied James Gee's (2000) analysis of four interrelated perspectives to understanding how the ADHD diagnostic entity functions as part of identity. He conceptualizes four perspectives and sources of identities: Nature, institution, discourse, and affinity. Each source of identity has a distinct process of recognition of what kind (of a person) one is. Nature identity becomes recognized through a process of development, institution identity through authorization, discourse identity through dialogue, and affinity identity through shared endeavors and practices. Although interrelated and eventually bound together in discourse practice, this division is illustrative of how the diagnostic entity is confined to identities of those categorized, diagnosed, and labelled.

Nature perspective on ADHD identities

The official and hegemonic discourse on ADHD formed in the DSM and similar manuals has globalized our perceptions of kinds of persons with problems in life. It portrays and construes ADHD as a fixed internal neurodevelopmental state affecting behaviors, performance, and functioning. Biological states (e.g., blood relation, cancer) are not meaningful parts of our identities outright unless they are recognized as such in portraying what kind of a person one is by themself and/or others. In other words, biological state, either assumed (e.g., ADHD) or identified (e.g., cancer), gains force as identities through discourse in institutional (e.g., diagnosis-bound support distribution) and social practices (e.g., social interactions).

Assuming and consuming ADHD as a nature identity materializes in through *the explanatory function* the ADHD diagnostic entity has in discourse practice. Recognizing that a person has a neurodevelopmental condition functions as an explanation to problems, experienced or perceived, related to behaviors, performance and functioning in everyday life. It communicates about recognition for the veracity of problems experienced by people of certain kinds, namely people with ADHD symptoms, and for taking these problems seriously.

DSM and similar 'identification' manuals and law and national care guidelines applying the text of these manuals are examples of top-down processes through which the idea that ADHD represents a (complex) neurodevelopmental state becomes naturalized. As a bottom-up process, this naturalization typically happens in interactions between and among school representatives and parents, in which the psycho-medical discourse of ADHD is distributed as an account for school failure resulting from a naturally occurring deficit in brain functioning. Once educators such as parents and teachers get hold of the psycho-medical discourse of ADHD as an explanation for lived experiences of and with the child, it starts forming the ways child's behaviors are recognized even before or without official diagnosis, thus imposing ADHD as nature identity (e.g., Hjörne & Säljö, 2004; 2014a; 2014b).

Institution perspective on ADHD identities

The idea that behaviors, performance, and functioning are explainable by neurobiological developmental deficits becomes legitimized in institutional practice, by which we refer to actions and meaning-making processes within institutions by authorities entitled with the power to authorize the kind of recognition in question, for instance, having the authority to diagnose (Gee, 2000). After an official diagnosis, the hypothesized natural state becomes legitimized by institutional authorities, strengthening the nature perspective of ADHD identity of the one diagnosed and adding an institutional perspective on identity negotiations. In other words, now the person has a neurodevelopmental condition that causes their neuropsychiatric disorder. The nature and institution identities mutually support and sustain each other.

An ADHD diagnosis communicates information about the veracity of needed professional support between authorities and institutions (e.g., home, school, psychiatric clinic). Institutional practice transforms ADHD from a natural state to an institutionally recognized position: Not only do individuals 'have' the condition but with the formal diagnosis they are *legally entitled* to societal and institutional recognition of certain kinds. The institutional perspective on ADHD identities plays a central role in the governance of 'normalcy' through the services that the diagnosis entitles one to.

Drawn from the critique we presented on DSM, it would be naïve to assert that diagnosing ADHD follows a logical identification trajectory of individual impairments followed by diagnosis-specific remedial social practices. ADHD diagnostic entity is an instrument of institutional governance resulting in a top-down process of distributing and directing societal and institutional resources (e.g., welfare, healthcare, education etc.) according to information communicated through the diagnosis. Although organizing support practice based on the psychiatric diagnosis has doubtful effectiveness (Koutsoklenis & Gaitanidis, 2017; Timimi, 2017), for resource providers and service providers the diagnosis signifies a legit cut-off of resource distribution between those entitled to support resources (i.e., diagnosed) and those who are not (i.e., non-diagnosed). Apart from the societal distribution of support, in many countries, remedial or special educational support at schools is diagnosis-bound. Thus, diagnosing ADHD, followed by special needs education resolution and/or medication at school, is a typical sequence of events in institutional practice (e.g., Koutsoklenis, 2020).

It has also been extensively and clearly pointed out how exclusive education policies leave educators (parents, teachers) with little choice but to find diagnostic categories for "disorderly" students (e.g., Hinshaw & Scheffler, 2014; Tomlinson, 2015). For example, in the USA, laws and policies related to school accountability and the push for performance give schools the incentive to direct parents to seek diagnoses in order to attract resources that help schools raise students' test scores and that allow schools to 'exempt a low achieving youth from lowering the district's overall achievement ranking' (Hinshaw & Scheffler, 2014, p. 79).

The relative age effect on diagnosing and medicating for ADHD provides perhaps the most tangible example of how schooling is intrinsically interconnected with diagnosing ADHD. Recent literature reviews have revealed a cross-national norm for the youngest children in a classroom to be more likely to be diagnosed with, and medicated for, ADHD than their older age classroom group peers (Koutsoklenis et al., 2020; Whitely et al. 2018). Regardless of whether countries have high rates of diagnosing or prescribing (like USA) or low rates (like Finland), this pattern is still evident, suggesting that relative immaturity in the class keeps emerging as a risk factor for being diagnosed and medicated. Children mature at different rates, raising an important question of whether a diagnosis of ADHD, even for the older in the class children, might also be reflective of their relative slower developmental trajectory. Thus, financial interests are embedded in top-down governance ranging from providing services to promoting and marketing them (e.g., Davies, 2013; Hinshaw & Scheffler, 2014).

For lay people, the diagnosis denotes an institutionally recognized psychiatric disorder followed by entitlement to a range of goods, support services and treatments. Thus, parents may actively seek a diagnosis for their children so that their so-called pedagogical "special needs," verified by the diagnosis, will be adequately met at schools. The diagnosis also serves as a *disclaimer* discharging them from liability. Tait (2005) provides an example of how a student who caused $40,000 worth of damage to two elementary schools in Wisconsin, USA, was not expelled, unlike his two accomplices, because his mother acquired a private psychologist's statement that he might have ADHD. The reassertion was that student's actions were caused by a compulsive medical condition that overruled the legal accountability of his actions.

Given the extent to which children and young people become subjected to certain levels of institutional and social monitoring, support and/or treatment after being diagnosed, it is unlikely for them to avoid forming their identities in relation to ADHD diagnostic entity in one way or another. The analysis by Honkasilta and Vehkakoski (2017) about how diagnosed young people and their parents negotiate identities in relation to their ideas about ADHD and medication use is revealing about how dynamically nature and institution identities are intertwined.

When ADHD was regarded as both authentic-self and preferred-self, it gained meaning as one's natural valued trait that medication threatened to alter or hinder. On the other hand, ADHD was also regarded as one's authentic-self, yet medicated-self was the preferred one. ADHD gained meaning as a natural deficit whereas medication enabled recreating one's identity. Medicated-self was also regarded as authentic-self and preferred-self, in which case ADHD-self was portrayed as a treatable disease entity overcome by medicine. The ways diagnosed children and youth voice their experiences, accounting for their behaviors, is likely to entail intertextuality with discourse by their parents, teachers, and the mental health professionals they have direct or indirect access to. The imposed nature identity is paired with the imposed institutional identity.

At an institutional level, the diagnostic entity serves as an explanation for problems experienced and the need for support, entitlement to receive support resources, and a potential disclaimer for legal liability. Therefore, the idea of a neuropsychiatric disorder called ADHD caused by neurodevelopmental condition is sustained and cultivated in discourses practiced by institutions and laypeople regardless of the lack of evidence supporting this idea; it has a pragmatic value. The diagnostic entity is an instrument of normalization that forms boundaries for identity negotiations for the subjects of the normalization process, or those subjected to them. However, the normalization process is not limited to institutional practice. In addition to political and legal spheres of recognition (i.e., institutional), the ADHD diagnostic entity entails a promise for social and psychological recognition of a certain kind. The psycho-medical discourse cultivates people being perceived differently by others and themselves in social and (intra)personal lives.

ADHD identity governance via social practices

Discursive perspective on ADHD identities

Gee (2000) calls the third perspective on ADHD identities the discursive perspective through which recognition emerges in a dialogue between people. Whereas institutions must rely on discursive practices to construct and sustain ADHD as nature and institution identities, ADHD identities can also be constructed and sustained through dialogue between people without them being sanctioned and sustained by clinical institutions and authorities.

The mobilization of ADHD-related stereotypes and lay diagnoses, or the act of lay or self-diagnosing, are examples of forming discursive ADHD identities without them being warranted by institutional authorities. Parents' active attempts to have their children recognized as 'disordered' to gain remedial support is an example of parents' *achieving* a certain kind of ADHD discourse identity for the child authorized by institutions. Parents tend to *receive a diagnosis* for their children. Children, on the other hand, play no active role in the process. They are *diagnosed*, and the basis for the ADHD discourse identities is *ascribed* to them.

The psycho-medical discourse is harnessed to counter normative assumptions and judgments regarding "normal" development, behavior, performance, functioning, parenting, teaching, and so on: broadly put, cultural blame. In and through this discourse, ADHD diagnosis is mobilized as an emancipation of moral liability, or as Reid and Maag (1997) conclude, a label of forgiveness, carrying psychological meanings. For parents, a child's diagnosis absolves the culture of blame of what may be seen as poor parenting, since asserting that a child 'suffers' from a neurobiological disorder is not as delicate a matter as asserting that the child manifests unwanted

ADHD-like symptoms in response to an unsteady home life (e.g., Frigerio & Montali, 2016; Wong et al., 2018). The diagnostic entity eases parents from self-blame or guilt against conventional beliefs of good or bad parenting, and protects them from being blamed, shamed, and held accountable for their child's doings in social interaction between home and education institution, for example (e.g., Dauman et al., 2019; Frigerio et al., 2013).

Similarly, diagnosed children and young people make use of neurobiological and diagnostic explanations dynamically and deliberately to minimize their own responsibility for behaviors, providing the means to excuse oneself from demanding self-control as well as to explain and neutralize behaviors in face-to-face interactions (Berger, 2015; Honkasilta et al., 2016; Singh 2011; Travell & Visser 2006). The diagnostic entity thus functions as a moral disclaimer for both parents and their diagnosed children. Not surprisingly, it also serves the same function for educators (e.g., Bailey, 2014; Hjörne & Säljö, 2004; Shallaby, 2017). The diagnosis serves as a rhetorical device that creates a common understanding of school difficulties for school staff, parents, and other actors, and simultaneously as a legitimate proof that these difficulties lay not within the social environment and its everyday praxis: the child is not the problem nor does the child have a problem, the problem lies *within* the child.

In addition to moral disclaimer, ADHD diagnostic entity is an instrument of humanizing used to evoke sympathy, empathy and/ or understanding for lived experiences and challenges experienced, challenging life situations and individual traits deemed deviant. Parents seek a diagnosis for their children not only to advocate for their children's so-called remedial or special needs being recognized and supported, but also as a response to perceiving their children as being misjudged and inadequately socioemotionally supported

(Bailey, 2014; Emerald & Carpenter, 2010, Honkasilta et al., 2015). The psycho-medical discourse of ADHD directs the focus from behaviors and performance that may be of concern to an individual characterized by so-called 'neurodiversity'. Furthermore, the humanizing function and how it interplays with that of moral emancipation from blame or guilt also extends to parents' negotiating an alternative form of recognition for themselves. The diagnostic entity normalizes parents, who can now establish their moral status as competent educators and caregivers through received/ internalized emotional reprieve from guilt and blame (Frigerio & Montali 2016; Honkasilta & Vehkakoski, 2019; Schubert et al., 2009; Singh, 2011, Wong et al., 2018).

Along with normalizing how individuals are viewed and treated by others – that is humanizing those living 'with' ADHD – the diagnosis also entails a promise of empathetically receiving and treating oneself. Hence, the diagnosis also takes form as an instrument of empowerment, serving as a means to come to terms with the idea of ADHD as an individual trait and characteristic and embrace it as such. ADHD is portrayed as an embodiment of certain ways of being, experiencing, doing, and interacting with social environments. The psycho-medical discourse provides people with liberty to express one's ADHD as part of self and empowers the claiming of ownership in ways subjectivities are recognized in social interactions. Harnessing the discourse as part of personal, and beyond dispute, social narratives provide a rationale for making sense of lived experiences and selves, and language to communicate these experiences and advocate for recognition of a certain kind. Metaphorically put, it breaks the chains of blame, shame and guilt and provides a chance to re-discover oneself .

For people diagnosed in adulthood, on the other hand, they will have likely started monitoring themselves according to the psycho-medical discourse of ADHD prior to official diagnosing. The discourse provides adults with heuristic understanding of their past and present – of themselves – now presenting them with a pathway to re-create themselves (with or without the help of medication) empowered by the discourse alone or by authorities through the diagnosis. It is noteworthy that this function is not limited to the subjectivities of those diagnosed. Instead, for parents of a diagnosed child, the empowering nature of the diagnosis may materialize in the form of claiming strong advocacy and expertise in the diagnosed child's schooling, after having gained a more in-depth understanding of the claimed condition, the manifestation of its so-called symptoms, and means of support (e.g., Frigerio et al., 2013; Honkasilta & Vehkakoski, 2019).

Discursive identities are dynamic and enable detachment from the official psycho-medical model of deficit, disorder, and disability by reconstructing what ADHD as an individual trait is about. Contemporary western zeitgeist is characterized by new emerging discourses aimed at changing the ways people 'with' ADHD are recognized. The neurodiversity movement[2] is an example of a social movement which reconstructs discourse identities for advocating social change. Mobilizing neuroscientific metaphors about 'differently wired brains,' the movement asserts that neurobiological differences are part of natural variation among the human population. Academia has further adopted this discourse and harnessed it to rebrand traits associated with ADHD, such as an entrepreneurial mindset (Moore et al., 2021) or character strengths and virtues (Sedgwick et al., 2019). Similarly, a quick online search illustrates that a range of advocacy groups has harnessed the

---

[2] The movement was originally coined by and for people labelled with what is currently described as the autism spectrum. (For a critical account, see e.g., Ortega, 2009; Runswick-Cole, 2014)

neuroscientific discourse to create entrepreneurial ADHD discursive identities with headlines such as "Why hiring upside-down thinkers is a competitive advantage."

The auspicious attempt here is to change the narrative and interpretation frames from disorder subject to rehabilitation and treatment to a difference worth embracing. The advocacy for social change by reforming discourse identities brings us to the last perspective on ADHD identities, the affinity identities (Gee, 2000).

Affinity perspective on ADHD identities

The recognition of affinity identities stems from the distinctive practices of a group of people, an affinity group, that shares allegiance to, access to, and participation in specific endeavors or social practices that create and sustain group affiliations. One does not need to own ADHD as part of natural or institutional identity to acquire ADHD as an affinity identity, that is, partly constitutive of the 'kind of person' they are, nor does an ADHD diagnosis lead to acquiring a meaningful affinity identity outright.

Take parents, clinicians, authors, scholars and (other) advocates with or without the diagnosis as an example. For them ADHD can become an affiliation, a matter of participating in a common cause, through actively sharing inside information or experiences on ADHD, or advocating for policies and changes in practices, values, and attitudes to improve lives of those 'with' ADHD. Furthermore, scholars representing different disciplines and paradigms, and perhaps sharing ADHD as their affinity identity, play their role in creating and strengthening the set of available ADHD discursive identities by communicating about the phenomenon as if it was an objective natural state, not a value-laden social category.

Normalization via labelling of difference

The ADHD diagnosis does not project a value-neutral self-image for those so-labelled. Although a label may provide resources to understand oneself (empowerment) and make oneself understandable (humanize), it simultaneously distances one from 'normalcy' and imposes a potential stigma (e.g., Honkasilta et al., 2016; Honkasilta & Vehkakoski, 2019; Laws & Davies, 2000; Wong et al., 2018). ADHD is an identity category that creates and fortifies the category memberships of *us* and *them/others*.

Psycho-medical discourse of ADHD forms the object of which it speaks, that is the person "with" ADHD and various traits associated with the label. It directs focus on individuals deemed different – *them* – and guides the kinds of action that should be targeted for *us* to intervene positively in their lives and potential life trajectories, ranging from treatments to taking a positive attitude toward human diversity. The well-meaning discourse also forms the subject of which it speaks, the certain kind of a person 'with' ADHD.

The governance of identities through the discourse dynamically takes shape in and between these spaces of us and them in the form of mobilizing and materializing the diagnostic entity. It enables a subject's maneuvering within the discourse for achieving certain kinds of recognition while simultaneously limiting subjects' access to other discourses (van Dijk, 1996). The psycho-medical discourse widens the gap between *us* and *them* rather than bridges it and closes the arbitrary boundaries of 'normalcy' rather than opens them (see, Runswick-Cole, 2014). It normalizes the ableist status quo, favoring and privileging assumed 'neurotypicals.'

Discussion – Making sense of ADHD

The ontology of the contemporary hegemonic idea on ADHD does not exist in nature nor does its epistemology point to clinical practices successfully "identifying" the alleged condition. Instead, the onto-epistemological premises of the cotemporary notion of ADHD are founded on pragmatism[3] (Sjöberg, 2019; Tait, 2005). As Gordon Tait (2005, 32, original emphasis) points out in his philosophical analysis of the notion of truth revolving around ADHD, pragmatism supports the theory that ADHD is a natural disorder within an individual, because the theory "provides a straightforward *workable* explanation as to why seemingly otherwise healthy and normal children are incapable of behaving well [...]."

This take on pragmatism highlights the ideology upon which contemporary praxis directed by the DSM – the so called 'bible' of modern psychiatry (Horwitz, 2021) – are premised. The policy level structures in place govern the pragmatic praxis in which people experiencing or being perceived as having problems in their everyday lives should be identified as 'having' ADHD. Regarding ADHD as a neurodevelopmental disorder does not reflect scientific progress but pragmatic utility for diagnoses and diagnostic explanations. The frequent changes in the diagnostic criteria of ADHD are done, among other reasons, to match better the maneuvers of individuals when navigating their social world(s) in the search for recognition, support, category membership, immunity, sympathy, and sense of belonging.

In this regard, Tait (2005) points out another theory supported by pragmatism that seems to be more appropriate for understanding the nature of ADHD as a diagnostic entity structuring our social lives. According to this theory, the idea of ADHD as a neurodevelopmental disorder within an individual is a product of *social governance*

[3] We refer to the commonsense pragmatism (thinking of or dealing with problems in a practical way, sometimes in a cynical manner), not the epistemology of pragmatism as a philosophical tradition.

through which "previously untapped areas of human conduct are being opened up to pathologization [...] at which point the organs of intervention and regulation will be put in place, and normalization will commence – more often than not pharmacologically" (Tait 2005, 32). This depiction of ADHD, he continues, also explains the emergence of the disorder almost exclusively in areas where associated behaviors and functioning are felt to pose a threat to effective social and educational management.

The act of naming and making sense of behaviors, experiences, or persons through psychiatric nomenclature such as ADHD is a moral goal-oriented discursive practice. Fighting for legal rights or for discharge from liability, explaining behaviors, performance and functioning, allocating, planning and implementing means of supports and treatments, involving parents in school, and cultivating sympathy, empathy and valued identities and agency are built on the idea of an ADHD as a neurobiological entity within an individual. This form of mobilizing and materializing the pragmatic approach to utilize the diagnostic entity is an example of the governance of identities through the psycho-medical discourse. It is revealing about the entangled ways that we are cultured to make meaning of human difference and diversity and the support structures in place that guide the institutional practices to react to the diversity of the support needs of people.

To conclude, diagnosis does not represent *having or being* ADHD but *becoming* and *performing* ADHD through deploying psycho-medical discourse provided in the DSM. The diagnostic label is a sociocultural means of making meaning of embodied, material, and social experiences that may conflict with social contexts, and a means of communicating about these experiences and reacting to them at societal, institutional, social, and individual levels. ADHD is better understood as a social category that eliminates human diversity and enforces the standard model of what an individual should be like and how to behave within the cultural boundaries of 'normalcy'.

References

American Psychiatric Association [APA] (2022). *Diagnostic and statistical manual of mental disorders*, 5th edn, Text Revision. Washington, DC: American Psychiatric Association.

Bailey, S. (2010). The DSM and the dangerous school child, Int. J. Incl. Educ., 14:6, 581-592. doi: 10.1080/13603110802527961

Bailey, S. (2014). Exploring ADHD: An ethnography of disorder in early childhood. London: Taylor & Francis.

Berger, N. P. (2015). The Creative Use of the ADHD Diagnosis in Probationers' Self-Narratives. Journal of Scandinavian Studies in Criminology and Crime Prevention 16:1, 122–139. doi:10.1080/14043858.2015.1024945.

Crowe, M. (2000). Constructing normality: a discourse analysis of the DSM-IV. *J. Psychiatr. Ment. Health Nurs.*, 7, 69–77. https://doi.org/10.1046/j.1365-2850.2000.00261.x

Danielson, M. L., Bitsko, R. H., Ghandour, R. M., Holbrook, J. R., Kogan, M. D., and Blumberg, S. J. (2018). Prevalence of Parent-Reported ADHD Diagnosis and Associated Treatment Among U.S. Children and Adolescents, 2016. Journal of Clinical Child & Adolescent Psychology. 47:2, 199-212, doi: 10.1080/15374416.2017.1417860

Dauman, N., Haza, M., and Erlandsson, S. I. (2019). Liberating Parents from Guilt: A Grounded Theory Study of Parents' Internet Communities for the Recognition of ADHD. International Journal of Qualitative Studies on Health and Well-Being. 14:1. doi: 10.1080/17482631.2018.1564520

Davies, J. (2013). *Cracked. The unhappy truth about psychiatry*. New York, NY: Pegasus Books.

DeRonda, A., Zhao, Y., Seymour, K. E., Mostofsky, S. H., and Rosch, K. S. (2021). Distinct patterns of impaired cognitive control among boys and girls with ADHD across development. *Res. Child Adolesc. Psychopathol.* 49, 835–848. doi: 10.1007/s10802-021-00792-2

Emerald, E., & Carpenter, L. (2010). ADHD, mothers, and the politics of school recognition. In L. J. Graham (Ed.), *(De)Constructing ADHD: Critical guidance for teachers and teacher educators* (pp. 99-118). New York: Peter Lang.

Fairclough, N. (2004). "Semiotic Aspects of Social Transformation and Learning", in *An introduction to critical discourse analysis in education,* ed. R. Rogers (Mahwah, NJ: Lawrence Erlbaum Associates), 225-236...

Freedman, J. E., and Honkasilta, J. (2017). Dictating the boundaries of Ab/normality: a critical discourse analysis of the diagnostic criteria for attention deficit hyperactivity disorder and hyperkinetic disorder. Disabil. Soc. 32, 565–588. doi: 10.1080/09687599.2017.1296819

Frigerio, A., and Montali, L. (2016). An Ethnographic-Discursive Approach to Parental Self-Help Groups: The Case of ADHD. Qualitative Health Research 26:7, 935–950, doi:10.1177/1049732315586553.

Frigerio, A., Montali, L., and Fine, M. (2013). Attention Deficit/Hyperactivity Disorder Blame Game: A Study on the Positioning of Professionals, Teachers and Parents. Health: An Interdisciplinary Journal for the Social Study of Health, Illness and Medicine. 17:6, 584–604. doi:10.1177/1363459312472083.

Gambrill, E. (2014). The diagnostic and statistical manual of mental disorders as a major form of dehumanization in the modern world. *Res. Soc. Work Pract.* 24, 13–36. doi: 10.1177/1049731513499411

Gee, J. P. (2000). Identity as an Analytic Lens for Research in Education. Review of Research in Education. 25:1, 99–125.

Hacking, I. (2006). Making Up People. *London Review of Books* 28 (16). https://www.lrb.co.uk/the-paper/v28/n16/ian-hacking/making-up-people

Hinshaw, S.P., and Scheffer, R.M. (2014). The ADHD Explosion: Myths, Medication, Money, and Today's Push for Performance. Oxford: Oxford University press.

Hjörne, E. & Säljö, R. (2004). "There is something about Julia": symptoms, categories, and the process of invoking attention deficit hyperactivity disorder in the Swedish school: a case study. J. Lang. Identity Educ., 3(1), 1–24. doi:10.1207/s15327701jlie0301_1

Hjörne, E. & Säljö, R. (2014a). Analyzing and preventing school failure: Exploring the role of multi-professionality in pupil health team meetings. Int J Educ Res, 63, 5–14.

Hjörne, E. & Säljö, R. (2014b). Defining student diversity: categorizing and processes of marginalization in Swedish schools. Emot Behav Diffic, 19(3), 251–265. doi: 10.1080/13632752.2014.883781

Honkasilta, J. (2016). Voices behind and beyond the label: The master narrative of ADHD (de)constructed by diagnosed children and their parents. Doctoral thesis, Jyväskylä Studies in Education, Psychology and Social Research 553. Jyväskylä: Jyväskylä University Printing House. Saatavilla

Honkasilta, J. and Koutsoklenis, A. (2022). The (un)real existence of ADHD—Criteria, functions, and forms of the diagnostic entity. *Front. Sociol.* 7:814763. doi: 10.3389/fsoc.2022.814763

Honkasilta, J. and Vehkakoski, T. (2017). Autenttisuutta Lääkitsemässä vai Lääkitsemällä? Adhd-lääkitykselle Annetut Merkitykset Nuorten Identiteettien Muokkaajana. (in Finnish) [Medicating Authenticity or Authenticity Through Medication? Meanings Given to ADHD Medication as a Means to Construct Identities of Young People]. Nuorisotutkimus. 35:4, 21-34.

Honkasilta, J., and Vehkakoski, T. (2019) The premise, promise and disillusion of the ADHD categorization – family narrative about the child's broken school trajectory. Emot Behav Diffic, 24:3, 273-286, DOI: 10.1080/13632752.2019.1609269

Honkasilta, J., Vehkakoski, T., and Vehmas, S. (2015). Power Struggle, Submission and Partnership: Agency Constructions of Mothers of Children with ADHD Diagnosis in their Narrated School Involvement. Scandinavian Journal of Educational Research. 59:6, 674-690. doi: 10.1080/00313831.2014.965794.

Honkasilta, J., Vehmas, S., and Vehkakoski, T. (2016). Self-Pathologizing, Self-condemning, Self-liberating: Youths' Accounts of their ADHD-Related Behavior. Social Science & Medicine. 150, 248–255. doi:10.1016/j.socscimed.2015.12.030.

Horwitz, A. V. (2021). DSM: A History of Psychiatry's Bible. Baltimore: Johns Hopkins University Press

Horwitz, A. V., and Wakefield, J. C. (2012). All We Have to Fear: Psychiatry's Transformation of Natural Anxieties into Mental Disorders. New York: Oxford University Press.

Jacobs, D. H., and Cohen, D. (2012). The end of neo-kraepelinism. Ethical Human Psychology and Psychiatry, 14, 2, 87-90. doi: 10.1891/1559-4343.14.2.87

Koutsoklenis, A., and Gaitanidis, A. (2017). Interrogating the Effectiveness of Educational Practices: A Critique of Evidence-Based Psychosocial Treatments for Children Diagnosed with Attention-Deficit/Hyperactivity Disorder. *Front. Educ.* 2:11. doi: 10.3389/feduc.2017.00011

Koutsoklenis, A. (2020). Functions of the ADHD Diagnosis in Educational Contexts. Metalogos. 36, 1-10.

Koutsoklenis, A., Honkasilta, J., and Brunila, K. (2020) Reviewing and Reframing the Influence of Relative Age on ADHD Diagnosis: Beyond Individual Psycho(patho)logy. Pedagogy, Culture & Society. 28:2, 165-181. doi: 10.1080/14681366.2019.1624599

Kirk, S. A., Cohen, D., and Gomory, T. (2015). "DSM-5: the delayed demise of descriptive diagnosis," in The DSM-5 in Perspective: Philosophical

Reflections of the Psychiatric Babel, eds S. Demazeux and P. Singy (London: Springer), 63–81. doi: 10.1007/978-94-017-9765-8_4

Kirk, S. A., Gomory, T., and Cohen, D. (2013). *Mad Science: Psychiatric Coercion, Diagnosis, and Drugs.* New Brunswick, NJ: Transaction.

Kirk, S. (2004). Are children's DSM diagnoses accurate? *Brief Treat Crisis Interv.* 4: 255-270. doi: 10.1093/brief-treatment/mhh022

Kofler, M. J., Irwin, L. N., Soto, E. F., Groves, N. B., Harmon, S. L., and Sarver, D. E. (2019). Executive functioning heterogeneity in pediatric ADHD. *J. Abnorm. Child Psychol.* 47, 273–286. doi: 10.1007/s10802-018-0438-2

Kohn, A. 1999. *Punished by Rewards. The Trouble with golden Stars, Incentive Plans, A's, Praise and Other Bribes*. Houghton Mifflin

Laws, C., and Davies, B. (2000). Poststructuralist Theory in Practice: Working with 'Behaviourally Disturbed' Children. International Journal of Qualitative Studies in Education. 13:3, 205–221.

Mills, C. (2014). *Decolonizing global mental health: The psychiatrization of the majority world.* London: Routledge. doi: 10.4324/9780203796757

Moore, C. B., McIntyre, N. H., and Lanivich, S. E (2021). ADHD- Related Neurodiversity and the Entrepreneurial Mindset. Entrepreneurship Theory and Practice. 45:1, 64–91. doi: 10. 1177/ 1042 2587 19890986

Ortega, F. (2009). The Cerebral Subject and the Challenge of Neurodiversity. Biosocieties. 4:4. doi: 10.1017/S1745855209990287.

Pérez-Álvarez, M. (2017). The Four Causes of ADHD: Aristotle in the Classroom. Front. Psychol. 8:928. doi: 10.3389/fpsyg.2017.00928

Reid, R. & Maag, J. (1997). Attention deficit hyperactivity disorder: over here, over there. Educ. Child Psychol, 14, 10–20.

Runswick-Cole, K. (2014). 'Us' and 'them': The Limits and Possibilities of a 'Politics of Neurodiversity' in Neoliberal Times. Disability & Society. 29. doi: 10.1080/09687599.2014.910107.

Sanders, S., Thomas, R., Glasziou, P., and Doust, J. (2019). A review of changes to the attention deficit/hyperactivity disorder age of onset criterion using the checklist for modifying disease definitions. *BMC Psychiatry* 19, 357. doi: 10.1186/s12888-019-2337-7

Schubert, S. J., Hansen, S. Dyer, K. R., and Rapley, M. (2009). 'ADHD Patient' or 'Illicit Drug User'? Managing Medico-Moral Membership Categories in Drug Dependence Services. Discourse & Society 20:4, 499–516. doi:10.1177/0957926509104025.

Sedgwick, J.A., Merwood, A., and Asherson, P. (2019). The Positive Aspects of Attention Deficit Hyperactivity Disorder: A Qualitative Investigation of Successful Adults with ADHD. ADHD Atten Def Hyp Disord. 11, 241–253 doi: https://doi.org/10.1007/s12402-018-0277-6

Shallaby, C. (2017). Troublemakers. Lessons in Freedom from Young Children at School. New York: The New Press.

Singh, I. (2011). A Disorder of Anger and Aggression: Children's Perspectives on Attention Deficit/Hyperactivity Disorder in the UK. Social Science & Medicine. 73:6, 889–896. doi:10.1016/j.socscimed.2011.03.049.

Sjöberg, M. N. (2019). Reconstructing truth, deconstructing ADHD: Badiou, onto-epistemological violence and the diagnosis of ADHD. *Critical Studies in Education* 62 (2): 243-257. doi: 10.1080/17508487.2019.1620818

Smith, M. (2014). *Hyperactive: the controversial history of ADHD*. Reaktion Books.

Solovieva, Y., and Rojas, L. Q. (2014). Syndromic analysis of ADHD at preschool age according to A.R. Luria concept. *Psychol. Neurosci.* 7, 443–452. doi:10.3922/j.psns.2014.4.03

Solovieva, Y., and Rojas, L. Q. (2015). Qualitative syndrome analysis by neuropsychological assessment in preschoolers with attention deficit disorder with hyperactivity. *Psychol. Russ.* 3, 112–123. doi:10.11621/pir.2015.0309

Tait, G. (2005). The ADHD Debate and the Philosophy of Truth. International Journal of Inclusive Education. 9:1, 17-38, doi: 10.1080/1360311042000299775

Tait, G. (2009). The logic of ADHD: a brief review of fallacious reasoning. Stud. Philo. Educ. 28, 239–254. doi: 10.1007/s11217-008-9114-2

Timimi, S. (2017). Non-diagnostic Based Approaches to Helping Children Who Could be Labelled ADHD and Their Families. *Int J Qual Stud Health Well-being*. 12:1298270. doi:10.1080/17482631.2017.1298270

Travell, C., and J. Visser. (2006). 'ADHD Does Bad Stuff to You': Young People's and Parents' Experiences and Perceptions of Attention Deficit Hyperactivity Disorder (ADHD). Emot Behav Diffic. 11:3, 205–216. doi:10.1080/13632750600833924.

van Dijk, T. A. (1996). "Discourse, Power, and Access" in Text and practices: Reading in critical discourse analysis, eds. R.C. Caldas-Coulthard and M. Coulthard (London: Routledge & Kegan Paul), 84-104.

Whitely, M., M. Raven, S. Timimi, J. Jureidini, J. Phillimore, J. Leo, J. Moncrieff, and P. Landman. 2018. "Attention Deficit Hyperactivity Disorder Late Birthdate Effect Common in Both High and Low Prescribing International Jurisdictions: A Systematic Review." *Journal of Child Psychology and Psychiatry* 60 (4): 380–391. doi:10.1111/jcpp.12991.

Wong, I. Y. T., Hawes, D. J., Clarke, S., Kohn, M. R., and Dar-Nimrod, I. (2018). Perceptions of ADHD Among Diagnosed Children and Their Parents: A Systematic Review Using the Common-Sense Model of Illness Representations. Clinical Child and Family Psychology Review. 21:1, 57–93. doi:10.1007/s10567-017-0245-2.

The Silencing of ADHD Critics

Gretchen LeFever Watson, David Antonuccio and David Healy

The German philosopher Arthur Schopenhauer is credited with having once said, "All truth passes through three stages. First, it is ridiculed. Second, it is violently opposed. Third, it is accepted as being self-evident." The truth about the over-diagnosis and over-treatment of ADHD may now be transitioning to Schopenhauer's third stage. But those who have tried to help us get to this stage have been regularly criticized, silenced, ridiculed, and attacked.

Orchestrated attacks on health researchers whose findings conflict with industry interests are not new or uncommon.[1] As detailed in the *New England Journal Medicine* (NEJM), there is a pattern of such attacks.[2] My own research came under attack for documenting high and rising rates of ADHD diagnosis and related drug use among American children. I was likely also attacked for presenting promising non-drug interventions. In an effort to shut down this work, I experienced every attack strategy outlined in the *NEJM*. Predictably, one of the attacks came in the form of an anonymous allegation of scientific misconduct.

Dr. Gretchen LeFever Watson is a developmental and clinical psychologist.

Updated and adapted from Watson G.L., Arcona A.P., Antonuccio D.O., Healy D., Shooting the Messenger: The Case of ADHD. *J Contemp Psychother.* 2014;44(1):43-52. doi: 10.1007/s10879-013-9244-x. PMID: 24532852; PMCID: PMC3918118.

My personal story is that in 2004 I had my research halted, my computers seized, and my staff prohibited from contacting me due to a malicious allegation of scientific misconduct. My story is a chilling account of how the public can be misled about health interventions that don't support the sale of drugs and I've documented that story in a number of places.

At the time that the improper allegation was filed against me, my research team had spent 10 years collecting data and developing alternatives to ADHD drugs in collaboration with local institutions, parents, and other concerned community members. Our successful community initiative, which was open to the public, had drawn attention across Virginia. Increasingly, our scientific evidence of ADHD overtreatment and effective non-drug interventions were gaining national and international attention, until the misconduct charge put an end to that work.

In my case, innovative research-to-action strategies with great potential for improving ADHD care across the U.S. and beyond were shut down. Today most parents and caregivers are not even aware that there are alternatives to a medical approach, and collecting information that our team gathered is not considered an option. In this chapter, rather than recounting those attacks on my work and me, I want to share some of our research findings, so as to add to the scientific record.

Typical of such research attacks, existing academic channels for handling it failed and contributed to a corruption of the scientific record.[3] Although I was eventually cleared of all wrongdoing,[4] the false allegation, coupled with press interference and over-reliance on views expressed by industry-biased key opinions leaders (KOLs), resulted in the suppression of information from my part of a multi-site, multi-million dollar study funded by the Centers for Disease

Control and Prevention (CDC)[5] and the total dismantling of a successful 10-year initiative that might otherwise have served as a national model for improving ADHD care.[6] Such actions played a role in the escalation and spread of excessive reliance on psychoactive drugs among ADHD-identified children and unnecessary iatrogenic harm—problems that continue unabated.

Documenting the ADHD epicenter

When I began documenting the prevalence and impact of ADHD in the early- to mid-1990s, the prevailing dogma was that no more than 3-5% of children suffered from ADHD, and that far fewer received a diagnosis or medical treatment for their condition. But my research findings painted a very different picture. Because the rigorous, robust, and externally valid nature of this body of work has been detailed elsewhere,[6] this chapter summarizes the work only to provide the context surrounding efforts to discredit and bury it.

Research I conducted while on the faculty at Eastern Virginia Medical School (EVMS) and its affiliated pediatric hospital (CHKD) indicated that by 2000, 14% of all elementary school students in southeastern Virginia had been diagnosed with ADHD. It also revealed that 33% of white boys in the region had been diagnosed with ADHD. Such figures went up with each grade. By middle school, for example, 38% of white boys had been ADHD-diagnosed.

All researchers who have studied the epidemiology of ADHD have consistently noted that white boys are most likely to be ADHD-diagnosed and ADHD-medicated. However, in my research, even among the demographic group least likely to be treated for ADHD (black girls), the rate of diagnosis was high (7%). In one city (Virginia Beach), children who were young relative to their grade placement were up to 23 times more likely than their classmates to be medicated for ADHD.

In every one of my studies, 84% to 90% of ADHD-diagnosed children had been medicated for the condition. Among ADHD-medicated children, up to 28% were simultaneously on two different types of psychiatric drugs (usually a stimulant and an antidepressant); 8% were simultaneously on three (often including an antipsychotic or sleep aid); and 1% were simultaneously on four different psychoactive drugs.[7, 8]

Despite such high rates of ADHD diagnosis and treatment, this body of research suggested that ADHD-diagnosed children had worse educational outcomes than their non-ADHD peers. Furthermore, ADHD-medicated children had even worse outcomes than ADHD-diagnosed children who had never been medicated.[8] At the time, virtually all these findings were in direct contrast to claims made by leading and highly esteemed ADHD authority figures—individuals whose careers and positions of authority had been built, often to a great extent, on the backs of money and support from the manufacturers of ADHD drugs.

Compared to all U.S. cities, the cities where my colleagues and I were conducting these epidemiologic investigations fell in the top one to five percent with respect to rates of ADHD-drug consumption.[9] Using stimulant distribution data provided to me from the Drug Enforcement Agency (DEA), I was able to document that a high rate of ADHD-related stimulant use was occurring in many other U.S. communities. The data suggested excessively high ADHD treatment patterns were emerging in 36 of the 50 states. According to the then Deputy Assistant Administrator for the DEA Office of Diversion Control, every state in the nation had at least one community with very high rates of ADHD-related stimulant consumption—a fact that was corroborated by other researchers who examined DEA data and an independent county-by-county investigation of per capita Ritalin distribution by the Cleveland Plain Dealer.[10, 11]

Around this time, the Editor of *Scientific Review of Mental Health Practice (SRMHP)* asked me if I would be willing to submit a paper justifying the position that ADHD was over-diagnosed, knowing a well-known ADHD subject matter expert would be submitting a paper taking the opposite view. I agreed.[1] *SRMHP* never published the opposing view. The article I published included the following summary statements in its abstract and conclusion:

The 700% increase in psychostimulant use that occurred in the 1990s justifies concern about potential over-diagnosis and inappropriate treatment of child behavior problems ... It is essential that mechanisms be established to track rates of child mental health diagnoses and psychotropic drug treatment and its outcomes among American children. Until we have a better understanding of these issues, it is appropriate to be judicious in our use of psychotropic medications and cautious about dismissal of concern about ADHD over-diagnosis.[7]

Such mechanisms have never been developed.

Unexpectedly, I had uncovered the most heavily psychiatrically drugged population of children in the U.S., and in the world. And while this problem first took hold around the use of stimulant drugs to treat ADHD in the southeastern region of Virginia (the ADHD epicenter), we observed signs indicating that it was spreading across the nation and mushrooming into a drug cocktail approach to addressing child mental health concerns. Virginia's regional epidemic predictably foreshadowed our nation's over-reliance on the medical model and the use of psychiatric drugs to address child mental health concerns. Today, per a 2022 report, it is not unprecedented for young people to be prescribed up to 10 psychiatric drugs.[12]

---

[1] Although my *SRMHP* article carries a 2003 publication date, it was not released until 2004.

A robust community response

When high rates of ADHD diagnosis and related drug treatment among children in southeastern Virginia were publicly reported, the community responded in healthy and novel ways. In partnership with diverse providers, policy makers, parents, and other community members, colleagues and I formed the School Health Initiative for Education (SHINE).[13]

Through regular meetings that were open to the public, the coalition facilitated and conducted parent, teacher, and provider surveys, focus groups, key informant interviews, and analysis of new and extant databases. Based on an extensive community needs assessment, the coalition identified four major gaps in ADHD care: (1) systematic behavior management, (2) school-provider communication, (3) teacher training and education, and (4) parent training and support.[9] I obtained local, state, and federal grant support to implement and evaluate the effectiveness of interventions for each of the community's self-identified gaps.

As detailed previously, this included (a) implementation of a school-wide positive discipline program, (b) a program to facilitate communication—with parent permission—between teachers and doctors, (c) a single-page checklist to remind or apprise parents, school personnel, and providers of the necessary steps to completing a comprehensive ADHD diagnostic assessment process, (d) a bill that was passed by the Virginia legislature that prohibited teachers from recommending ADHD medication to parents, (e) an annual legislative forum to ensure high-level awareness of the community's needs and progress, (f) many other community-based educational offerings and teacher training sessions, (g) and the spearheading of the first-ever public health psychology internship in the country.

Interestingly, parents in the region reported greater satisfaction with behavioral interventions than drug treatment, although their children were far more likely to receive drug treatment than other interventions.[14] To expand participation in parent training, I used local, state, and federal funding to develop and implement a unique approach to marketing parenting classes. The program experienced unprecedented levels of parent participation. It was so well received that five school districts in southeastern Virginia arranged for their psychologists to participate in a train-the-trainer program to ensure its availability in every elementary school across the region.

Our various community-oriented interventions appeared to be making a difference. Between 1998 and 2004, southeastern Virginia witnessed a significant (32%) decrease in the rate of ADHD diagnosis. This was remarkable, especially because ADHD diagnoses were on the rise in the rest of the country.[6]

The fallout

The rate of ADHD drug use has been on an almost continual rise ever since the American Pediatric Association sanctioned its use in 1960. In the years following the shutdown of my work, ADHD drug treatment soared.[15, 16] In 2013, C. Keith Conners, an eminent scholar who helped create the modern concept of ADHD and authored the most widely used ADHD rating scales, told an audience of other industry-funded key opinion leaders [KOLs], that rising ADHD rates reflected a "false epidemic" that had become "a national disaster of dangerous proportions."[17] ADHD drug promotion, however, did not stop. The latest CDC figures reveal yet another uptick, with the rate of ADHD diagnosis having increased by four percent from 2013-2015 to 2016-2018.[18] This relentless rise in ADHD drug treatment has occurred despite mounting and definitive evidence that long-term benefits of ADHD drug treatment conveys no benefits and leads to a *worsening of symptoms and/or deterioration in functioning*.[19-26] The ever-rising rates of ADHD also have contributed to ever-increasing rates of ADHD-related stimulant abuse, addiction, and deaths.[27]

Widespread use of ADHD drug treatment may have contributed to an outbreak of "pediatric bipolar disorder." Prior to the 1990s, virtually nobody believed bipolar disorder existed among children. Then, abruptly, between 1995 and 2003, pediatric bipolar diagnoses increased by 4,000%.[28] During this time, industry-funded clinicians had been "enlightening" clinicians and the public about this newly recognized disorder. Industry funding, and even small gifts from drug reps, invariably biases researchers expressed views[29]—a phenomenon potentially worsened when industry marketing specialists polish their presentation materials and delivery style. But what KOLs touted as symptoms of pediatric bipolar disorder were often side effects of ADHD stimulants.[29] Millions of children have now been bipolar-diagnosed and prescribed many untested drug combinations that often include powerful antipsychotic drugs.

Prescriptions for powerful antipsychotic drugs—drugs like risperidone/Risperdal and many other second-generation antipsychotics that historically had been reserved for treatment of adults with schizophrenia and other psychotic disorders—increased eight-fold among children between the years 1993 and 2009.[30] Between 2005 and 2007, the state of Florida witnessed a 250% increase in the prescription of antipsychotic drugs for children.[31] This included 1,100 Medicaid children as young as 3 years of age.

Many such prescriptions were specifically for children carrying a diagnosis of ADHD;[32] others are likely prescribed for iatrogenic effects of ADHD drug treatment.[33] Data collected between 2005 and 2009 reveal that, of all children's physician office visits, almost 2% resulted in the prescription of an antipsychotic drug. The rate was almost 4% for adolescents and skyrocketed to 30% when the visit involved a psychiatrist.[30] In 2022, researchers reported a high rate of adverse events among children treated with antipsychotic drugs. Most of the events were "serious." Close to half (42%) were for ADHD or related problems of "disruptive, impulse-control, and conduct problems." More than 25% occurred in children who were treated specifically for ADHD. Another 14% occurred in children treated for bipolar disorders.[34]

To wit, emergency departments in southeastern Virginia cannot manage the number of children and teens being admitted for serious psychiatric symptoms—a problem that emerged prior to the COVID pandemic, beginning around 2010, according to the director of mental health at CHKD.[35] In response, CHKD—the pediatric hospital serving the ADHD epicenter that foreshadowed the national explosion of psychiatric care and its fallout—has responded by building a $224M pediatric psychiatric hospital and hiring many more child psychiatrists. Spending hundreds of millions of dollars to increase the amount of psychiatric "treatment" available in southeastern Virginia is a questionable strategy because excessive psychiatric "treatment" likely contributed to the deterioration of child mental health in the region (and the nation).[36, 37] In any event, such developments reaffirm the need for communities to demand mechanisms for tracking and reporting on psychiatric diagnoses and psychoactive prescriptions, especially among their pediatric populations.

Countless numbers of ADHD-diagnosed and bipolar-diagnosed children who have exhibited drug-induced problems have been "treated" by switching up and piling on psychiatric drugs. Prescriptions for antidepressants, which are often added to psychostimulant treatment regimens for children with ADHD, increased over 400% in a recent time period.[38] By 2000, children in many parts of the U.S. were being treated with more than one psychotropic drug at a time.[39, 40] A 2022 news story about a teenage girl that had been prescribed 10 psychiatric drugs now represents a national trend rather than an anomaly:

> A study published in 2020 in the journal *Pediatrics* found that 40.7 percent of people ages 2 to 24 who were prescribed a drug for attention deficit hyperactivity disorder [ADHD] were also prescribed at least one other medication for depression, anxiety, or another mood or behavioral disorder. The study found more than 50 different psychotropic medicines prescribed in such combinations, and a review by The New York Times found that roughly half of the drugs were not approved for use in adolescents, although doctors have discretion to prescribe as they see fit.[12]

Consistent with the *NYT's* apparent tentative and emerging openness toward including perspectives of researchers whose views are contrary to those of KOLs,[41] the article quoted Lisa Cosgrove, a clinical psychologist who co-authored a book detailing the "institutional corruption" driving modern psychiatry practices[42] as saying, "You can very cogently argue that we don't have evidence about what it means to be on multiple psychotropic medications. This is a generation of guinea pigs."

The fact that children in foster care have been the recipients of liberal and lax use of powerful psychoactive drugs and drug combinations drew the attention of public health officials and legislators. According to the *NYT*, "Legislative reforms were passed to curb the practice in those settings, but it has since widened to include affluent and middle-class families."[12] The more a drug is prescribed, the more it is available for diversion and abuse—a problem that has been well documented with respect to ADHD stimulants on high school and college campuses.[27, 43]

An ongoing challenge is sorting out scientific fact from marketing "spin." It is well documented that drug industry marketing strategies include "paying consultants [KOLs] to speak at scientific meetings in which it is possible to circumvent FDA guidelines that require disclosure of side effects" and "offering pre-packaged information for journalists in the form of video and news releases that give the appearance of having been independently developed."[45]

Unfortunately, history has shown that neither penalties levied by the U.S. Department of Justice (DOJ) on companies that have engaged in misbranding and false advertising of psychiatric drugs nor clinical practice guidelines have stemmed the tide of America's ever-expanding use of psychiatric drugs to treat ADHD or other DSM diagnoses. Dr. Carl Elliott, professor in the Center for Bioethics and the Department of Pediatrics at the University of Minnesota, studies medical research scandals. He has learned that most such scandals have little negative consequence to their perpetrators unless the press catches wind of them. In fact, one of the most unusual outcomes is for the wrongdoers to be punished, which has been the track record for KOLs involved in misbranding scandals. According to Elliott:

> *When social scientists ask witnesses to corruption or safety violations why they remained silent, they usually get one of two answers. First, many people are afraid that blowing the whistle will be futile; second, they're afraid of retribution. With medical research scandals, unfortunately, both of those fears appear well-founded ... Many researchers who mistreat human subjects escape unscathed, while the whistle-blowers who spoke out against them are vilified.*[3]

Elliott's objective observations are in sync with my personal experience, as well as the case of Dr. Nadie Lamber, a UC Berkley researcher who was falsely accused of scientific misconduct after reporting evidence that the use of ADHD stimulant drugs in childhood increased the likelihood of later tobacco and cocaine use.[46] My "wrongdoing" (undoing) was "having the courage to be among the first to sound the alarm about high and escalating rates of ADHD drug use."[4] I will continue to sound the alarm and I hope that others will be brave enough to do likewise.

Summary and conclusion

Industry-funded ADHD thought leaders, also known as key opinion leaders (KOLs) have contributed to the corruption of the scientific record. Their biased views have been over-represented in the media and leveraged to shut down unwelcome scientific findings. Such actions have interfered with evidence-based medicine and accurately informed clinical practice, and they have needlessly exposed millions of children to ADHD diagnoses and addictive and psychoactive drugs. Widespread use of ADHD drug treatment has contributed to epidemic-level ADHD drug abuse and addiction among American teens and young adults. Neither pending federal prosecutions nor new ADHD guidelines are likely to curb this problem.

At a minimum, improvement will require that citizens demand mechanisms be established to enable routine tracking and public reporting on psychiatric diagnoses and psychoactive drug prescriptions among pediatric populations, especially in communities with pediatric psychiatric hospitals. Allegations of scientific/research misconduct should be investigated by institutionally unaffiliated scientists who are free of conflicts of interest. Media outlets should demand and enable their journalists do a better job vetting views expressed by KOLs and routinely include countervailing voices from scientists free of inherent conflicts of interest.

Journalists must not shy away from reporting on research scandals; however, they must take precautions not to interfere with ongoing investigations. Until the weak firewalls between industry and academia are strengthened,[44] doctors and allied healthcare providers, schoolteachers, and others responsible for protecting children suffering from mental and emotional distress ought to consider limiting their participation in educational programs sponsored by drug companies or delivered by KOLs and their associates while also maintaining a healthy skepticism about their claims and clinical recommendations regardless of how scientific or reasonable they may sound.

References

1. Healy D. Conflicting interests in Toronto: anatomy of a controversy at the interface of academia and industry. *Perspect Biol Med.* 2002;45(2):250-263.

2. Deyo R, Psaty B, Simon G, Wagner E, Omenn G. The messenger under attack -- intimidation of researchers by special interest groups. *New England Journal of Medicine`*. 1997;336:1176-1180.

3. Elliott C. The Anatomy of Research Scandals. *Hastings Cent Rep.* 2017;47(3):inside back cover-inside back cover.

4. Lenzer J. Research cleared of misconduct charges. *The British Medical Journal.* 2005b;331: 865.2.

5. Lenzer J. Research to be sacked after reporting high rates of ADHD. *Br Med J.* 2005a;330:691.1.

6. Watson GL, Arcona AP, Antonuccio DO, Healy D. Shooting the Messenger: The Case of ADHD. *Journal of Contemporary Psychotherapy*. 2014;44(1):43-52.

7. LeFever G, Arcona A, Antonuccio D. ADHD among American schoolchildren: evidence of overdiagnosis and overuse of medication. *Scientific Review of Mental Health Practice*. 2003;2(1):49-60.

8. LeFever G, Villers M, Morrow A, Vaughn E. Parental perceptions of adverse educational outcomes among children diagnosed with ADHD: A call for improved school/provider collaboration. *Psychol Sch*. 2002;39(1):63-71.

9. LeFever G, Parker J, Morrow A, Villers M. Understanding ADHD issues in a community with a high ADHD prevalence rate: parent, teacher, and provider prespectives. 128th Annual Meeting of the American Public Health Association; November 15, 2000, 2000; Boston, MA.

10. Eaton S, Marchak E. Ritalin prescribed unevenly in US. *Cleveland Plain Dealer*. 2001:1.

11. Morrow R, Morrow, AL, and Haslip, AL. Methylphenidate in the United States, 1990 through1995. *American Journal of Public Health* (Research Letter). 1998;88:1121.

12. Richtel M. This teen was prescribed 10 psychiatric drugs. She's not alone. *The New York Times*. August 27, 2022.

13. LeFever G, Butterfoss F, N V. High prevalence of attention deficit hyperactivity disorder: catalyst for development of a school health coalition. *Fam Community Health*. 1999;22(1):38–49.

14. LeFever G. Overcoming the ADHD research to practice gap. Virginia Academy of Special Education; 2008; Regent University.

15. Centers for Disease Control and Prevention. Increasing prevalance of parent-reported attention-deficit/hyperactivity disorder among children -- United States, 2003 and 2007. *Morbidity and Mortality Weekly*. 2010;59(44):1439-1443.

16. Centers for Disease Control and Prevention. Mental health surveillance among children: United States, 2005-2011. *Morbidilty and Mortality Weekly* Report. 2013;62(02):1-35.

17. Schwarz A. The selling of attention deficit disorder. *The New York Times*. December 14, 2013.

18. Centers for Disease Control and Prevention. *Data and Statistics About ADHD.* National Center on Birth Defects and Developmental Disabilities;2022.

19. Currie J, Stabile M, Jones L. Do stimulant mediations improve educational and behavioral outcomes for children with ADHD? In: Research NBoE, ed. Vol Working paper No. 19105. Cambridge, MA: NBER Publications; 2013.

20. Molina B, Flory K, Hinshaw S, et al. Delinquent behavior and emerging substance use in the MTA at 36 months: prevalence, course, and treatment effects. *J Am Acad Child Adolesc Psychiatry.* 2007;46(8):1028-1040.

21. Molina B, Hinshaw S, Swanson JM, et al. The MTA at 8 years: prospective follow-up of children treated for combined-type ADHD in a multisite study. *J Am Acad Child Adolesc Psychiatry.* 2009;48(5):484-500.

22. Pelham W. The NIMH multimodal treatment study for attention-deficit/ hyperactivity disorder: Just say yes to drugs alone? *Canadian Journal of Psychiatry.* 1999;44:765-775.

23. Pelham W, Fabiano G. Evidence-based psychosocial treatments for attention-deficit/hyperactivity disorder. *J Clin Child Psychol.* 2008;37(1):184214.

24. Pelham WE, Wheeler T, Chronis A. Empirically supported psychological treatments for attention deficit hyperactivity disorder. *J Clin Child Psychol.* 1998`;27(2):190-205.

25. Jensen P, Arnold L, Swanson J, et al. 3-year follow-up of the NIMH MTA study. *J Am Acad Child Adolesc Psychiatry.* 2007;46(8):989-1002.

26. Molina B, Flory K, Hinshaw S, et al. Delinquent behavior and emerging substance use in the MTA at 36 months: prevalence, course, and treatment effects. *J Am Acad Child Adolesc Psychiatry.* 2007;46(8):1028-1040.

27. Watson GL, Arcoan AP, Antonuccio DO. The ADHD drug abuse crisis on American college campuses. *Ethical Hum Psychol Psychiatry.* 2015;17(1):5-21.

28. Moreno C, Laje G, Blanco C, Jiang H, Schmidt AB, Olfson M. National Trends in the Outpatient Diagnosis and Treatment of Bipolar Disorder in Youth. *Arch Gen Psychiatry*. 2007;64(9):1032-1039.

29. Olfman SE. *Bipolar Children: Cutting-Edge Controversy, Insights, and Rsearch Westport*, CT: Praeger Publishers; 2007.

30. Olfson M, Blanco C, Liu S-M, Wang S, Correll CU. National Trends in the Office-Based Treatment of Children, Adolescents, and Adults With Antipsychotics. *Arch Gen Psychiatry*. 2012;69(12):1247-1256.

31. Farley R. The "atypical" dilemma: skyrocketing numbers of kids are prescribed powerful antipsychotic drugs. 2007. http://www.sptimes.com/2007/07/29/news_pf/Worldandnation/The__atypical__dilemm.shtml.

32. Matone M, Localio R, Huang Y, DdosReis S, Feudtner C, Rubin D, Pilar. The relationship between mental health diagnosis and treatment with second-generation antipsychotics over time: a national study of U.S. Medicaid-enrolled children. *Health Serv Res*. 2012;47(5):1836-1860.

33. Whitaker R. *Anatomy of an Epidemic: Magic Bullets, Psychiatric Drugs, and the Astonishing Rise of Mental Illness in America*. New York: Random House; 2010.

34. Rafaniello C, Sullo MG, Carnovale C, et al. We really need clear guidelines and recommendations for safer and proper use of aripiprazole and risperidone in a pediatric population: real-world analysis of EudraVigilance database. *Frontiers in Psychiatry*. 2020;2(December).

35. Old Dominion University. The Kids Are Not All Right: Youth Mental Health In Hampton Roads. The State of the Region: *Hampton Roads 2020*. 2020. https://digitalcommons.odu.edu/cgi/viewcontent.cgi?article=1178&context=sor_reports.

36. The Virginian-Pilot & Daily Press Editorial Board. Improving kids' mental health. *The Virginian-Pilot*. January 17, 2022;Editorial.

37. Murphy V. Protecting Youth Mental Health: The U.S. Surgeon General's Advisory. In. Rockville, MD: U.S. Department of Health and Human Services; 2021.

38. Pratt L, Brody DJ, Gu Q. *Antidepressant use in persons aged 12 and over: United States,* 2005-2008. Hyattsville, MD: National Center for Health Statistics;2011.

39. Mojtabai R, Olfson M. National Trends in Psychotropic Medication Polypharmacy in Office-Based Psychiatry. *Arch Gen Psychiatry*. 2010;67(1):26-36.

40. Zonfrillo M, Penn J, Leonard H. Pediatric psychotropic polypharmacy. *Psychiatry*. 2005;2(8):14-19.

41. Leo J, Lacasse JR. The New York Times and the ADHD Epidemic. *Society*. 2015;52(1):3-8.

42. Whitaker R, Cosgrove L. *Psychiatry Under the Influence: Institutional Corruption, Social Injury, and Prescriptions for Reform*. New York: Palgrave MacMillan; 2015.

43. Watson G, Arcona A. 8 ways to respond to student ADHD drug abuse. In. *Campus Safety*. Vol April/May2014:34-37.

44. Antonuccio D, Danton W, McLanahan T. Building a firewall between marketing and science. *Am Psychol*. 2003;58(12):1028-1043.

For Professionals and For Parents

Eric Maisel

We've come to the end of this book. So, how are we to think about this thing called ADHD?

Surely it is impossible to buy the vision promulgated by the mental disorder establishment. Lumping some behaviors together, providing a pseudo-medical-sounding label for the lump you created, and then throwing addictive chemicals at your creation, is both absurd and an abomination. The mental disorder establishment should be ashamed of itself—but of course, it is hard to find time for shame when you are busy counting your profits.

The trouble with trying to make sense of ADHD or any other so-called mental disorder is that there are too many things to consider when it comes to "what's going on." What in fact is going on? Well, a given child's fundamental temperament and personality. The demands of his intelligence. The nervousness of his mother and the anger of his father. The boring nature of school. His vivid imagination. A relentless, pulsating energy—his chi, his life force. His trickster nature. His desire to act out, make a scene, get noticed. His difficulties with a given subject. His ease with a given subject. His rebellious nature. That his friends are restless, too. That it is hot, that it is almost summer, that it is three in the afternoon and that no human child should still be sitting at his desk. That the history of

---

Eric Maisel is a retired family therapist, and active creativity coach, based in California, USA.

California missions is a thousand times less interesting than a video game. That …

We understand the extent to which both parents and mental health professionals are pressured to buy the mental disorder view. Both are bombarded by the mainstream view, promoted by pharmaceutical companies, academic researchers, other mental health professionals, professional organizations, a naïve or indifferent media, and their own friends and family members, that "mental disorders" exist in the same way that "physical disorders" exist. Likewise, they are told that if their child is afflicted with one of these "mental disorders," the only real help available are chemicals and, in a secondary way, tactics from the world of behavior modification and/or the "expert talk" called psychotherapy.

Advocates of a critical psychology approach suggest that there are other ways to conceptualize what's going on and other helpful approaches to take. If you are a professional helper, you can present various alternative views to your clients. That isn't to say, however, that your client, whether parent or child, will be pleased with what you're suggesting. Some parents may be very happy that, for example, their "disruptive" child has "finally" received a mental disorder diagnosis—that they now "know what's going on"—and they may likewise be very happy that "doctors are now doing something for my child."

They may swear by the chemicals that their child is being given, grateful for the short-term ameliorating effects, and not overly concerned about any lasting side effects or about opening up pathways to addiction. Your client may be one of these and may strongly oppose any other point of view and reject the information you're providing. So, not only am I asking a lot of you, the progressive helper, that you actively paint a picture of alternatives to the current paradigm—your client may be anything but grateful when you do so.

Nevertheless, I think that it is our job and our duty to invite the parents we work with to think about their child's distress from a "critical" point of view. Does this amount to a certain sort of activism? Yes, it does. Is this you being rather directive? Yes, it is. Is this you functioning in part as a teacher? Yes, indeed. Might you have to tell clients some hard truths about their part in the problem? Yes, you might. Does this require that you craft talking points about the current faulty diagnostic system and about the use and abuse of psychiatric medication? Yes, it does. But if you would like to help your clients who are also parents, I hope that you'll agree that all of this is required of you. Parents are under siege—and you are in a position to help them.

Here is what I would like to see:

1. I would want the very ideas of "mental disorder" and "mental disease" widely critiqued and deconstructed. I would want a new picture painted of distress occurring as a result of being human and because of problems in living and not because of mental viruses, chemical imbalances, ghostly genetics, or faulty plumbing. We would drop the game of "diagnosing" and "treating" and ask ourselves, "What makes human beings human and what can we do to help people who are suffering?"

2. We might likewise change our thinking from considering so-called psychiatric medication "medications used to treat mental illness" to the more accurate view that they are powerful, often addictive chemicals that may or may not produce some desired effect. I would want far fewer human beings on these chemicals, especially far fewer children.

3. I would want all that we do not know much more honored, so that we can finally really get at, insofar as it is possible to do so,

cause-and-effect in human matters and a better sense of what actually helps. There would also need to be a way of speaking about "all that we don't know" that prevents the mental disorder establishment from retorting, "Look, you say that you don't know and we say that we do know, so we win!" One of the challenges in moving forward is finding language that allows us to announce that there is a lot that we do not know without allowing that "not knowing" to become a decisive factor is dismissing us and any reform initiatives that we might propose.

4. I would want us to carefully avoid a proliferation of new manuals, catalogues, lists, menus, and other systems that might be thought to be better than the DSM method but that do not do the real (and hard and maybe impossible) work required of some truly better manual. For example, some new "manual of concerns" would prove no improvement, since the same faulty transaction as presently occurs would continue to occur. You come in and say that you are sad, I look up your concern in my manual of concerns, I find it, and I agree, "You are concerned that you are sad." This isn't much of an improved transaction over the current one.

5. I would want us to think through how institutions that currently exist might be improved and how different institutions—for example, therapeutic communities of care—might be supported. The current institutional approach has mainly to do with society's need to warehouse dangerous and difficult people and keep society safe from and segregated from folks who, for example, are hearing voices or threatening to kill themselves. In the current model, the number one goal is not "treatment" but "difficult person management." Naturally, we would expect coercive methods to flourish in institutions with this mandate, just as we would expect them to flourish in prisons, and that is exactly what we see.

6. We desperately need a clear picture of what actually helps. In fact, we already know many things that help. We know that the warmth and humanness of the mental health service provider helps. There is tremendous evidence on that score. The warmer and more human the provider, the better the outcome. Doesn't it also seem likely that teaching helps, that skill-building helps, that providing useful homework helps, that holding a sufferer accountable for taking action helps, that inquiring into what's going on helps, that providing basic information helps, that pointing the way to resources and making referrals help, that creating a spirit of cooperation and collaboration helps, that the provider being calm and caring helps, and so on? Don't we need a smart, sensible "guide to helping strategies and when to use them"? Are there, for instance, better times to listen, better times to inquire, better times to interrupt, better times to instruct, better times to comfort, better times to confront? Wouldn't such a guide, whatever its flaws and shortfalls, go a long way toward arming helpers with an arsenal of genuinely helpful helping strategies?

7. We need to stop using words like "normal" and "abnormal." We need to distinguish between medications and chemicals. We need to look carefully at the empty, meaningless definitions of "mental disorder" promulgated by the various DSMs, definitions that have changed radically from one edition to the next according to taste and whim and for pocketbook reasons. We need to stop claiming that "mental disorders" are "biopsychosocial" in nature, as if by saying that we are saying anything true or useful. We need more honesty and better thinking than that.

8. We need top thinkers, who perhaps currently rightly shy away from the world of mental health as a too muddy, too soft, and too difficult a place in which to do real science, to inquire of themselves, "Yes, that would prove a truly difficult place to be.

But isn't having a say about the future of the emotional health of our species more important than participating in the creation of a new phone?" We need strong, smart people who know a thing or two about being human to help foment and manage a revolution away from the current pseudo-medical approach to mental health. We need strong, smart people to begin to really help the billions of people who experience emotional distress and who might love to have some real help offered to them.

9. We could, even in the absence of any agreement about what we meant by "mental health," affirm that certain life skills are good things and begin to teach them in our schools in addition to and side-by-side academic subjects. We could teach our children how to align their thoughts and their behaviors with their intentions, how to retain their individuality in a group setting, how to self-regulate and tolerate ambiguity and difference, how to seize meaning opportunities and make meaning investments, and so on. All of this could be taught.

10. For children and for adults both, we could provide stress reduction techniques, anxiety management techniques, recovery techniques, and other helpful techniques as part of a nationwide and worldwide effort at preventative health care, since everyone knows that ineffectively handling stress, anxiety, addictive impulses, and other common human challenges lead inexorably to medical problems that come with substantial costs and that are bound to tax our health care systems.

11. We could launch all sorts of initiatives and public service advertising campaigns that in simple language and through clear messages underline the challenges that human beings face and made suggestions as to how to handle those challenges. Spectacularly simple messages could begin to appear on the

sides of buses and in between television shows, just as powerful anti-smoking messages have previously appeared. These campaigns might announce that being human comes with predictable, painful challenges and that help is available. As a small relief from the constant barrage of pharmaceutical ads, maybe an occasional public service announcement of this sort might appear.

12. We could educate our children about the demanding nature of life and the likelihood that they will experience difficulties. At the same time, we could teach them humanistic values, encourage them not to let their personality become their destiny, and paint a clear, simple picture of value-based meaning-making. These life lessons could be taught in schools; but, since that is rather unlikely to ever happen, teachers could at least point students to cyberspace resources and embrace cyber-education as a great adjunctive tool to brick-and-mortar rote education.

We need a fundamental shift—nowadays typically called a "paradigm shift"—in our basic orientation, one away from the ideas of "mental disorder" and "mental disease" and toward a more rounded, sophisticated and truer vision of what it means to be human: how living naturally produces distress, how our formed personality locks in that distress, and what helps to relieve that distress. We likewise need a new professional to help with human problems, someone who knows more than pharmacology, who doesn't see himself as an expert with a "talking cure," and who knows an awful lot about being human and about negotiating life's challenges.

We need all these changes. We especially need them because our children are under siege. It is one thing for an adult to accept that his despair is a "mental disorder" that can be "treated" with a chemical. He is an adult, after all, and entitled to make that choice. It is another thing for a seven-year-old to find himself on three or four psychiatric chemicals for his "ADHD." There are many reasons why we require a mental health revolution but let's underline just one of these many: to spare our children from the labels and chemicals that the mental disorder establishment is blithely and perniciously offering.

A 14-Point Checklist for Parents

If your child is experiencing difficulties or causing difficulties, here are a few questions to ask yourself, your child, the people in your circle, and, once they enter the picture, mental health service providers. These aren't the only questions you might consider—I hope you'll add your own questions to this list. But these are some of the more important questions and each is worth pondering.

1. *Is there a problem?*

Let's say that your child is exhibiting some sort of behavior or having certain thoughts or feelings. First of all, is it a problem? Is it a problem that your child waits two months longer to speak than did Jane across the street? Why is that a problem as opposed to a natural difference? Is it a problem that he enthusiastically signs up for violin lessons and then wants to stop them after two weeks? Why is that a problem as opposed to a simple change of heart? Is it a problem that he doesn't want to sit at the dinner table where you and your mate are fighting? Why is that a problem as opposed to good common sense? You can label any of these a problem—a developmental delay, a lack of discipline, a refusal to obey—but where is the love, charity, or logic in that?

2. *Has my child always been like this?*

If your child has always been shy, why is it suddenly surprising that he or she is still shy? If your child has always been bursting with energy and bouncing off the walls, why is it suddenly surprising that he or she is still full of energy and still bouncing off the walls? If your child has always been the quiet, brooding one, why is it suddenly surprising that he or she is still quiet and brooding? These may be features of your child's natural endowment and original personality or these may be features of his or her formed personality acquired so early on that they are quite baked in now. Either way, there is no reason to treat your child's unique ways of being as suddenly surprising. His or her ways of being may create difficulties and those difficulties certainly must be addressed; but that isn't to say that your child suddenly "came down" with shyness, restlessness or brooding tendencies. Nor are there any good or fair reasons to treat those qualities or behaviors as markers of a "mental disorder."

3. *Have there been any big (or small) changes recently?*

If a child's circumstances change, he or she is likely to react to those changes. Is your child in a new school? Doing new, harder schoolwork? In a class with older children? Dealing with your separation or divorce? Living in a new town? Dealing with a new sibling? Did he or she move from a single room to a shared room? Have there been any changes in his diet or in his exercise patterns? Maybe there's been more junk food intake than usual or less exercise during a long winter? Changes in circumstances really do matter and you should think through if there have been any changes in your child's circumstances or your family's circumstances that may be contributing to or causing your child's current distress or difficulties.

4. *Is your child under stress?*

You might not think that your child having a prominent part in the school play might prove a source of serious stress for him or her. But it might. The same might hold true for an upcoming piano recital, spelling bee, or other public event or competition. Is your child taking a harder math class than last year or a history or language class that requires massive memorization? Challenges of this sort and many of the other challenges of childhood and the school years produce stress and that stress is likely to play itself out as distress and difficulty. Consider the link between stress and distress in your child's life.

5. *Has your child been abused or traumatized?*

Trauma and abuse produce distress. If your child comes home from summer camp and seems not to be his or her usual self, wouldn't it make sense to check in with your child to see if something abusive or traumatic occurred at camp? Has there been a death in the family, the death of one of your child's friends, or the death of a pet? Is your family life so chaotic as to rise to level of trauma? Has a difficult, aging parent recently moved into your home? Might there be issues of abuse or trauma that your child is trying to deal with (and maybe keep secret about)?

6. *Who has the problem?*

If your mate belittles your child and your child grows sad and withdrawn, your child certainly has a problem. But isn't your mate the real problem? If you are highly anxious and vigilant and your child becomes highly anxious and vigilant, your child certainly has a problem. But what's your part in the equation? If yours is a rigid and dogmatic household and your child rebels against your house rules, your child certainly has a problem. But isn't the family rigidity its own sort of problem? The question isn't about assigning blame or making anyone feel guilty. Rather it's a matter of appraising the situation honestly, so that genuine answers can be found.

7. *What does your child say?*

Have you asked your child what's going on? Asking is very different from accusing or interrogating. Have you had a quiet, compassionate, heart-to-heart conversation with your child in which you express your worry, announce your love, listen to your child's concerns, and collaborate with him on creating some strategies and tactics that might help your child deal with the problems he is experiencing? Are you in the habit of checking in with your child to understand what he or she is thinking and feeling? If you haven't gotten into that habit, wouldn't that be a great habit to cultivate?

8. *What do other people say?*

Have you checked in with the people in your circle: your mate, your other children, your parents, and anyone else who knows your child well? What are their thoughts about what's going on? They may have nothing useful or productive to offer or they may have some very important insights into what's happening. Ask the people who know your child well what they think. Make a special effort to check in with those people who seem the most levelheaded and whose opinions you respect the most.

9. *Do you feel kindly toward your child?*

Human beings do not automatically love other human beings. Nor is love a stable, impregnable sort of thing. You may have lost patience with your child, feel oppressed by him or her, or in some other way have lost that loving feeling. Do you soften in his or her presence and want to hug your child or do you harden in his or her presence and start scolding? What child wouldn't grow sadder or angrier if he or she felt that what he or she got from a parent wasn't love but criticism or even revulsion? Think whether a softening and a more loving attitude might amount to great medicine.

10. Are you quick to accept labels for yourself?

How do you describe your own difficulties to yourself and to others? Do you say things like, "Oh, I have ADD and Bobby does too," "Depression runs in our family," or "We can't seem to get Sally's anxiety meds right—but I have the same problem myself"? If this is the way you speak and the way you conceptualize your difficulties and the difficulties of others, I would suggest that you educate yourself about alternate visions that reject the idea that because you have a certain experience, say of anxiety, you have a "mental disorder" and must take "medication" for that so-called mental disorder. I would ask you to be a little less quick to accept such labels for yourself or for your children and do your "due diligence" in researching alternatives to the current ubiquitous mental disorder labelling paradigm.

11. Has your child had a full medical workup recently?

What if your child's school difficulties have to do with poor eyesight or poor hearing? What if his or her lethargy, pain complaints, or sleeplessness are symptoms of a medical condition? Make sure that you rule out genuine organic and biological causes for the "symptoms" that your child is displaying before supposing that they are "symptoms" of a "mental disorder." Of course, the root causes of human behaviors are not so easily traced back to medical conditions even when such conditions exist. Nevertheless, make sure that a medical workup is part of your plan to help your child with his or her current distress or difficulties.

12. What sort of help are you looking for?

You may decide that you alone can't do enough to help your child reduce his or her experience of distress. Where should you turn for help? It amounts to a very different decision to take your child to a child psychologist whose specialty is talk and who uses techniques like play therapy or to a psychiatrist who routinely "diagnoses mental disorders" and who then "prescribes medication." There are many types of helpers out there, from peer counselor to school counselor to mentor to dietician to family therapist to residential treatment specialist to clinical psychologist to psychiatrist, and each comes at human challenges from a different angle. Educate yourself as to what these different service providers actually provide and decide which sort of service makes the most sense to you.

13. *A question to ask a mental health service provider: what is your rationale for labeling my child with a mental disorder and prescribing chemicals?*

If a mental health professional would like to give your child a mental disorder label, for instance the label ADHD, inquire as to his or her rationale for doing so. Ask questions like, "By 'mental disorder' do you mean 'medical issue'? If you do not mean 'medical issue,' why do you want to prescribe medicine to my child? If you do mean 'medical issue,' please explain to me what the medical issue is and what the evidence for it is." And, of course, there are many more questions than these that you would want to ask before deciding to believe that the idea of "diagnosing and treating mental disorders" makes sense to you.

14. *Is my child actually getting better?*

Say that your child is placed on so-called psychiatric medication and his or her situation worsens. You will then be faced with the following very difficult questions. Is your child's condition actually worsening and is the so-called medication proving ineffective (and therefore perhaps ought to be changed or increased, which is likely what your child's psychiatrist will recommend)? Or is it the case that the so-called medication is actually causing the worsening (there is ample evidence that this can happen, as you've read about in this book)? If your child's situation doesn't improve, you are caught in the predicament of trying to figure out what's going on with your child and also caught needing to appraise the effectiveness or the dangerousness of the help being offered your child.

The above fourteen questions are a sizeable number of questions and, if you tackle them, may involve you in some painful self-reflection and a lot of investigating. But endeavoring to answer them will help you better understand what's really going on with your child and what will genuinely help her deal with her distress or difficulties. My fingers are crossed that you will make that effort.

Whether you're a researcher, academic, service provider, parent, or interested layperson, I hope that this volume has added to your understanding of the thing called ADHD. And remember: there's more great information in other volumes of the Ethics International Press Critical Psychology and Critical Psychology Series. I recommend those volumes to you.

About the Contributors

Thomas Armstrong

Thomas Armstrong, Ph.D. is an educator, psychologist, and the author of 19 books in learning and human development, including *The Myth of the ADHD Child, The Power of Neurodiversity, and 7 Kinds of Smart*. His first novel entitled *Childless*, about a plot to remove childhood from the human genome, was published in September, 2022.

Ben Bernstein

Ben Bernstein, Ph.D., is a psychologist and educator. Known as the "Stress Doctor," he is the author of four books on how stress affects performance and works with physicians, dentists, athletes, parents and people of all ages taking tests. Originally trained as a teacher in London, in the progressive British infant schools in the late '60s, he has received major grants from the American and Canadian governments for his work. He lectures worldwide, live and online, to audiences of teachers, business executives, professors, parents, and healthcare professionals as well as at universities, colleges, schools and hospitals. Ben has a parallel career as a composer and director of opera and is the founder of the nonprofit arts organization "The Singer's Gym."

Soly Erlandsson

Soly Erlandsson is a licensed clinical psychologist and senior professor of Psychology (Ph.D.) at University West, Sweden. Her main interests in research are health and disability issues (among children, adolescents and adults), psychodynamic/psychoanalytical perspectives on human suffering, and qualitative research methodology (Grounded Theory, discourse analysis, and narrative approaches).

Robert Foltz

Dr. Robert Foltz is a clinical psychologist and associate professor of clinical psychology at the Chicago School of Professional Psychology, Chicago campus. Dr. Foltz has over 30 years of experience in the field, starting his career working in inpatient settings with adults diagnosed with schizophrenia and other severe conditions. From there, he transitioned into residential treatment centers working as a clinician, and then administrator, providing services to some of the most complicated clinical presentations in youth within the state of Illinois. During this residential work of over 15 years, Dr. Foltz began his private practice, largely working with clients who had not found success down the typical path of mental health care (e.g., medications with a side of therapy). Now in academia, Dr. Foltz teaches graduate courses related to psychiatric disorders, evidence-based treatments and the integration of psychotherapy within a medical-model-dominated field, pediatric psychopharmacology, trauma-informed care, and foundations in research and practice. Dr. Foltz has multiple publications and presentations related to evidence-based care and the use (and misuse) of psychotropic medications in youth.

Al Galves

Al Galves is a psychologist who lives in Las Cruces, New Mexico. For the past 20 years he has been exposing the flaws in biopsychiatry and advocating for safe, humane, life-enhancing approaches to helping people who are diagnosed with mental illnesses. He is a past Executive Director of the International Society for Ethical Psychology and Psychiatry (ISEPP) and a member of the Board of Directors of ISEPP and MindFreedom International. He is the author of *Lighten Up: Dance with Your Dark Side and Harness Your Dark Side: Mastering Jealousy, Rage, Frustration and Other Negative Emotions* (New Horizon Press, 2012). Website www.algalves.com.

Patrick Hahn

Patrick D. Hahn is the author of three books: *Madness and Genetic Determinism: Is Mental Illness in Our Genes?* (Palgrave McMillan); *Prescription for Sorrow: Antidepressants, Suicide, and Violence* (Samizdat Health Writer's Cooperative); and *Obedience Pills: ADHD and the Medicalization of Childhood* (Samizdat). Dr. Hahn is an affiliate professor of Biology at Loyola University Maryland.

Juho Honkasilta

Juho Honkasilta, PhD, currently works as a University Lecturer at the Department of Education, University of Helsinki, Finland. He is an in-service and pre-service teacher educator at the Special Education study program. Honkasilta has researched how ADHD as a diagnostic entity structures institutional, social and personal lives, and the role of school institutions in this process. He has published about Inclusion in Education from the Disability Studies perspectives.

Christoffer Hornborg

Christoffer Hornborg is a licensed clinical psychologist, holds an M.A. in medical anthropology, and Is currently a licentiate candidate in sociology at the University of Gothenburg, and Campus Västervik, Västervik municipality, Sweden. His research interests include anthropological and sociological perspectives on psychiatric disorder, identity, and theories of modernity.

Erica Komisar

Erica Komisar, LCSW, is a clinical social worker, psychoanalyst, and parent guidance expert who has been in private practice in New York City for over 30 years. A graduate of Georgetown and Columbia

Universities and The New York Freudian Society, Ms. Komisar is a psychological consultant bringing parenting workshops to clinics, schools, corporations, and childcare settings. She is a contributor to *The Wall Street Journal, The Washington Post* and *The New York Daily News*. She is also a Contributing Editor to *The Institute for Family Studies* and appears regularly on *Fox and Friends* and *Fox 5 News*. Erica is the author of *Being There: Why Prioritizing Motherhood in the First Three Years Matters* and *Chicken Little the Sky Isn't Falling: Raising Resilient Adolescents in the New Age of Anxiety.*

Athanasios Koutsoklenis

Athanasios Koutsoklenis has studied at the Department of Educational and Social Policy, University of Macedonia (BA), the School of Education, University of Birmingham (MA) and the Department of Educational and Social Policy, University of Macedonia (PhD). He currently works as an assistant professor of Inclusive Education at the Department of Primary Education, Democritus University of Thrace, Greece.

Judy Kupchan

Judy Kupchan is a clinical psychology doctoral student at the Chicago School of Professional Psychology, Chicago campus. Judy is in the second year of her doctoral training program, currently completing her diagnostic externship at Streamwood Behavioral Healthcare System's inpatient hospital. In this position, Judy conducts psychodiagnostic assessments and facilitates group therapy with a population of children, adolescents, and adults with severe psychopathology. Judy has also worked at a day-treatment center for children with autism spectrum disorder and at an after-school program as a behavioral aide for children with behavioral issues. Judy's clinical and research interests revolve around complex childhood trauma and its impact on development, the efficacy of trauma-informed care, the use (and misuse) of psychotropic medications in youth, and systemic issues in psychiatric care. Judy was recently involved in a review of the American Psychological Association's curriculum requirements for Clinical Psychology doctoral training programs, specifically as the requirements relate to coursework in psychopharmacology and trauma-informed care. This review provided an analysis of best practices and recommendations for modifying curricula to improve the ability of clinicians to provide their clients with competent, informed, and ethical care. This work has been submitted for publication.

Eric Maisel

Eric Maisel, retired family therapist and active creativity coach, is the author of 50+ books. His books include *Unleashing the Artist Within* (Dover, 2020), *Lighting the Way* (Crossways Press, 2020), *The Power of Daily Practice* (New World Library, 2020), *Redesign Your Mind* (Conari, 2021), *Why Smart Teens Hurt* (Conari, 2022), and *The Coach's Way* (New World Library, 2023). His other books include *The Future of Mental Health, Rethinking Depression, Fearless Creating, Coaching the Artist Within, Managing Creative Anxiety, Why Smart People Hurt, The Van Gogh Blues,* and many more. Dr. Maisel is the creator of and lead editor for the Ethics International Press Critical Psychology and Critical Psychiatry series. In 2022 the first two volumes in that series, *Critiquing the Psychiatric Model and Humane Alternatives to the Psychiatric Model*, appeared. In 2023, additional volumes in the series will appear, to include *Deconstructing ADHD*.

Lexi Pope

Lexi Pope is a member of the International Society for Ethical Psychology & Psychiatry and a doctoral student in clinical psychology at the Chicago School of Professional Psychology, Chicago campus. She is currently working as a diagnostic neuropsychology extern at The Family Institute at Northwestern University where she conducts neuropsychological assessments with clients across the lifespan. Lexi is a part of the Association of Neuropsychology Students & Trainees (ANST) at The Chicago School of Professional Psychology and has led journal club on the topic of ADHD and the impact of the spreading of false diagnostic information via social media platforms such as TikTok. Lexi's interests include the conceptualization and transdiagnostic nature of ADHD, the use (and misuse) of psychotropic medications, and substance use disorders. She has been involved in work submitted for publication which includes a review of Clinical Psychology Doctoral programs, accredited by the American Psychological Association, in their provision of courses related to psychopharmacology and trauma-informed care. This review also included an analysis of best practices and recommendations for modifying curricula to improve the ability to respond to the needs of clients.

Burton Seitler

Burton Norman Seitler, Ph.D. is a psychoanalyst/clinical psychologist in private practice. He is the former Director of Counseling and Psychotherapy Services in Ridgewood and Oakland, NJ; former Director of the Child and Adolescent Psychotherapy Studies Program, and Supervising Training Analyst; and current Chair of the Board of Trustees of the New Jersey Institute for Training in Psychoanalysis and Psychotherapy, Teaneck, NJ. Dr. Seitler is the Founder and Editor-in-Chief of the International Journal for the Advancement of Scientific Psychoanalytic Empirical Research (*JASPER*). He is also a Faculty member of the Gordon Derner Postdoctoral Program at Adelphi University. Dr. Seitler has presented and published over 100 combined articles, chapters, book reviews and an edited book nationally and internationally. Topics covered include ADHD, soma psyche, ethnic humor, Randomized Controlled Trials, artificial intelligence, racism, psychosis, dreams, resilience, altruism, suicide, child abuse, autism, and forced hospitalization and medicating. An article on research in psychoanalysis recently won the prestigious Gradiva Award.

Mattias Nilsson Sjoberg

Mattias Nilsson Sjöberg has a Ph.D. in Education and works at Malmö University in the department Childhood-Education-Society. He is a reader in critical theory and his research primarily focuses on inclusive and exclusive educational processes from a critical pedagogical standpoint.

Jeanne Stolzer

Dr. Jeanne Stolzer is professor of Family Science at the University of Nebraska-Kearney. She currently teaches infant, child, adolescent, and lifespan development classes and is a prolific researcher. Dr. Stolzer has published numerous peer-reviewed scientific articles and has presented her research at the national and international levels. She has won numerous prestigious research and teaching awards and has been a passionate child advocate for over 35 years. Dr. Stolzer's research interests include Attention Deficit Hyperactivity Disorder (ADHD), the biocultural implications of attachment theory, bioevolutionary theory, the meteoric rise of psychiatric diagnoses in infant, child, and adolescent populations, the multivariational effects of labeling children, and challenging the existing medical model which seeks to pathologize normal-range human behaviors.

David Walker

David Edward Walker is a liberation psychologist, writer, musician, and Missouri Cherokee descendent. His new book, *Coyote's Swing: A Memoir & Critique of Mental Hygiene in Native America* is slated to be published by Washington State University Press in fall 2022. His critical essays on the U.S. mental health system in Native America for Indian Country Today (ICT) in 2015 and 2016 were both well received and controversial. ICT also praised Dr. Walker's Medicine Valley novels, *Tessa's Dance* and *Signal Peak*, for dealing "with all the issues of tragedy, psychological healing, and cultural and language revitalization. . . necessary in the wake of centuries of genocidal efforts to destroy our Nations and Peoples." An established singer-songwriter, Music Hound's Essential Guide to Folk Music calls David "a singer-songwriter with a special ability to reach listeners" via "rich metaphors, spiritual themes, moving ballads, and ambitious fingerstyle guitar work."

Gretchen LeFever Watson

Dr. Gretchen LeFever Watson is a developmental and clinical psychologist with postdoctoral training in pediatric psychology. She has served as a professor of multiple disciplines at universities and medical schools in the U.S. and the Caribbean, director of public health psychology at a pediatric research center, and patient safety director for a large healthcare system. She secured millions of dollars of federal, state, and private funding to study the epidemiology of psychiatric drug use and develop community-based strategies to reduce over-reliance on psychiatric labels and drugs, including a school-wide behavioral initiative that reduced ADHD symptoms and classroom discipline problems while significantly improving educational outcomes. Her projects and publications have received extensive national media coverage. In 2008, a leading medical journal vetted her for a list of 100 international scientists that journalists can count on for unbiased reviews of health research. In 2012, Watson's local business community selected her for its *Health Care Hero Award* for her corporate innovations in patient safety technology. She is president of a safety and change management consulting firm in Virginia Beach.